Study Guide for

Essentials of Nursing Research

APPRAISING EVIDENCE FOR NURSING PRACTICE

SEVENTH EDITION

Denise F. Polit, PhD

President, Humanalysis, Inc., Saratoga Springs, New York
and Adjunct Professor, Griffith University School of Nursing
Gold Coast, Australia
(www.denisepolit.com)

Cheryl Tatano Beck, DNSc, CNM, FAAN

Distinguished Professor, School of Nursing
University of Connecticut
Storrs, Connecticut

Wolters Kluwer | Lippincott Williams & Wilkins
Health

Philadelphia • Baltimore • New York • London
Buenos Aires • Hong Kong • Sydney • Tokyo

Acquisitions Editor: Annette Ferran
Director of Nursing Production: Helen Ewan
Senior Managing Editor / Production: Erika Kors
Manufacturing Coordinator: Karin Duffield
Production Editor: Mary Kinsella
Production Services / Compositor: Aptara, Inc.

Seventh Edition

9 8 7 6 5 4

Printed in China

Care has been taken to confirm the accuracy of the information presented and to describe generally accepted practices. However, the authors, editors, and publisher are not responsible for errors or omissions or for any consequences from application of the information in this book and make no warranty, expressed or implied, with respect to the currency, completeness, or accuracy of the contents of the publication. Application of this information in a particular situation remains the professional responsibility of the practitioner; the clinical treatments described and recommended may not be considered absolute and universal recommendations.

The authors, editors, and publisher have exerted every effort to ensure that drug selection and dosage set forth in this text are in accordance with the current recommendations and practice at the time of publication. However, in view of ongoing research, changes in government regulations, and the constant flow of information relating to drug therapy and drug reactions, the reader is urged to check the package insert for each drug for any change in indications and dosage and for added warnings and precautions. This is particularly important when the recommended agent is a new or infrequently employed drug.

Some drugs and medical devices presented in this publication have Food and Drug Administration (FDA) clearance for limited use in restricted research settings. It is the responsibility of the health care provider to ascertain the FDA status of each drug or device planned for use in his or her clinical practice.

RRS1008

Preface

This Study Guide has been prepared to complement the seventh edition of *Essentials of Nursing Research: Appraising Evidence for Nursing Practice.* As is true for the textbook, this Study Guide retains many features that have made it a useful learning tool in the past, and we have introduced new material designed to further bridge the gap between the passive reading of abstract materials and the active development of skills needed to critique studies and use their findings in practice.

The guide provides you with opportunities to reinforce the acquisition of basic research skills through systematic learning exercises—some of which are designed to be "fun." For example, we have included a crossword puzzle for every chapter, using key new terms that were introduced in the textbook. Another important feature is that the appendices include research reports in their entirety. In this edition, we deliberately selected some studies that are geared to evidence-based practice (EBP), such as a study on the results of an EBP implementation project, and two systematic reviews. There are activities in each chapter of this Study Guide (the Application Exercises) geared around these studies.

The Study Guide consists of 19 chapters—one chapter corresponding to every chapter in the textbook. Each of the 19 chapters (with a few exceptions) consists of four sections:

- **Crossword Puzzle**. Terms and concepts presented in the textbook are reinforced by having you complete a crossword puzzle. All answers are in the back of the book for easy reference and cross-checking.
- **Matching Exercises**. Further reinforcement for key new terms is offered in a matching exercise, which often involves matching the concrete (for example, an actual research hypothesis) with the abstract (e.g., the term for a specific type of hypothesis). Again, answers are at the back of the book.
- **Study Questions**. Each chapter contains two to five short individual exercises relevant to the materials in the textbook.
- **Application Exercises**. These exercises are geared specifically to helping you to read, comprehend, and critique nursing studies. In each chapter, the application exercises focus on two of the studies in the appendices—typically one qualitative and one quantitative study. For each study, there are two sets of questions— *Questions of Fact* and *Questions for Discussion*. The Questions of Fact will help you to read the report and find specific types of information, related to the content covered in the textbook. For these questions, there are "right" and "wrong" answers, which we provide at the back of the book. For example, a question might ask: How many people participated in this study? The Questions for Discussion, by contrast, require an assessment of the merits of various features

of the study. For example, a question might ask: Were there *enough* people participating in this study? The second set of questions can be the basis for classroom
discussions.

We hope that you will find these activities rewarding, enjoyable, and useful in your
effort to develop skills for evidence-based nursing practice.

Contents

PART 5
Data Analysis and Interpretation   105

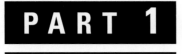
PART 1

Overview of Nursing Research and Its Role in Evidence-Based Practice

PART 1

Introduction to Nursing Research in an Evidence-Based Practice Environment

■ A. Crossword Puzzle

Complete the crossword puzzle below, which uses terms and concepts presented in Chapter 1.

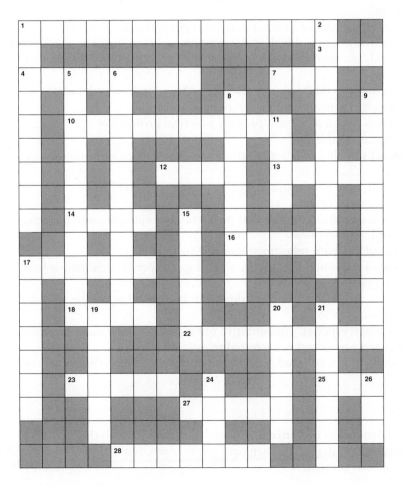

There is a crossword puzzle in each chapter of this *Study Guide*. We hope they will be a "fun" way for you to review key terms used in each chapter. However, we are not professional puzzle designers and so there are some oddities about the puzzles. These oddities are not intended to be trick questions, but rather represent liberties we took in trying to get as many terms as possible into the puzzle. So, for example, you will find a lot of acronyms (e.g., evidence-based practice = EBP) and abbreviations (e.g., evidence = evid), and even a few words that are written backwards (e.g., evidence = ecnedive). Two-word answers sometimes appear with a space (e.g., evidence-based) and sometimes they are just run together (e.g., evidencebased). The crossword puzzle answers are at the back of this *Study Guide,* in case our intent is too obscure!

ACROSS

1. Nurses are increasingly encouraged to develop a practice that is _____ (hyphenated).
3. The clinical learning strategy developed at the McMaster School of Medicine (acronym).
4. A worldview, a way of looking at natural phenomena.
7. The worldview that holds that there are multiple interpretations of reality (abbr.).
10. The worldview that assumes that there is an orderly reality that can be studied objectively.
12. The precursor to the National Institute of Nursing Research (acronym).
13. Successively trying alternative solutions is known as _____ and error.
14. Research designed to solve a pressing practical problem is _____ (not basic) research (abbr.).
16. Nurses get together in practice settings to critique studies in the context of journal _____.
17. Research designed to inform nursing practice is referred to as _____ nursing research (abbr.).
18. The U.S. government agency that promotes and sponsors nursing research (acronym).
22. A source of evidence reflecting ingrained customs.
23. The type of reasoning that involves developing specific predictions from general principles (abbr.).
25. The degree to which research findings can be applied to people who did not participate in a study (abbr.).
27. Many studies, especially quantitative ones, seek to understand determinants of phenomena and are sometimes referred to as _____-probing.
28. A principle that is believed to be true without proof or verification (abbr.).

DOWN

1. Evidence rooted in objective reality and gathered through the senses
2. The assumption that phenomena are not random, but rather have antecedent causes.

5. The repeating of a study to determine if findings can be upheld with a new group of people
6. A purpose of doing research, involving a portrayal of phenomena as they exist
8. A scheme for ordering the utility of evidence for practice is an evidence _____.
9. A purpose of doing research, often linked to theory in quantitative studies
11. The techniques used by researchers to structure a study are called research _____ (abbr.).
15. The type of research that analyzes narrative, subjective materials is _____ research (abbr.).
17. Purposes primarily associated with quantitative research are prediction and _____.
19. An EBP-related purpose of research is to develop and evaluate treatments or _____ (abbr.).
20. The scientific method involves procedures to enhance objectivity and reduce _____ that could distort the results.
21. An EBP-related purpose of research is to rigorously develop and test instruments to make assessments or _____ of nursing clients (abbr.).
24. An EBP-related purpose of research concerns examining the etiology of _____ (i.e., health care problems and adverse consequences of exposures).
26. The major U.S. federal agency that addresses health issues and funding for health research, within which NINR is housed (acronym).

■ B. Matching Exercises

Match each statement in Set B with one of the paradigms in Set A. Indicate the letter corresponding to the appropriate response next to each entry in Set B.

SET A

a. Positivist or postpositivist paradigm

b. Naturalist paradigm

c. Neither paradigm

d. Both paradigms

SET B   RESPONSES

1. Assumes that reality exists and that it can be objectively studied and known   _____

2. Subjectivity in inquiries is considered inevitable and desirable   _____

3. Inquiries rely on external, empirical evidence collected through human senses   _____

4. Assumes reality is a construction and that many constructions are possible _____

5. Method of inquiry relies primarily on collecting and analyzing quantitative information _____

6. Method of inquiry relies primarily on collecting and analyzing narrative, qualitative information _____

7. Provides an overarching framework for inquiries undertaken by nurse researchers _____

8. Inquiries give rise to emerging interpretations that are grounded in people's experiences _____

9. Inquiries are not constrained by ethical issues _____

10. Inquiries focus on discrete, specific concepts while attempting to control others _____

■ C. Study Questions

1. Why is it important for nurses who will never conduct their own research to understand research methods?

2. What are some potential consequences to the nursing profession if nurses stopped conducting their own research?

3. Below are descriptions of several research problems. Indicate whether you think the problem is best suited to a qualitative or quantitative approach, and explain your rationale.
   a. What is the decision-making process of AIDS patients seeking treatment?
   b. What effect does room temperature have on the colonization rate of bacteria in urinary catheters?
   c. What are sources of stress among nursing home residents?
   d. Does therapeutic touch affect the vital signs of hospitalized patients?
   e. What is the meaning of *hope* among stage IV cancer patients?
   f. What are the effects of a formal exercise program on high blood pressure and cholesterol levels of middle-aged men?
   g. What are the health care needs of the homeless, and what barriers do they face in having those needs met?

4. What are some of the limitations of quantitative research? What are some of the limitations of qualitative research? Which approach seems best suited to address problems in which you might be interested? Why is that?

5. Scan the titles in the table of contents of a recent issue of a nursing research journal (e.g., *Nursing Research, Research in Nursing & Health, Journal of Advanced Nursing*). Find the title of a study that you think is basic research and another that you think is applied research. Read the abstracts for these studies to see if you can determine whether your original supposition was correct.

■ D. Application Exercises

EXERCISE 1: STUDY IN APPENDIX A

Read the Abstract and Introduction to the report by Hill and colleagues ("Chronically Ill Rural Women") in Appendix A. Then answer the following questions:

Questions of Fact

a. Does this report describe an example of "disciplined research?"
b. Is this a qualitative or quantitative study?
c. What is the underlying paradigm of the study?
d. Does the study involve the collection of empirical evidence?
e. Is this study applied or basic research?
f. Could this study be described as *cause probing?*
g. Is the specific purpose of this study identification, description, exploration, prediction/control, and (or) explanation?
h. Does this study have an EBP-focused purpose, such as a one related to treatment, diagnosis, prognosis, and so forth?

Questions for Discussion

a. How relevant is this study to the actual practice of nursing?
b. Could this study have been conducted as *either* a quantitative or a qualitative study? Why or why not?

EXERCISE 2: STUDY IN APPENDIX B

Read the Abstract and Introduction to the report by Rasmussen and colleagues ("Young Women with Type 1 Diabetes") in Appendix B. Then answer the following questions:

Questions of Fact

a. Does this report describe an example of "disciplined research?"
b. Is this a qualitative or quantitative study?
c. What is the underlying paradigm of the research?
d. Does the study involve the collection of empirical evidence?
e. Is this study applied or basic research?
f. Could this study be described as *cause probing?*

g. Is the specific purpose of this study identification, description, exploration, prediction/control, and (or) explanation?

h. Does this study have an EBP-focused purpose, such as one related to treatment, diagnosis, prognosis, and so forth?

Questions for Discussion

a. How relevant is this study to the actual practice of nursing?

b. Could this study have been conducted as *either* a quantitative or a qualitative study? Why or why not?

c. Which of the two studies cited in these exercises (the one in Appendix A or Appendix B) is of greater interest and/or relevance to you personally? Why?

CHAPTER 2

Evidence-Based Nursing Practice: Fundamentals

■ A. Crossword Puzzle

Complete the crossword puzzle below, which uses terms and concepts presented in Chapter 2.

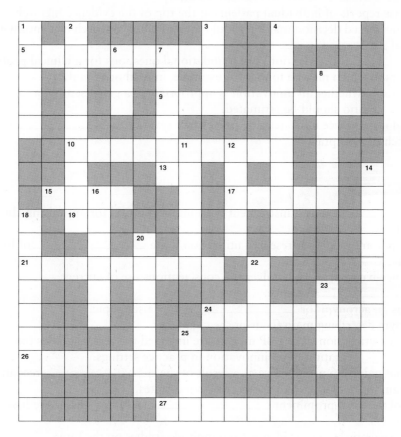

ACROSS

4. Earliest large-scale research utilization project by nurses (acronym)
5. A clinical practice _____ based on rigorous systematic evidence is an important tool for evidence-based care.
9. *Environmental readiness* for an innovation concerns it implementation _____ in a given setting.
10. _____ reviews of randomized controlled trials (RCTs) are at the pinnacle of most evidence hierarchies.
13. The Cochrane Collaboration is a cornerstone of the evidence-based practice (EBP) _ _vement.
15. _ _ _ _ground questions are ones that can be answered based on current best research evidence.
17. When a new protocol or guideline is developed in an EBP project, it must be _____ tested to evaluate its utility.
19. Are case reports of individual patients at the top of the evidence hierarchy?
21. Evidence-based decision making should integrate best research evidence with clinical _____.
24. _____ questions are foundational questions for a clinical problem, answers to which may be found, for example, in textbooks (abbr.).
26. In assessing whether an innovation is appropriate in a given setting, a _____/ _____ ratio should be estimated.
27. Abundant evidence indicates that nurses face several _____ to using research in their practice.

DOWN

1. The _____ instrument is an important tool for appraising clinical guidelines.
2. An important model for research utilization is the _____ of Innovations Theory.
3. Evidence-based practice involves the conscientious use of current _____ evidence.
4. CAT is an acronym for _____ appraised topic.
6. Acronym describing main focus of the chapter
7. Research utilization (RU)/EBP models are intended to serve as guides for the _ _ _ _ _ _entation of an innovation in practice settings.
8. EBP has gained in prominence as a result of the _____ recognition program for nursing excellence in the United States.
11. Two of the most prominent _____ of EBP for nurses are Iowa and Stetler.
12. In a systematic review, evidence from multiple studies on the same _____ is integrated.
14. One trigger in the Iowa Model, which involves an origin in the research literature, is called _____-focused.

16. Originator of a prominent theory on how new ideas are diffused and adopted
18. An arrangement of the worth of various types of evidence
20. The earliest model of research utilization in nursing was developed by
    _____.
22. Acronym for the five-component scheme for asking EBP questions
23. One trigger in the Iowa Model, stemming from practice issues, is called
    _____-focused (abbr.).
25. A statistical method of combining evidence is a systematic review known as
    _____-analysis.

■ B. Matching Exercises

Match each of the statements in Set B with the appropriate phrase in Set A. Indicate the letter(s) corresponding to your response next to each of the statements in Set B.

SET A

a. Research utilization (RU)

b. Evidence-based practice (EBP)

c. Neither RU nor EBP

d. Both RU and EBP

SET B	**RESPONSES**
1. Has been easily achieved in nursing	_____
2. Systematic reviews play a prominent role	_____
3. Emphasis on translating knowledge to practical applications	_____
4. Integrates research findings with clinical expertise and client input	_____
5. Has given rise to several models by nurses	_____
6. Specifically begins with a knowledge-focused trigger	_____
7. The CURN project focused on this	_____
8. Sackett and Cochrane were prominent proponents	_____

■ C. Study Questions

1. Identify the factors in your own practice setting that you think facilitate or inhibit research utilization and evidence-based practice (or, in an educational setting, the factors that promote or inhibit a climate in which RU or EBP is valued).

2. Think about a nursing procedure that you have learned. What is the basis for this procedure? Determine whether the procedure is based on scientific evidence indicating that the procedure is effective. If it is not based on scientific evidence, on what is it based, and why do you think scientific evidence was not used?

3. Read one of the following articles and identify the steps of the Iowa Model (or an alternative model of EBP) that are represented in the RU or EBP projects described.

   a. Clarke, H. F., Bradley, C., Whytock, S., Handfield, S., van der Wal, R., & Gundry, S. (2005). Pressure ulcers: Implementation of evidence-based nursing practice. *Journal of Advanced Nursing, 49*(6), 578–590.

   b. Hatler, C., Mast, D., Corderella, J., Mitchell, G., Howard, K., Aragon, J., & Bedker, D. (2006). Using evidence and process improvement strategies to enhance healthcare outcomes for the critically ill: A pilot project. *American Journal of Critical Care, 15,* 549–555.

   c. Kavanagh, D., Connolly, P., & Cohen, J. (2006). Promoting evidence-based practice: Implementing the American Stroke Association's acute stroke program. *Journal of Nursing Care Quality, 21,* 135–142.

■ D. Application Exercises

EXERCISE 1: STUDY IN APPENDIX E

Read the Abstract and Introduction (everything before the subheading "Step 1") to the report by Tracy and colleagues ("Translating Best Practices") in Appendix E. Also re-read the project summary in Chapter 2 of the textbook. Then answer the following questions:

Questions of Fact

a. Who were the team members in this study, and what were their affiliations?
b. What did Tracy and her coauthors say about the need for this EBP project?
c. Did the article indicate that there were existing pain management guidelines for non-drug pain management? Were these guidelines described, and were they used in the development of the project's protocols?
d. What types of barriers to research translation did Tracy and her colleagues discuss?
e. What aspect of the Collaborative Research Utilization (CRU) model was described as being unique?
f. What criteria did the team use in selecting a study site for this project?
g. Did this project involve the collection of empirical evidence?

Questions for Discussion

a. What might be some clinical foreground questions that were used in seeking relevant evidence in preparing for this project? Identify components of these questions (e.g., population, intervention).
b. What are some of the praiseworthy aspects of this project? What could the team members have done differently to improve the project?

EXERCISE 2: STUDY IN APPENDIX F

Read the abstract and introduction (from the beginning to the "Methods" section) to the report by Lee and colleagues ("Interventions for Informal Stroke Caregivers") in Appendix F. Then answer the following questions:

Questions of Fact

a. Does this report summarize a systematic review? If yes, what type of systematic review was it? Is this an example of preappraised evidence?
b. Where on the evidence hierarchy shown in Figure 2.1 of the textbook would this study belong?
c. What is the stated purpose of this study?
d. What was the stated research question? Which parts of the "PICOT" scheme are represented in this question?

Questions for Discussion

a. Could a clinical practice guideline be developed based on the findings from this study? Why or why not?
b. What are some of the steps you would need to undertake if you were interested in using this study as a basis for an EBP project in your own practice setting?

CHAPTER 3

Key Concepts and Steps in Qualitative and Quantitative Research

■ A. Crossword Puzzle

Complete the crossword puzzle below, which uses terms and concepts presented in Chapter 3.

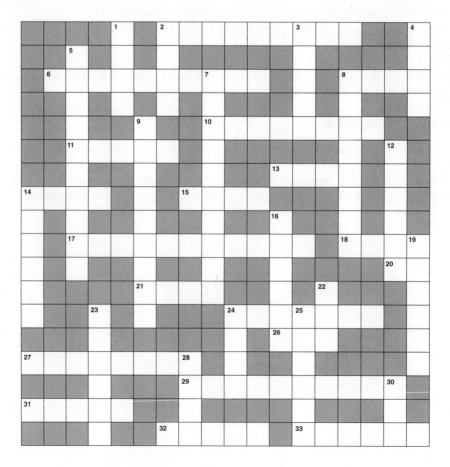

ACROSS

2. Another name for outcome variable is _____ variable.
6. An individual with whom a researcher must negotiate to get access into a site
8. To get access to a site and its inhabitants is to _____ entrée into the site.
10. A step in experimental research involves the development of an intervention _____ .
11. In "What is the effect of radon on health?" the independent variable is_____ .
13. During the design phase of a quantitative study, researchers must develop a data collection _____ that they will implement in the empirical phase of the project.
14. Pieces of information gathered in a study
15. A subset of a population from whom data are gathered (abbr.)
17. The _____ definition indicates how a variable will be measured or observed.
18. Qualitative researchers use in_ _ _ _ive reasoning in analyzing their data.
20. A systematic, abstract explanation of phenomena (first two letters)
21. A type of fieldwork done to enhance the value of a study for practicing nurses (abbr.)
24. The type of analysis used by quantitative researchers (abbr.)
26. Some qualitative researchers do not undertake an upfront _____ . review to avoid having their conceptualization influenced by the work of others (abbr.).
27. The type of design used in qualitative studies
29. The type of research that involves an intervention is a(n) _____ .
31. In medical literature, a study that tests the effect of an intervention is a clinical _____ .
32. A research investigation
33. The procedure of translating data into numerical values (backwards!)

DOWN

1. The qualitative research tradition that focuses on lived experiences (abbr.)
2. In "What is the effect of a cancer patient's diet on pain levels?" the independent variable is: _____ .
3. The qualitative tradition that focuses on the study of cultures (abbr.)
4. The abstractions in which researchers are interested (abbr.)
5. A principle used to decide when to stop sampling in a qualitative study
7. The entire aggregate of units in which a researcher is interested
8. A qualitative tradition that focuses on social psychological processes within a social setting is _____ theory.
9. A somewhat more complex abstraction than a concept

12. If the independent variable is the cause, the dependent variable is the
_____.

14. The research _____ is the basic architecture of a study.

16. A relationship in which one variable directly induces changes in another is a(n)
_____ relationship.

19. Qualitative analyses usually involve a search for recurrent _____.

22. Quantitative researchers develop a knowledge context by doing a
_____ review early in the project (abbr.).

23. In quantitative research a concept is usually referred to as a _____
(abbr.).

24. The first _____ in a project involves formulating a research problem.

25. In terms of _____, the independent variable occurs before the dependent variable.

28. In some studies, the design and plans are not finalized until a pilot
_____ has been undertaken.

30. A relationship expresses a bond between at least _____ variables.

■ B. Matching Exercises

1. Match each statement in Set B with one of the paradigms in Set A. Indicate the letter
corresponding to the appropriate response next to each entry in Set B.

SET A

a. Term used in quantitative research

b. Term used in qualitative research

c. Term used in either qualitative or quantitative research

SET B	**RESPONSES**
1. Subject	_____
2. Study participant	_____
3. Informant	_____
4. Variable	_____
5. Phenomena	_____
6. Construct	_____
7. Theory	_____
8. Data	_____
9. Emergent design	_____
10. Data analysis	_____

2. Match each term in Set B with one of the terms in Set A. Indicate the letter corresponding to your response next to each item in Set B.

SET A

a. Independent variable
b. Dependent variable
c. Either or both
d. Neither

SET B   **RESPONSES**

1. The variable that is the presumed effect   _____

2. The variable involved in a cause-and-effect relationship   _____

3. The variable that is the presumed cause   _____

4. The variable, "length of hospital stay"   _____

5. The variable that requires an operational definition   _____

6. The variable that is the main outcome of interest in the study   _____

7. The variable that is constant   _____

8. The variable in a grounded theory study   _____

3. Match each activity in Set B with one of the options in Set A. Indicate the letter corresponding to your response next to each item in Set B.

SET A

a. An activity in quantitative research
b. An activity in qualitative research
c. An activity in both qualitative and quantitative research
d. An activity in neither quantitative nor qualitative research

SET B   **RESPONSES**

1. Choosing between an experimental or nonexperimental design   _____

2. Ending data collection once saturation has been achieved   _____

3. Developing or evaluating measuring instruments   _____

4. Doing a literature review   _____

5. Gaining entrée into a site   _____

6. Taking steps to ensure protection of human rights   _____

7. Developing strategies to avoid data collection   _____

8. Disseminating research results   _____

9. Analyzing the data for major themes or categories   _____

10. Developing hypotheses to be tested statistically   _____

4. Match each activity relating to quantitative studies in Set B with an option in Set A. Indicate the letter corresponding to your response next to each item in Set B.

SET A

a. Conceptual phase

b. Planning phase

c. Empirical phase

d. Analytic phase

e. Dissemination phase

SET B   **RESPONSES**

1. Distributing questionnaires to a group of nursing home residents   _____

2. Deciding what type of design to use   _____

3. Conducting a literature review   _____

4. Identifying a suitable theoretical framework   _____

5. Deciding to collect data from 300 alcoholics in treatment   _____

6. Computing the percentage of subjects clinically depressed   _____

7. Presenting a paper at a meeting of the Eastern Nursing Research Society   _____

8. Designing a training session for data collectors   _____

9. Coding data for entry of information onto a computer file   _____

10. Interpreting findings that were contrary to the hypotheses   _____

■ C. Study Questions

1. Suggest operational definitions for the following concepts.
   a. Stress
   b. Prematurity of infants
   c. Fatigue
   d. Pain
   e. Prolonged labor
   f. Dyspnea

2. In each of the following research questions, identify the independent and dependent variables.

   a. Does assertiveness training improve the effectiveness of psychiatric nurses?

   Independent: _____

   Dependent: _____

   b. Does the postural positioning of patients affect their respiratory function?

   Independent: _____

   Dependent: _____

   c. Is the psychological well-being of patients affected by the amount of touching received from nursing staff?

   Independent: _____

   Dependent: _____

   d. Is the incidence of decubitus reduced by more frequent turning of patients?

   Independent: _____

   Dependent: _____

   e. Are people who were abused as children more likely than others to abuse their own children?

   Independent: _____

   Dependent: _____

   f. Is tolerance for pain related to a patient's age and gender?

   Independent: _____

   Dependent: _____

   g. Is the number of prenatal visits of pregnant women associated with labor and delivery outcomes?

   Independent: _____

   Dependent: _____

   h. Are levels of depression higher among children who experience the death of a sibling than among other children who do not?

   Independent: _____

   Dependent: _____

   i. Is compliance with a medical regimen higher among women than among men?

      Independent: _____

      Dependent: _____

   j. Does participating in a support group enhance coping among family caregivers of patients with AIDS?

      Independent: _____

      Dependent: _____

   k. Is hearing acuity of the elderly affected by the time of day?

      Independent: _____

      Dependent: _____

   l. Does home birth affect the parents' satisfaction with the childbirth experience?

      Independent: _____

      Dependent: _____

   m. Does a neutropenic diet in the outpatient setting decrease the positive blood cultures associated with chemotherapy-induced neutropenia?

      Independent: _____

      Dependent: _____

3. Below is a list of variables. For each, think of a research question for which the variable would be the independent variable, and a second for which it would be the dependent variable. For example, take the variable "birth weight of infants." We might ask, "Does the age of the mother affect the birth weight of her infant?" (dependent variable). Alternatively, our research question might be, "Does the birth weight of infants (independent variable) affect their sensorimotor development at 6 months of age?" HINT: For the dependent variable problem, ask yourself, "What factors might affect, influence, or cause this variable?" For the independent variable, ask yourself, "What factors does *this* variable influence, cause, or affect?

   a. Body temperature

      Independent: _____

      Dependent: _____

   b. Amount of sleep

      Independent: _____

      Dependent: _____

c. Frequency of practicing breast self-examination

Independent: _____

Dependent: _____

d. Level of hopefulness in cancer patients

Independent: _____

Dependent: _____

e. Stress among victims of domestic violence

Independent: _____

Dependent: _____

4. Look at the table of contents of a recent issue of *Nursing Research* (available at www.nursingcenter.com/library) or *Research in Nursing & Health* (available at www.interscience.wiley.com). Pick out a study title (not looking at the abstract) that implies that a relationship between variables was studied. Indicate what you think the independent and dependent variable(s) might be, and what the title suggests about the nature of the relationship (i.e., causal or not).

5. Describe what is wrong with the following statements:

   a. Opitz's experimental study was conducted within the ethnographic tradition.

   b. Brusser's experimental study examined the effect of relaxation therapy (the dependent variable) on pain (the independent variable) in cancer patients.

   c. Ball's grounded theory study of the caregiving process for caretakers of patients with dementia was a clinical trial.

   d. In Rossi's phenomenologic study of the meaning of futility among patients with AIDS, subjects received an intervention designed to sustain hope.

   e. In her experimental study, Gabris developed her data collection plan after she introduced her intervention to a group of patients.

6. Which qualitative research tradition do you think would be most appropriate for the following research questions? Justify your response:

   a. How do the health beliefs of Chinese immigrants influence their health-seeking behavior?

   b. What is it like to be a recovering alcoholic?

   c. What is the process by which a husband adapts to the sudden loss of his wife?

■ D. Application Exercises

EXERCISE 1: STUDY IN APPENDIX C

Read the abstract and introduction (the material before "Methods") to the report by Vollman and colleagues ("Coping and Depressive Symptoms") in Appendix C. Then answer the following questions:

Questions of Fact

a. Who were the researchers and what are their credentials and affiliation?
b. Who were the study participants?
c. What were the site and setting for this study?
d. What is the independent variable (or variables) in this study? Is this variable(s) *inherently* an independent variable?
e. What is the dependent variable (or variables) in this study? Is this variable(s) *inherently* a dependent variable?
f. Did the report actually use the terms "independent variable" or "dependent variable"?
g. How was *depression* operationally defined? Was a conceptual definition provided?
h. Were the data in this study quantitative or qualitative?
i. Were any relationships under investigation? What type of relationship?
j. Is this an experimental or nonexperimental study?
k. Was there any intervention? If so, what is it?
l. Did the study involve statistical analysis of data? Did it involve the qualitative analysis of data?

Questions for Discussion

a. How relevant is this study to the actual practice of nursing?
b. How good a job did the researchers do in summarizing their study in the abstract?
c. How long do you estimate it took for this study to be completed?
d. Do you think the study might have been strengthened if it were a multisite study? Why or why not?

EXERCISE 2: STUDY IN APPENDIX D

Read the Abstract and Introduction to the report by Ward-Griffin and colleagues ("Perspectives of Women with Dementia") in Appendix D. Then answer the following questions:

Questions of Fact

a. Who were the researchers and what are their credentials and affiliation?
b. Who were the study participants?
c. In what type of setting did the study take place?

d. What were the key concepts in this study?
e. Were there any *independent variables* or *dependent variables* in this study?
f. Were the data in this study quantitative or qualitative?
g. Were any relationships under investigation?
h. Could the study be described as an ethnographic, phenomenologic, or grounded theory study?
i. Is this an experimental or nonexperimental study?
j. Does the study involve an intervention? If so, what is it?
k. Did the study involve statistical analysis of data? Did the study involve qualitative analysis of data?

Questions for Discussion

a. How relevant is this study to the actual practice of nursing?
b. How good a job did the researchers do in summarizing their study in the abstract?
c. How long do you estimate it took for this study to be completed?
d. Which of the two studies cited in these exercises (the one in Appendix C or the one in Appendix D) is of greater interest and/or relevance to you personally? Why?

EXERCISE 3: STUDY IN APPENDIX E

Read the Abstract, Introduction, and the first part of the "Approach" section (everything before the subheading "Analysis of Substudy Data") of the report by Tracy and colleagues ("Translating Best Practices") in Appendix E. Then answer the following questions:

Questions of Fact

a. Does this appear to be a *collaborative* project?
b. For the substudy described in the report, who were the study participants?
c. In the substudy, what was the independent variable? What was the dependent variable?
d. How much time on the project timetable was devoted to the actual implementation of the protocol and the collection and analysis of project data?

Questions for Discussion

a. Compare the flow of steps on this project with the five phases for a study described in this chapter. In what ways are the activities similar and different?
b. Do you think the project might have been strengthened if it had been undertaken in multiple sites? Why or why not?

CHAPTER 4

Reading and Critiquing Research Reports

■ A. Crossword Puzzle

Complete the crossword puzzle below, which uses terms and concepts presented in Chapter 4.

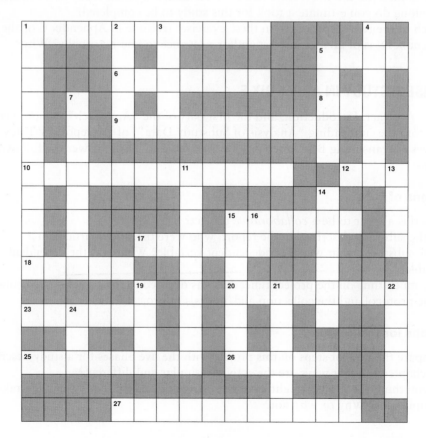

ACROSS

1. Type of tests used by quantitative researchers to test hypotheses and assess how likely the results are real
5. An influence that results in a distortion or error
6. Section of the report that summarizes the findings
8. Qualitative researchers use th_ _ _ description to enhance the transferability of their findings.
9. Section of the report that presents interpretations
10. The first major section of a research report
12. Confounding variable in the example of research control in the book (regarding the effect of urinary incontinence [UI] on depression)
15. Technical terminology that often makes research reports difficult to read
17. Section of the report that describes what the researcher did to answer the research question
18. "The lived experience of caring for a dying spouse" is an example of this part of the report
20. Process of reflecting critically on one's self, used by many qualitative researchers (abbr.)
23. Readers who check to ensure comprehension are _____ readers.
25. The analyses of research data yield _____.
26. One conventional _____ of significance is .05.
27. Qualitative researchers strive to ensure that their findings are _____.

DOWN

1. If the results of a statistical test indicated a probability of .001, the results would be highly _____.
2. Format used to structure most research reports (acronym)
3. Dozens of statistical _____ are available for analyzing quantitative data.
4. To address biases stemming from *awareness*, researchers may use this procedure.
5. Type of review in which reviewers and researchers do not know each other's identity
7. A summary of a study appearing at the beginning of a report
11. Journal editors rely on these to make decisions about publishing submitted manuscripts
13. A confounding variable is a variable that is _____ to the research question, but that is related to the dependent variable and needs to be controlled (abbr.).
14. One of two types of sessions at conferences at which researchers present their findings
15. Research reports are most likely to be accessed as _____ articles.
16. Nursing research began in the 19th century _____ (Latin acronym!)
19. The discussion section presents a researcher's ideas about what the findings _____.
21. Qualitative reports typically include many verbatim excerpts that give readers a _____ of the actual data.

22. Quantitative researchers strive for findings that are reliable and _____.
24. A manuscript for a research report is typically between _____ and 20 pages double-spaced.

■ B. Matching Exercises

Match each statement in Set B with one of the report sections in Set A. Indicate the letter corresponding to the appropriate response next to each entry in Set B.

SET A

a. Abstract
b. Introduction
c. Method
d. Results
e. Discussion

SET B   **RESPONSES**

1. Describes the research design   _____

2. In quantitative studies, presents outcomes of statistical analyses   _____

3. Identifies the research questions or hypotheses   _____

4. Presents a brief summary of the major features of the study   _____

5. Provides information on how study participants were selected   _____

6. Offers an interpretation of the study findings   _____

7. In qualitative studies, describes the themes that emerged from the data   _____

8. Offers a rationale for the study and describes its significance   _____

9. Describes how the research data were collected   _____

10. Identifies the study's main limitations   _____

11. This sentence would appear there: "The purpose of this study was to explore the process by which patients cope with a cancer diagnosis."   _____

12. Includes raw data, in the form of excerpts, in qualitative reports   _____

■ C. Study Questions

1. Why are qualitative research reports generally easier to read than quantitative research reports?

2. Read the following Abstract and rewrite it as a "new style" abstract with specific headings: Van Riper, M. (2007). Families of children with Down syndrome: Responding to a "change in plans" with resilience. *Journal of Pediatric Nursing, 22,* 116–128.

   The purpose of the present investigation, which was guided by the Resiliency Model of Family Stress, Adjustment, and Adaptation, was twofold: (*a*) to describe maternal perceptions of parental and family adaptation in families raising a child with Down syndrome, and (*b*) to examine linkages between family demands, family resources, family problem-solving and coping, and family adaptation in families of children with Down syndrome. Of mothers, 76 completed mailed questionnaires; 70% of the mothers rated their family's overall functioning as either a 4 or a 5 on a 5-point scale (1 = poor; 5 = excellent). In their written comments, most mothers reported that their family was doing well or very well. Three family variables (i.e., family demands, family resources, and family problem-solving communication) were significantly associated with family adaptation. These results provide support for the belief that many families of children with Down syndrome respond to "a change of plans" with resilience. That is, they are able to endure, survive, and even thrive in the face of ongoing challenges associated with raising a child with Down syndrome.

3. Read the titles of the journal articles appearing in the December 2008 issue of *Applied Nursing Research* (or some other issue of this or another nursing journal). Evaluate the titles of the articles in terms of length and adequacy in communicating essential information about the studies.

4. Below is a brief Abstract of a fictitious study, followed by a critique. Do you agree with the critique? Can you add other comments relevant to issues discussed in Chapter 4 of the textbook?

   Fictitious Study. Guslander (2008) prepared the following Abstract for her study:

   Abstract. Family members often experience considerable anxiety while their loved ones are in surgery. This study examined the effectiveness of a nursing intervention that involved providing oral intraoperative progress reports to family members. Surgical patients undergoing elective procedures were selected either to have family members receive the intervention or to not have them receive it. The findings indicated that the family members in the intervention group were less anxious than family members who received the usual care.

   Critique. This brief Abstract provides a general overview of the nature of Guslander's study. It indicates a rationale for the study (the high anxiety level of surgical patients' family members) and summarizes what the researcher did. However, the Abstract could well have provided more information while still staying within a 100- or 125-word guideline (the Abstract contains only 77 words). For example, the Abstract could have better described the nature of the intervention (e.g., at what point during the operation was information given to family members? How much detail was provided?). For a reader to have a preliminary assessment of the worth of the study—and, therefore, to make a decision about whether to read the entire report—more information about the methods used would also have been helpful. For example, the Abstract should have indicated such methodological features as how the researcher measured anxiety and how many surgical patients were in the sample. Some indication of the study's implications might also have enhanced the usefulness of the Abstract.

■ D. Application Exercises

EXERCISE 1: STUDY IN APPENDIX A

Read the Abstract and Introduction to the report by Hill and colleagues ("Chronically Ill Rural Women") in Appendix A. Then answer the following questions:

Questions of Fact

a. Does the structure of this article follow the IMRAD format?
b. Is this Abstract a traditional narrative or is it a "new style" abstract?
c. Does this Abstract include information about the study purpose, how the study was conducted, what the findings were, and what the findings mean?
d. Skim the Method section. Is the presentation in the active or passive voice?
e. Is this study experimental or nonexperimental?
f. Was the principle of *randomness* used in this study?

Questions for Discussion

a. What parts of this Abstract were most difficult to understand? Identify words that you consider to be research "jargon."
b. Comment on the organization *within* the Method section of this report.

EXERCISE 2: STUDY IN APPENDIX B

Read the Abstract and Introduction to the report by Rasmussen and colleagues ("Young Women with Type 1 Diabetes") in Appendix B. Then answer the following questions:

Questions of Fact

a. Does the structure of this article follow the IMRAD format?
b. Is this Abstract a traditional narrative or is it a "new style" abstract?
c. Does this Abstract include information about the study purpose, how the study was conducted, what the findings were, and what the findings mean?
d. Skim the Design and Methods section. Is the presentation in the active or passive voice?
e. Is the study in one of the three main qualitative traditions described in Chapter 3? If so, which tradition?

Questions for Discussion

a. What parts of the Abstract were most difficult to understand?

b. Comment on the organization *within* the Results section of this report.

c. Compare the level of difficulty of the Abstracts for the two studies used in these exercises (i.e., the studies in Appendix A and B). Why do you think the level of difficulty differs?

d. Which type of abstract do you prefer—the traditional one or the "new" style? Why?

CHAPTER 5

Ethics in Research

■ A. Crossword Puzzle

Complete the crossword puzzle below, which uses terms and concepts presented in Chapter 5.

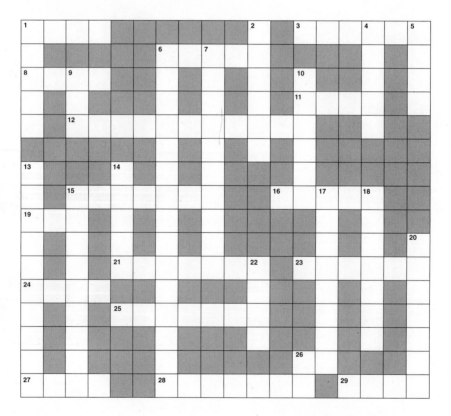

ACROSS

1. A fundamental right for study participants is freedom from _____.
3. Misconduct that involves changing data or distorting results (abbr.)
6. Most disciplines have developed _____ of ethics.
8. Anonymity is a method of protecting this (abbr.).

11. Researchers should conduct a _____-benefit assessment.
12. Major ethical principle concerning maximizing benefits of research
15. Type of consent procedure that may be required in qualitative research
16. A young _____ is considered a vulnerable subject.
19. Debriefings give participants an opportunity to _____ complaints.
21. Payment sometimes offered to participants as an incentive to take part in a study
23. Data collection without participants' awareness, using concealment
24. Procedure for collecting data without linking data to individual participants (abbr.)
25. Report that is the basis for ethical regulations for studies funded by the U.S. government
26. Numbers used in place of names to protect individual identities (abbr.)
27. Fraud and misrepresentations are examples of research _____ (abbr.).
28. A major ethical principle involves respect for human _____ (backwards!).
29. The return of a questionnaire is often assumed to demonstrate _ _ _ _ied consent (abbr.).

DOWN

1. Legislation passed in the U.S. in 1996 concerning privacy of health information (acronym)
2. Informal agreement to participate in a study (e.g., by minors)
4. The Declaration of Hel_ _ _ _ _ , the code of ethics of the World Medical Association
5. The ethical principle of *justice* includes the right to _____ treatment.
6. Participants' privacy is often protected by these procedures, although the researchers know participants' identities.
7. People can make informed decisions about research participation when there is full
   _____.
9. A committee (in the U.S.) that reviews the ethical aspects of a study (acronym)
10. Situation in which private information is divulged is a _____ of confidentiality.
13. Appropriation of someone's ideas without proper credit
14. Documents used to record consent are called informed consent _____.
15. A vulnerable, institutionalized group with diminished autonomy
17. Adequate consent procedures document that study participation is voluntary and that participants are fully _____ about possible costs and benefits.
18. A conflict between the rights of participants and the demands for rigorous research creates an ethical _____.
20. _____ guidelines help to protect the rights of research participants.
22. Mismanagement of _____ can result in a type of research misconduct.
26. Numbers used in place of names to protect individual identities (abbr.)

■ B. Matching Exercises

Match each description in Set B with one of the procedures used to protect human subjects listed in Set A. Indicate the letter corresponding to the appropriate response next to each entry in Set B.

SET A

a. Freedom from harm or exploitation

b. Informed consent

c. Anonymity

d. Confidentiality

SET B   RESPONSES

1. A questionnaire distributed by mail bears an identification number in one corner. Respondents are assured their responses will not be individually divulged.   _____

2. Hospitalized children included in a study, and their parents, are told the study's aims and procedures. Parents are asked to sign an authorization.   _____

3. Respondents in a study in which the same respondents will participate twice by completing questionnaires are asked to place their own four-digit identification number on the questionnaire and to memorize the number. Respondents are assured their answers will remain private.   _____

4. Study participants in an in-depth study of family members' coping with a natural disaster renegotiate the terms of their participation at successive interviews.   _____

5. Women who recently had a mastectomy are studied in terms of psychological consequences. In the interview, sensitive questions are carefully worded. After the interview, debriefing with the respondent determines the need for psychological support.   _____

6. Women interviewed in the above study (question 5) are told that the information they provide will not be individually divulged.   _____

7. Subjects who volunteered for an experimental treatment for AIDS are warned of potential side effects and are asked to sign a waiver.   _____

8. After determining that a new intervention resulted in subject discomfort, the researcher discontinued the study.   _____

9. Unmarked questionnaires are distributed to a class of nursing students. The instructions indicate that responses will not be individually divulged.   _____

10. The researcher assures subjects that they will be interviewed as part of the study at a single point in time and adheres to this promise. _____

11. A questionnaire distributed to a sample of nursing students includes a statement indicating that completion and submission of the questionnaire will be construed as voluntary participation in a study. _____

12. The names, ages, and occupations of study participants whose interviews are excerpted in the research report are not divulged. _____

■ C. Study Questions

1. Below are brief descriptions of several research studies. Suggest some ethical dilemmas that could emerge for each.
   a. A study of coping behaviors among rape victims
   b. An unobtrusive observational study of fathers' behaviors in the delivery room
   c. An interview study of the determinants of heroin addiction
   d. A study of dependence among autistic children
   e. An investigation of verbal interactions among schizophrenic patients
   f. A study of the effects of a new drug on humans
   g. A study of the relationship between sleeping patterns and acting-out behaviors in hospitalized psychiatric patients

2. Evaluate the ethical aspects of one or more of the following studies using the critiquing guidelines in Box 5.2 of the textbook (available as a Word document in the Toolkit of the CD-ROM that accompanies the textbook), paying special attention (if relevant) to the manner in which the subjects' heightened vulnerability was handled.
   • El-Mallakh, P. (2007). Doing my best: Poverty and self-care among individuals with schizophrenia and diabetes mellitus. *Archives of Psychiatric Nursing, 21,* 49–60.
   • Hinsley, R., & Hughes, R. (2007). "The reflections you get": An exploration of body image and cachexia. *International Journal of Palliative Nursing, 13,* 84–89.
   • McFarlane, J., Groff, J., O'Brien, J., & Watson, K. (2006). Behaviors of children following a randomized controlled treatment program for their abused mothers. *Issues in Comprehensive Pediatric Nursing, 28,* 195–211.
   • Zieber, C., Hagen, B., Armstrong-Esther, C., & Alo, M. (2005). Pain and agitation in long-term care residents with dementia: Use of the Pittsburgh Agitation Scale. *International Journal of Palliative Nursing, 11,* 71–78.

3. In the textbook, several actual studies with ethical problems were described (e.g., the study of syphilis among black men and the study in which live cancer cells were injected in elderly patients). Identify which ethical principles were transgressed in these studies.

4. In the following study, the authors indicated that informed consent was not required because there was "no deviation from the standard of care or risk to the subjects" (p. 108). Skim the Introduction and Method section of this paper and comment on the researchers' decision not to obtain informed consent:

- Byers, J. F., et al. (2006). A quasi-experimental trial on individualized, developmentally supportive family-centered care. *Journal of Obstetric, Gynecologic, & Neonatal Nursing, 35*(1), 105–115.

■ D. Application Exercises

EXERCISE 1: STUDY IN APPENDIX C

Read the Method section of the report by Vollman and colleagues ("Coping and Depressive Symptoms") in Appendix C. Then answer the following questions:

Questions of Fact

a. Does the report indicate that the study procedures were reviewed by an IRB or other similar institutional human subjects group?
b. Would the participants in this study be considered "vulnerable subjects?"
c. Were participants subjected to any physical harm or discomfort or psychological distress as part of the study? What efforts did the researchers make to minimize harm and maximize good?
d. Were participants deceived in any way?
e. Were participants coerced into participating in the study?
f. Were appropriate informed consent procedures used? Was there full disclosure?
g. Does the report discuss steps that were taken to protect the privacy and confidentiality of study participants? Were data collected anonymously?

Questions for Discussion

a. Do you think the benefits of this research outweighed the costs to participants? What is the overall risk-to-benefit ratio?
b. Do you consider that the researchers took adequate steps to protect study participants? If not, what else could they have done?
c. The report did not indicate that the participants were paid a stipend. Do you think they should have been?
d. Is there any evidence of discrimination in this study, with regard to people recruited to participate?
e. How comfortable would you feel about having a parent or grandparent participate in this study?

EXERCISE 2: STUDY IN APPENDIX D

Read the Method section of the report by Ward-Griffin and colleagues ("Perspectives of Women with Dementia") in Appendix D. Then answer the following questions:

Questions of Fact

a. Does the report indicate that the study procedures were reviewed by an IRB or other similar institutional human subjects group?
b. Would the study participants in this study be considered "vulnerable subjects?"
c. Were participants subjected to any physical harm or discomfort or psychological distress as part of this study? What efforts did the researchers make to minimize harm and maximize good?
d. Were participants deceived in any way?
e. Were participants coerced into participating in the study?
f. Were appropriate informed consent procedures used? Was there full disclosure? Was process consent used?
g. Does the report discuss steps that were taken to protect the privacy and confidentiality of study participants?

Questions for Discussion

a. Do you think the benefits of this research outweighed the costs to participants: What is the overall risk-to-benefit ratio?
b. Do you consider that the researchers took adequate steps to protect the study participants? If not, what else could they have done?
c. Comment on the fact that some of the interviews with the mothers were conducted in the presence of other family members.

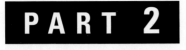

PART 2

Preliminary Steps in the Appraisal of Evidence

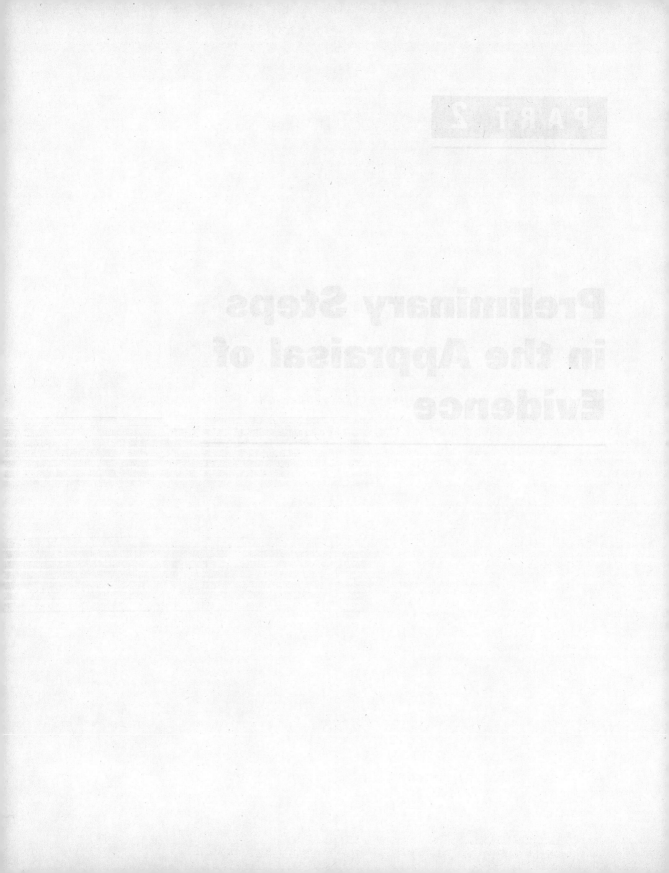

CHAPTER 6

Research Problems, Research Questions, and Hypotheses

■ A. Crossword Puzzle

Complete the crossword puzzle below, which uses terms and concepts presented in Chapter 6.

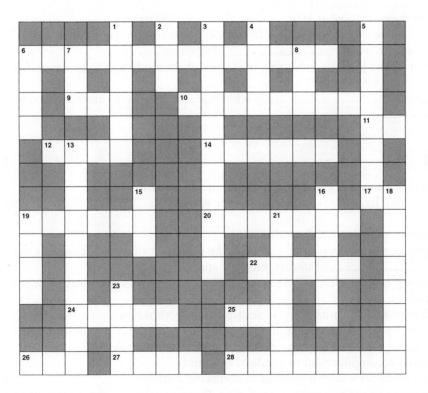

ACROSS

6. Hypothesis in which the specific nature of the predicted relationship is not stipulated
9. Statement of purpose in a quantitative study indicates the key study variables and the _____ of interest (abbr.).

Study Guide for Essentials of Nursing Research: Appraising Evidence for Nursing Practice, 7e

10. Researchers express the disturbing situation in need of study in their problem
_____.

11. Hypothesis that stipulates the expected relationship between an _____
and a DV (abbr.).

12. One phrase that indicates the relational aspect of a hypothesis is
_____ than

14. Topic for a research problem that might arise from global _____ or
political issues.

17. A popular television series based on a hospital drama.

19. One source of research problems, especially for hypothesis-testing research.

20. Hypothesis with two or more independent and/or dependent variables.

22. Hypothesis testing results never constitute _____ that the hypotheses
are or are not correct.

24. The purpose of a study is often conveyed through the judicious choice of
_____.

25. Hypotheses involve at least _____ variables.

26. In the question, "What is the effect of daily exercise on mood and weight?", mood
and weight are the _____ (acronym).

27. Statement of purpose indicating the intent of the study was to *prove* or *demonstrate*
something suggests a(n) _____.

28. A research _____ is what researchers wish to answer through systematic study.

DOWN

1. Hypothesis with one independent and one dependent variable.

2. The *actual* hypothesis of an investigator is the _____ hypothesis
(abbr.).

3. Another name for *null* hypothesis

4. A practical consideration in assessing the feasibility of a study concerns the
_____ of undertaking the study.

5. In complex hypotheses, there are _____ independent or dependent
variables.

6. Hypothesis that posits no relationship between variables

7. The independent variable in the research question, "Does a midafternoon
_____ improve evening mood state in the elderly?"

8. Desired accomplishment in conducting a study

13. The researcher's overall goals of undertaking a study.

15. Statement of the researcher's prediction about variables in the study (abbr.)

16. The study hypotheses should be stated _____ collecting the research
data, not after.

18. Hypotheses must predict a _____ between the independent and
dependent variables (abbr.).

19. Hypotheses are typically put to a statistical _____.

21. A statement of _____ is a declaration that communicates the general direction of the inquiry.

23. A research _____ is an enigmatic or troubling condition (abbr.).

■ B. Matching Exercises

1. Match each sentence in Set B with one of the phrases listed in Set A. Indicate the letter corresponding to the appropriate response next to each entry in Set B.

SET A

a. Statement of purpose—qualitative study

b. Statement of purpose—quantitative study

c. Not a statement of purpose for a research study

SET B   **RESPONSES**

1. The purpose of this study is to test whether the removal of physical restraints affects behavioral changes in elderly patients.   _____

2. The purpose of this project is to facilitate the transition from hospital to home among women who have just given birth.   _____

3. The goal of this project is to explore the process by which an elderly person adjusts to placement in a nursing home.   _____

4. The investigation was designed to document the incidence and prevalence of smoking, alcohol use, and drug use among adolescents aged 12 to 14.   _____

5. The study's purpose is to describe the nature of touch used by parents in touching their preterm infants.   _____

6. The goal is to develop guidelines for spiritually related nursing interventions.   _____

7. The purpose of this project is to examine the relationship between race or ethnicity and the use of over-the-counter medications.   _____

8. The purpose of this study is to develop an in-depth understanding of patients' feelings of powerlessness in hospital settings.   _____

2. Match each sentence in Set B with one of the phrases listed in Set A. Indicate the letter corresponding to the appropriate response next to each entry in Set B.

SET A

a. Research hypothesis—directional

b. Research hypothesis—nondirectional

c. Null hypothesis

d. Not a testable hypothesis as stated

SET B   **RESPONSES**

1. First-born infants have higher concentrations of estrogens and progesterone in umbilical cord blood than do later-born infants.   _____

2. No relationship exists between participation in prenatal classes and the health outcomes of infants.   _____

3. Nursing students are increasingly interested in obtaining advanced degrees.   _____

4. Nurse practitioners have more job mobility than do other registered nurses.   _____

5. A person's age is related to his or her difficulty in accessing health care.   _____

6. Glaucoma can be screened effectively by tonometry.   _____

7. Increased noise levels result in increased anxiety among hospitalized patients.   _____

8. Media exposure regarding the health hazards of smoking is unrelated to the public's smoking habits.   _____

9. Patients' compliance with their medication regimens is related to their perceptions of the consequences of noncompliance.   _____

10. The primary reason that nurses participate in continuing education programs is for professional advancement.   _____

11. Nursing graduates from the United States and Canada differ with respect to their level of job satisfaction in their first nursing jobs.   _____

12. A cancer patient's degree of hopefulness regarding the future is unrelated to his or her religiosity.   _____

13. The degree of attachment between infants and their mothers is associated with the infant's status as low birth weight or normal birth weight.   _____

14. The presence of homonymous hemianopia in stroke patients negatively affects the length of their hospitalization.   _____

15. Adjustment to hemodialysis does not vary by the patient's gender.   _____

■ C. Study Questions

1. Below is a list of general topics that could be investigated. Develop at least one research question for each, making sure that some are questions that could be addressed through qualitative research and others are ones that could be addressed through quantitative research. It may be helpful to use the question template in the Toolkit for Chapter 2 on the CD-ROM that accompanies the textbook. (HINT: For quantitative research questions, think of these concepts as potential independent or dependent variables, then ask, "What might cause or affect this variable?" and "What might be the consequences or effects of this variable?" This should lead to some ideas for research questions.)

   a. Patient comfort _____.

   b. Psychiatric patients' readmission rates _____.

   c. Anxiety in hospitalized children _____.

   d. Elevated blood pressure _____.

   e. Incidence of sexually transmitted diseases (STDs) _____.

   f. Patient cooperativeness in the recovery room _____.

   g. Caregiver stress _____.

   h. Mother–infant bonding _____.

   i. Menstrual irregularities _____.

2. Below are five nondirectional hypotheses. Restate each one as a directional hypothesis. Your hypotheses do not need to be "right"—this exercise is designed to encourage familiarity with wording hypotheses.

NONDIRECTIONAL	DIRECTIONAL
a. Tactile stimulation is associated with comparable physiologic arousal as verbal stimulation among infants with congenital heart disease.	a.
b. The risk of hypoglycemia in term newborns is related to the infant's birth weight.	b.
c. The use of isotonic sodium chloride solution before endotracheal suctioning is related to oxygen saturation.	c.
d. Fluid balance is related to degree of success in weaning older adults from mechanical ventilation.	d.
e. Nurses administer the same amount of narcotic analgesics to male and female patients.	e.

3. Below are five simple hypotheses. Change each one to a complex hypothesis by adding either a dependent or independent variable.

SIMPLE HYPOTHESIS	COMPLEX HYPOTHESIS
a. First-time blood donors experience greater anxiety during the donation than donors who have given blood previously.	a.
b. Nurses who initiate more conversation with patients are rated as more effective in their nursing care by patients than those who initiate less conversation.	b.
c. Surgical patients who give high ratings to the informativeness of nursing communications experience less preoperative stress than do patients who give low ratings.	c.
d. Appendectomy patients who are pregnant are more likely to experience peritoneal infection than female patients who are not pregnant.	d.
e. Women who give birth by cesarean delivery are more likely to experience postpartum depression than women who give birth vaginally.	e.

4. In study questions 2 and 3 above, 10 research hypotheses were provided. Identify the independent and dependent variables in each.

INDEPENDENT VARIABLE(S)	DEPENDENT VARIABLE(S)
2a	
2b	
2c	
2d	
2e	
3a	
3b	
3c	
3d	
3e	

5. Below are five statements that are *not* testable research hypotheses as currently stated. Suggest modifications to these statements that would make them testable hypotheses.

ORIGINAL STATEMENT	HYPOTHESIS
a. Relaxation therapy is effective in reducing hypertension.	a.
b. The use of bilingual health care staff produces high utilization rates of health care facilities by ethnic minorities.	b.
c. Nursing students are affected in their choice of clinical specialization by interactions with nursing faculty.	c.
d. Sexually active teenagers have a high rate of using male methods of contraception.	d.
e. In-use intravenous solutions become contaminated within 48 hours.	e.

■ D. Application Exercises

EXERCISE 1: STUDY IN APPENDIX A

Read the Abstract and Introduction to the report by Hill and colleagues ("Chronically Ill Rural Women") in Appendix A. Then answer the following questions:

Questions of Fact

a. In which paragraph(s) of this report is the research problem stated? Summarize the problem in three to four sentences.
b. Did the researchers present a statement of purpose? If so, what *verb* did they use in the purpose statement, and is that verb consistent with the type of research that was undertaken?
c. Did the researchers specify a research question? If so, was it well stated? If not, indicate what the question was.
d. Did Hill and colleagues specify hypotheses? If there are hypotheses, were they appropriately worded? Are they directional or nondirectional? Simple or complex? Research or null?
e. If no hypotheses were stated, what would one be?
f. Were any hypotheses *tested*?

Questions for Discussion

a. Did the researchers do an adequate job of describing the research problem? Suggest ways in which the problem statement could be improved.

b. Comment on the significance of the study's research problem for nursing.
c. Did the researchers adequately explain the study purpose, research questions, and/or hypotheses?

EXERCISE 2: STUDY IN APPENDIX B

Read the Abstract and Introduction to the report by Rasmussen and colleagues ("Young Women with Type 1 Diabetes") in Appendix B. Then answer the following questions:

Questions of Fact

a. In which paragraph(s) of this report is the research problem stated? Summarize the problem in three to four sentences.
b. Did the researchers present a statement of purpose? If so, what *verb* did they use in the purpose statement, and is that verb consistent with the type of research that was undertaken?
c. Did the researchers specify a research question? If so, was it well stated? If not, indicate what the question was.
d. Did Rasmussen and colleagues specify hypotheses? If there are hypotheses, were they appropriately worded? Are they directional or nondirectional? Simple or complex? Research or null?
e. Were any hypotheses *tested*?

Questions for Discussion

a. Did the researchers do an adequate job of describing the research problem? Suggest ways in which the problem statement could be improved.
b. Comment on the significance of the study's research problem for nursing.
c. Did the researcher adequately explain the study purpose, research questions, and/or hypotheses?

CHAPTER 7

Literature Reviews: Finding and Reviewing Research Evidence

■ A. Crossword Puzzle

Complete the crossword puzzle below, which uses terms and concepts presented in Chapter 7.

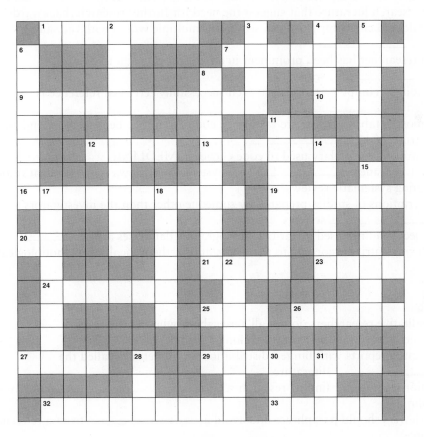

ACROSS

1. A good way to organize information when writing a complex literature review is to use a(n) _____.
7. A careful appraisal of the strengths and weaknesses of a study
9. The _____ approach is a search strategy that involves finding a pivotal early study and then searching for subsequent citations to it.
10. A common abbreviation for "literature"
12. Use of quotation _ _ _ _s around a search phrase can change the search results.
13. Most important bibliographic database for nurses
16. A thorough literature review includes a careful _____ of the methodological limitations of the body of existing studies.
19. The MEDLINE database can be accessed for free through _____.
20. A Boolean operator
21. In summarizing the literature, it is important to point out the _____ in the research literature that suggest the need for further research (backwards!).
23. A wildcard character permits a search for multiple words with the same _____.
24. If a researcher has been prominent in an area, it is useful to do a(n) _____ search.
25. In doing a computerized search, each successfully retrieved reference is sometimes called a "_____."
26. In most databases, there are "wildcard codes" that can be used to extend and search for truncated _____.
27. Controlled vocabulary used to code entries in MEDLINE
29. The Cochrane _____ of Systematic Reviews is an excellent resource for locating systematic reviews.
32. Descriptions of studies prepared by someone other than the investigators are _____ sources.
33. Subject headings used in various bibliographic databases are _____ for indexing entries according to their substantive, theoretical, or methodological focus

DOWN

2. Qualitative researchers do not all agree about whether the _____ should be reviewed before undertaking a study.
3. Research reports with limited distribution are sometimes called the _____ literature.
4. Major resource for finding research reports are _____ databases (abbr.).
5. Reviewers should paraphrase and avoid a _____ from a reference source.
6. A very important bibliographic database for health care professionals around the world

Study Guide for Essentials of Nursing Research: Appraising Evidence for Nursing Practice, 7e

8. Research literature reviews should contain few (if any) clinical _____.
11. Mechanism through which computer software translates topics into appropriate subject terms for a computerized literature search
14. Literature searches can be done on one's own or with the assistance of a _____ (abbr.).
15. When doing an electronic database search, one usually begins with one or more _____.
17. In launching a search for quantitative studies, the keywords are usually key _ _ _ _ _ _ _ _s.
18. An upfront literature review may not be undertaken by researchers doing a grounded _____ study.
22. A report written by researchers who conducted a study is a _____ source in a research review.
28. In writing a review, reviewers should paraphrase information in their _____ words.
30. A search strategy sometimes called "footnote chasing" is the _____ approach (abbr.).
31. A Boolean operator

■ B. Matching Exercises

Match each statement in Set B with one of the phrases in Set A. Indicate the letter corresponding to the appropriate response next to each entry in Set B.

SET A

a. CINAHL
b. MEDLINE
c. Neither CINAHL nor MEDLINE
d. Both CINAHL and MEDLINE

SET B	**RESPONSES**
1. An important bibliographic database for nurses	_____
2. Covers written materials from 1982 to present	_____
3. Can be accessed on the Internet through PubMed	_____
4. Permits a restriction (limit) to research reports (i.e., nonresearch reports can be excluded)	_____
5. Does not allow the use of wildcard characters	_____
6. Uses MeSH to index entries	_____
7. Can be accessed through proprietary search software	_____

8. Does not provide abstracts, only citations   _____

9. Has more than 15 million records   _____

10. The articles in the appendices to this *Study Guide* could be retrieved in this database   _____

■ C. Study Questions

1. Below are several research questions. Indicate one or more keywords that you would use to begin a literature search on this topic.

RESEARCH QUESTIONS	KEY WORDS
a. What is the lived experience of being a survivor of a suicide attempt?	_____
b. Does contingency contracting improve patient compliance with a treatment regimen?	_____
c. What is the decision-making process for a woman considering having an abortion?	_____
d. Do children raised on vegetarian diets have different growth patterns than other children?	_____
e. Is a special intervention for patients with spinal cord injury effective in reducing the risk of pressure ulcers?	_____
f. What is the course of appetite loss among cancer patients undergoing chemotherapy?	_____
g. What is the effect of alcohol skin preparation before insulin injection on the incidence of local and systemic infection?	_____
h. Are bottle-fed babies introduced to solid foods sooner than breastfed babies?	_____

2. Below are fictitious excerpts from research literature reviews. Each excerpt has a stylistic problem. Change each sentence to make it acceptable stylistically.

ORIGINAL	REVISED
a. Most elderly people do not eat a balanced diet.	_____
b. Patient characteristics have a significant impact on nursing workload.	_____
c. A child's conception of appropriate sick role behavior changes as the child grows older.	_____

   d. Home birth poses many potential dangers.   _____

   e. Multiple sclerosis results in considerable anxiety to the family
   of the patients.   _____

   f. Studies have proved that most nurses prefer not to work the night shift.   _____

   g. Life changes are the major cause of stress in adults.   _____

   h. Stroke rehabilitation programs are most effective when they involve
   the patients' families.   _____

   i. It has been proved that psychiatric outpatients have higher than
   average rates of accidental deaths and suicides.   _____

   j. The traditional pelvic examination is sufficiently unpleasant to
   many women that they avoid having the examination.   _____

   k. Most tonsillectomies performed three decades ago were unnecessary.   _____

   l. Few smokers seriously try to break the smoking habit.   _____

   m. Severe cutaneous burns often result in hemorrhagic gastric erosions.   _____

3. Read the following research report (or another article of your choosing). Complete as
   much information as you can about this report using the protocol in Figure 7.4,
   which is included as a Word document in the Toolkit on the CD-ROM that
   accompanies the textbook:

   • Bennett, J., et al. (2008). A telephone-only motivational intervention to increase
     physical activity in rural adults. *Nursing Research, 57*(1), 24–32.

4. Read the literature review section from a research article appearing in a nursing
   journal in the 1990s (some possibilities are suggested below). Search the literature for
   more recent research on the topic of the article and update the original researchers'
   review section. If possible, use the descendancy approach as one of your search
   strategies. (Do not forget to incorporate in your review the findings from the cited
   research article itself.) Here are some possible articles:

   • Long, K. A., & Boik, R. J. (1993). Predicting alcohol use in rural children. *Nursing
     Research, 42,* 79–86.
   • Morse, J. M., & Hutchinson, E. (1991). Releasing restraints: Providing safe care
     for the elderly. *Research in Nursing & Health, 14,* 382–396.
   • Quinn, M. M. (1991). Attachment between mothers and their Down syndrome
     infants. *Western Journal of Nursing Research, 13,* 382–396.
   • Singer, N. (1995). Understanding sexual risk behavior from drug users' accounts of
     their life experiences. *Qualitative Health Research, 5,* 237–249.

■ D. Application Exercises

EXERCISE 1: STUDY IN APPENDIX F

Read the Abstract, Introduction, and the first subsection under "Methods" of the report by Lee and colleagues ("Interventions for Informal Stroke Caregivers") in Appendix F. Then answer the following questions:

Questions of Fact

a. What type of research review did the investigators undertake?
b. Did the researchers begin with a problem statement? Summarize the problem in two or three sentences.
c. Did the researchers provide a statement of purpose? If so, what was it?
d. Which bibliographic databases did the researchers search? Were any other methods used in the search?
e. What keywords were used in the search? Were the keywords related to the independent or dependent variable of interest?
f. Did the researchers restrict their search to English-language reports?
g. How many citations were initially identified by the search?
h. What are some of the reasons the researchers cited for eliminating some of the retrieved studies from further consideration?
i. How many studies ultimately were included in the review?
j. Were the studies included in the review qualitative, quantitative, or both?

Questions for Discussion

a. Did the researchers do an adequate job of explaining the problem and their purpose in undertaking the review?
b. Did the researchers appear to do a thorough job in their search for relevant studies?
c. Certain studies that were initially retrieved were eliminated. Do you think the researchers provided a sound rationale for their decisions?

EXERCISE 2: STUDY IN APPENDIX G

Read the following Abstract, Introduction, and Study Design and Methods sections of the report by Xu ("Strangers in Strange Lands") in Appendix G. Then answer the following questions:

Questions of Fact

a. What type of research review did Xu undertake?
b. Did Xu begin with a problem statement? Did he articulate research questions? If yes, what were they?
c. How many different databases did Xu search? Were the searches of electronic databases? Were any manual methods used in the search?

d. What keywords were used in the search?
e. Did Xu restrict his search to English-language reports?
f. How many citations were initially identified by the search? How many studies were used in the review?
g. Were the studies included in the review qualitative, quantitative, or both?
h. Which qualitative research traditions were represented in the review?

Questions for Discussion

a. Did Xu do an adequate job of explaining the problem and the study purpose?
b. Did he appear to do a thorough job in his search for relevant studies?

Theoretical and Conceptual Frameworks

■ A. Crossword Puzzle

Complete the crossword puzzle below, which uses terms and concepts presented in Chapter 8

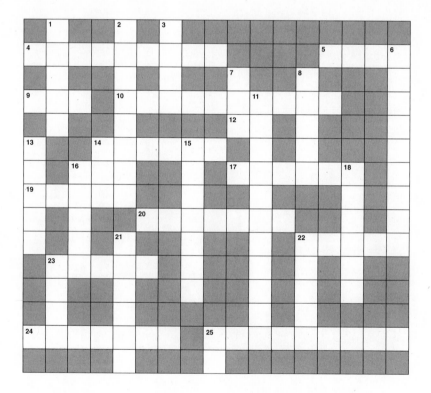

ACROSS

   4. Conceptual underpinnings of a study
   5. Originator of the Health Promotion Model (abbr.)
   9. One of the four elements in conceptual models of nursing (abbr.)

10. Abstractions assembled because of their relevance to a core theme form a _____ model.
12. Psychiatric nurse researchers sometimes obtain funding from an institute within the National Institutes of Health (NIH) with the acronym NI_ _.
14. Theory that focuses on an aspect of human experience is sometimes called _____-range.
16. Another term for a schematic model is conceptual _____.
17. Originator of the Science of Unitary Human Beings
19. Roy conceptualized the _____ Model of nursing (abbr.).
20. The Theory of _____ Behavior is sometimes used in nursing research.
22. Originator of the Theory of Human Becoming
23. A schematic _____ is a mechanism for representing concepts with a minimal use of words.
24. The development of theoretically sound definitions of constructs sometimes occurs in a _____ analysis.
25. A construct that was fully conceptualized by Bandura, which is a key mediator in many models of health behavior (abbr.).

DOWN

1. Theory aimed at explaining large segments of behavior or other phenomena
2. Theory that thoroughly accounts for or describes a phenomenon (abbr.)
3. A social psychological theory often used in nursing research is the Social _____ Theory (abbr.).
6. As classically defined, theories consist of concepts logically arrayed in an interrelated _____ system.
7. Acronym for Pender's model
8. Theory that focuses on a single aspect of human experience is sometimes called middle-_____.
11. In a study based on a specific theory, the framework is called the _____ framework.
13. *Stages of change* is the core construct in the _ _ _ _ _ theoretical Model.
14. A schematic model is also called a conceptual _____.
15. One of the originators of the Theory of Stress and Coping
16. Another name for a grand theory is a _____ theory.
18. Type of theory originally from another discipline used productively by nurse researchers
21. HBM is an acronym for the Health _____ Model.
22. The development of a theoretical context for a study typically takes place during the conceptual _____ of a project.
23. Originator of the Self-Care Deficit Theory (backwards!)
25. Theoretical underpinning of a grounded theory study (acronym)

■ B. Matching Exercises

1. Match each statement from Set B with one of the phrases in Set A. Indicate the letter corresponding to your response next to each of the statements in Set B.

SET A

a. Classic theory

b. Conceptual model

c. Schematic model

d. Neither a, b, nor c

e. a, b, and c

SET B   **RESPONSES**

1. Makes minimal use of language   _____

2. Uses concepts as building blocks   _____

3. Is essential in the conduct of good research   _____

4. Can be used as a basis for generating hypotheses   _____

5. Can be proved through empirical testing   _____

6. Incorporates a system of propositions that assert relationships
   among variables   _____

7. Consists of interrelated concepts organized in a rational scheme
   but does not specify formal relationships among the concepts   _____

8. Exists in nature and is awaiting scientific discovery   _____

2. Match each model from Set B with one of the theorists in Set A. Indicate the letter corresponding to your response next to each of the statements in Set B.

SET A

a. Orem

b. Pender

c. Roy

d. Watson

e. Rogers

f. Lazarus-Folkman

g. Mishel

h. Azjen

SET B	**RESPONSES**
1. Adaptation Model	_____
2. Theory of Caring	_____
3. Uncertainty in Illness Theory	_____
4. Self-Care Deficit Theory	_____
5. Theory of Stress and Coping	_____
6. Health Promotion Model	_____
7. Theory of Planned Behavior	_____
8. Science of Unitary Human Beings	_____

■ C. Study Questions

1. Read some recent issues of a nursing research journal. Identify at least three different theories cited by nurse researchers in these research reports.

2. Choose one of the conceptual models of nursing described in this chapter. Do some reading about the model in one of the cited references. Develop a research hypothesis based on this model.

3. Select one of the research questions or problems listed below. Could the selected problem be developed within one of the models or theories discussed in this chapter? Defend your answer.
   a. How do men cope with a diagnosis of prostate cancer?
   b. What are the factors contributing to perceptions of fatigue among patients with congestive heart failure?
   c. What effect does the presence of the father in the delivery room have on the mother's satisfaction with the childbirth experience?
   d. The purpose of the study is to explore why some women fail to perform breast self-examination regularly.
   e. What are the factors that lead to poorer health among low-income children than higher-income children?

4. Suggest an important health outcome that could be studied using the Health Promotion Model. Identify another theory described in this chapter that could be used to explain or predict the same outcome. Which theory or model do you think would do a better job? Why?

5. Read the following article and then answer these questions: (a) What evidence do the researchers offer to substantiate that their grounded theory is a good fit with their data? and (b) To what extent is it clear or unclear in the article that symbolic interactionism (or some other theoretical perspective) was the theoretical underpinning of the study?

- Rempel, G., & Harrison, M. (2007). Safeguarding precarious survival: Parenting children who have life-threatening heart disease. *Qualitative Health Research, 17,* 824–837.

■ D. Application Exercises

EXERCISE 1: STUDY IN APPENDIX C

Read the Introduction and Methods section of the report by Vollman and colleagues ("Coping and Depressive Symptoms") in Appendix C. Then answer the following questions:

Questions of Fact

a. Did this study involve a conceptual or theoretical framework? What is it called?
b. Did the authors explain features of the theory or model?
c. Is the framework one of the models of nursing cited in the textbook? Is it related to one of those models?
d. Is the theory or framework a *shared* theory?
e. Did the report include a schematic model? If so, what are the key concepts in the model?
f. Did the report present conceptual definitions of key concepts of the study?
g. Did the authors formally state a hypothesis deduced from the theory? Did they undertake hypothesis-testing statistical analyses?
h. According to the theory, what type of coping might be expected to result in depressive symptoms?

Questions for Discussion

a. Do the research problem and hypotheses (if any) naturally flow from the theory or framework? Does the link between the problem and the framework seem contrived?
b. Do you think any aspects of the research would have been different without the framework?
c. Would you describe this study as a model-testing inquiry or do you think the model was used more as an organizing framework?
d. Are the operational definitions of key constructs appropriate for the theoretical framework?
e. Develop a schematic model (conceptual map) that captures key aspects of this study. Then state the hypotheses that your model implies.

EXERCISE 2: STUDY IN APPENDIX D

Read the report by Ward-Griffin and colleagues ("Perspectives of Women with Dementia") in Appendix D. Then answer the following questions:

Questions of Fact

a. Did this article describe a conceptual or theoretical framework for the study? If so, what is it called?
b. Did the authors explain features of the theory or model?
c. Is the framework one of the models of nursing cited in the textbook? Is it related to one of those models?
d. Is the theory or framework a *shared* theory?
e. Did the report include a schematic model? If so, what are the key concepts in the framework?
f. Did the report explicitly present hypotheses deduced from the framework? Did they undertake hypothesis-testing statistical analyses?

Questions for Discussion

a. Does the research problem naturally flow from the framework? Does the link between the problem and the framework seem contrived?
b. Do you think any aspects of the research would have been different without the framework?
c. How good a job do you feel the researchers did in tying the perspectives of the framework to the presentation of the findings and the discussion of the results?

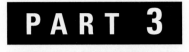

PART 3

Designs for Nursing Research

CHAPTER 9

Quantitative Research Designs

■ A. Crossword Puzzle

Complete the crossword puzzle below, which uses terms and concepts presented in Chapter 9.

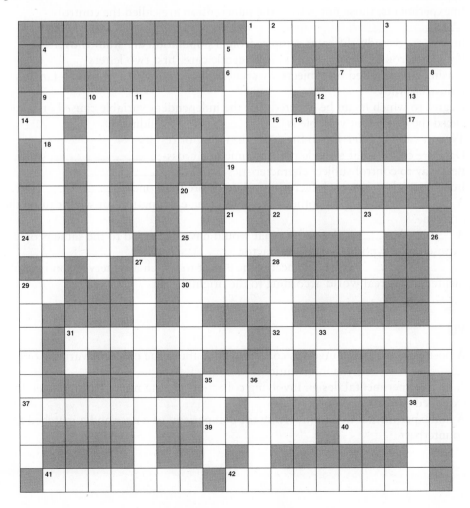

ACROSS

1. Good research design in quantitative studies involves four types of
   _____.
4. A design in which the same subjects are exposed to two or more conditions, in random order
6. Loss of subjects from a study over time (abbr.)
9. Threat to internal validity stemming from pre-existing group differences
12. In a factorial design, each independent variable is called a _____.
14. Design involving an intervention, but not randomization (acronym)
15. Allocation of subjects to groups by chance (acronym)
17. Design in which the independent variable is not manipulated (acronym)
19. Threat to internal validity stemming from differential loss of subjects from groups
22. Design in which data about presumed causes are collected before data about hypothesized effects (abbr.)
24. In experiments, those not getting the intervention are called the control
    _____.
25. In a _ _ _ _d study, different samples from a population are studied over time.
29. Popular acronym for a certain kind of gentle care (first two letters)
30. Biasing effect caused by subjects' awareness of being in a study, from a famous industrial study
31. Degree to which it can be inferred that the independent variable caused or influenced the dependent variable is _____ validity.
32. Type of validity referring to the generalizability of results
35. Data are collected at a single point in time in a cross-_____ study.
37. Best way to control subject characteristics is to _____.
39. In a factorial design, each factor must have more than one _____.
40. A _____ hypothesis is a competing explanation for what caused the outcome.
41. A _____ factual is what would have happened to the same people not exposed to a hypothesized causal factor.
42. _____ fidelity concerns the extent to which an intervention is implemented in the real world according to the original plan.

DOWN

2. A posttest-only design involves collecting data about the outcome variable only _____ the intervention.
3. A quasi-experimental design involving collection of data multiple times over an extended period (acronym)
4. A nonexperimental design involving the comparison of a *case* and a matched counterpart

5. A true experiment involves assignment of subjects to groups or conditions at
_____.

7. Type of longitudinal study that gathers data from the same people at multiple points in time

8. A _____ test involves the collection of baseline data on the dependent variable.

10. Study designed to collect data over an extended period (abbr.)

11. Type of nonexperimental design that focuses on relationships between variables (abbr.)

13. An experimental design that collects data after (but not before) the intervention is a posttest-_____ design.

16. An experimental design that collects baseline and outcome data is a before-_____ design.

20. Pairing of subjects in different groups as a method of controlling confounding variables

21. Designs involving comparisons of different people are _____-subjects designs (abbr.)

23. Statistical _ _ _ _r involves the strength of the design to detect true relationships among variables.

26. Study designed so that neither subjects nor agents know who got the intervention is _____-blind.

27. Another name for a randomized controlled trial (RCT) is a(n) _____.

28. A potential internal validity problem is the history _____, which concerns the effect of other things co-occurring with the independent variable.

29. A criterion for inferring causality is lack of _____ ambiguity.

31. Experiments offer greater corroboration than other designs approach that _ _ the independent variable is manipulated, *then* certain consequences may be expected to ensue.

33. In factorial designs, there must be at least _____ manipulated independent variables.

35. A main concern in nonexperimental research is the bias known as _____ selection into groups being compared.

36. One statistical method of controlling confounding variables is called analysis of _____ (abbr.).

38. In a delayed treatment situation, control group members are _____ listed for the intervention.

■ B. Matching Exercises

Match each research question from Set B with one (or more) of the phrases from Set A that indicates a potential reason for using a nonexperimental design. Indicate the letter(s) corresponding to your response next to each statement in Set B.

SET A

a. Independent variable cannot be manipulated

b. Possible ethical constraints on manipulation

c. Practical constraints on manipulation

d. No constraints on manipulation

SET B   **RESPONSES**

1. Does the use of certain tampons cause toxic shock syndrome? _____

2. Does heroin addiction among mothers affect Apgar scores of infants? _____

3. Is the age of a hemodialysis patient related to the incidence of the disequilibrium syndrome? _____

4. What body positions aid respiratory function? _____

5. Does the ingestion of saccharin cause cancer in humans? _____

6. Does a nurse's attitude toward the elderly affect his or her choice of a clinical specialty? _____

7. Does the use of touch by nursing staff affect patient morale? _____

8. Does a nurse's gender affect his or her salary and rate of promotion? _____

9. Does extreme athletic exertion in young women cause amenorrhea? _____

10. Does assertiveness training affect a psychiatric nurse's job performance? _____

■ C. Study Questions

1. Suppose you wanted to study self-efficacy among successful dieters who lost 20 or more pounds and maintained their weight loss for at least 6 months. Specify at least two different types of comparison strategies that might provide a useful comparative context for this study. Do your strategies lend themselves to experimental manipulation? If not, why not?

2. Refer to the 10 hypotheses in Exercises C.2 and C.3 of Chapter 6. Indicate on the following chart whether these hypotheses could be tested using an experimental or quasi-experimental approach, a nonexperimental approach, or both.

Question No.	Experimental/ Quasi-experimental	Nonexperimental	Both
2a			
2b			
2c			
2d			
2e			
3a			
3b			
3c			
3d			
3e			

3. In the following study, the researchers conducted a double-blind experiment. Review the design for this study, and comment on the appropriateness of the double-blind procedures. What biases were the researchers trying to avoid? Do you think they were successful?

   • McDonald, D. D., Amendola, M. G., Interlandi, E., Wall, K., Lewchik, B., Polouse, L., et al. (2007). Effect of reading additional safety information on planned use of over-the-counter analgesics. *Public Health Nursing, 24,* 230–238.

4. Suppose that you are studying the effects of range-of-motion exercises on patients who have had a radical mastectomy. You start your experiment with 50 experimental subjects and 50 control subjects. Your intervention requires the experimental subjects to come for daily sessions over a 2-week period, whereas control subjects come only once at the end of 2 weeks. Your final group sizes are 40 for the experimental group and 49 for the control group. The results of your study indicate that the experimental group did better in raising the arm of the affected side above head level. What effects, if any, do you think the subject attrition might have on the internal validity of your study?

5. Suppose you were interested in testing the hypothesis that regular ingestion of aspirin reduced the risk of colon cancer. Describe how such a hypothesis could be tested using a retrospective case-control design. Now describe a prospective cohort design for the same study. Compare the strengths and weaknesses of the two approaches.

■ D. Application Exercises

EXERCISE 1: STUDY IN APPENDIX A

Read the Methods section of the report by Hill and colleagues ("Chronically Ill Rural Women") in Appendix A. Then answer the following questions:

Questions of Fact

a. Was there an intervention in this study?
b. Is the design for this study experimental, quasi-experimental, or nonexperimental?
c. What were the independent and dependent variables?
d. Was randomization used? If yes, what method was used to assign subjects to groups?
e. In terms of the control group strategies described in the textbook, what approach did the researchers use?
f. What is the specific name of the research design used in this study?
g. Is the overall design a within-subjects or between-subjects design?
h. Was any masking or blinding used in this study?
i. Would this study be described as longitudinal?
j. Which of the methods of research control described in this chapter were used to control confounding variables?
k. What confounding variables were controlled?
l. Was there any attrition in this study?
m. Is there evidence that constancy of conditions was achieved?
n. Were group treatments as distinct as possible to maximize power? If not, why not?

Questions for Discussion

a. What was the intervention? Comment on how well the intervention was described, including a description of how it was developed and refined.
b. Comment on the researchers' counterfactual strategy. Could a more powerful or effective strategy have been used?
c. Discuss ways in which this study achieved or failed to achieve the criteria for making causal inferences.
d. Comment on the researchers' masking strategy.
e. Comment on the timing of postintervention data collection.
f. Discuss issues relating to the intervention fidelity in this study.
g. Is this study strong in internal validity? What, if any, are the threats to the internal validity of this study?
h. Is this study strong on external validity? What, if any, are the threats to the external validity of this study?

EXERCISE 2: STUDY IN APPENDIX C

Read the Methods section of the report by Vollman and colleagues ("Coping and Depressive Symptoms") in Appendix C. Then answer the following questions:

Questions of Fact

a. Was there an intervention in this study?
b. Is the design for this study experimental, quasi-experimental or nonexperimental?
c. What were the independent and dependent variables in this study?
d. Was the independent amenable to manipulation?
e. What comparison group strategy was used in this study?
f. What is the specific name of the research design used in this study?
g. Was randomization used to control confounding variables in this study? Was matching used? Was homogeneity used?
h. Was any masking or blinding used in this study?
i. Is the design retrospective or prospective?
j. Would this study be described as longitudinal or cross-sectional?
k. Could this study be described as cause-probing? What did the researchers themselves say about a possible causal connection between coping styles and depressive symptoms?

Questions for Discussion

a. Discuss ways in which this study achieved or failed to achieve the criteria for making causal inferences.
b. Comment on the comparison strategy that the researchers used.
c. Comment on the timing of data collection.
d. Is this study strong in internal validity? What, if any, are the threats to the internal validity of this study?
e. Is this study strong on external validity? What, if any, are the threats to the external validity of this study?

CHAPTER 10

Qualitative Designs and Approaches

■ A. Crossword Puzzle

Complete the crossword puzzle below, which uses terms and concepts presented in Chapter 10.

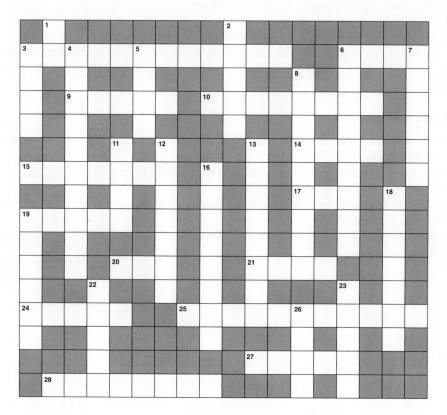

ACROSS

3. Leininger's phrase for research at the interface between culture and nursing
6. Type of phenomenology that includes the step of bracketing (abbr.)
9. In narrative analysis, the focus is on a(n)_____
10. Research that focuses on gender denomination
14. Type of psychological research that studies the environment's influence on behavior (abbr.)
15. One of the two originators of grounded theory
17. A type of action research (acronym)
19. Knowledge that is so embedded in a culture that people do not talk about it
20. The outsider's view is called the e_ _ _ perspective
21. In a(n) _____ ethnography, researchers study their own culture or subculture
24. Traditional qualitative research does not adopt a strong political point of view or _____ perspective (abbr.)
25. Ethnographers typically engage in _____ observation during their fieldwork
27. Grounded theory research often identifies the _____ social process that explains how people resolve a problem
28. Qualitative research design is typically a(n) _____ design

DOWN

1. A qualitative tradition concerned with social processes and social structures (acronym)
2. Phenomenologists study _____ experiences
3. Perspective that is the insider's view
4. Systematic collection and analysis of materials relating to the past is _____ research
5. Burke's pentadic dramatism is one approach to _____ analysis (abbr.)
6. Type of analysis designed to understand the rules and structure of conversations
7. The nurse researcher who worked with an originator of grounded theory to develop an alternative approach
8. A type of phenomenology focusing on the *meaning* of experiences (abbr.)
11. The second step in descriptive phenomenology is to in_ _ _ _
12. A phenomenologic question is: What is the _____ of this phenomenon?
13. Grounded theorists use an analytic strategy called _____ comparison
16. Research that seeks to be transformative is based on _____ theory
18. Hermeneutics focuses on the _____ of human experiences
19. An approach to classifying qualitative research design is according qualitative _____ (abbr.)
22. Descriptive qualitative studies involve a(n) _ _ _ _ _nt analysis of narrative data to search for key themes and patterns

23. One aspect of experience that phenomenologists study is spatiality or lived
_____

26. In a(n) _____ study, a single person or group is at center stage

■ B. Matching Exercises

Match each descriptive statement from Set B with one of the research traditions from Set A. Indicate the letter corresponding to your response next to each item in Set B.

SET A

a. Ethnography
b. Phenomenology
c. Grounded theory
d. Ethnography, phenomenology, and grounded theory

SET B   RESPONSES

1. Is rooted in a philosophical tradition developed by Husserl
   and Heidegger   _____

2. Studies both broadly defined cultures and more narrowly
   defined ones   _____

3. Uses qualitative data to address questions of interest   _____

4. Is an approach to the study of social processes and social structures   _____

5. Is concerned with the lived experiences of humans   _____

6. Strives to achieve an emic perspective on the members of a group   _____

7. Is closely related to a research tradition called hermeneutics   _____

8. Uses a procedure referred to as constant comparison   _____

9. Stems from a discipline other than nursing   _____

10. Developed by the sociologists Glaser and Strauss   _____

11. Is a tradition that is particularly well suited to a critical theory
    perspective   _____

12. Typically involves interviews with study participants   _____

■ C. Study Questions

1. For each of the research questions below, indicate what type of qualitative research tradition would likely guide the inquiry, and why you think that would be the case.
   a. What is the social psychological process through which couples deal with the sudden loss of an infant through SIDS?
   b. How does the culture of a suicide survivors' self-help group adapt to a successful suicide attempt by a former member?
   c. What are the "hidden agendas" that underlie conversations between nurses and bed-ridden nursing home patients?
   d. What is the lived experience of the spousal caretaker of an Alzheimer patient?

2. Skim the following two studies, which are examples of ethnographic and phenomenological studies that focused on the elderly. What were the central phenomena under investigation? Compare and contrast the methods used in these two studies (e.g., how were data collected? How many study participants were there? To what extent did the design unfold while the researchers were in the field?)
   • *Ethnographic Study*: Tutton, E., & Seers, K. (2004). Comfort on a ward for older people. *Journal of Advanced Nursing, 46*, 380–389.
   • *Phenomenological Study*: Hinck, S. (2007). The meaning of time in oldest-old age. *Holistic Nursing Practice, 21*, 35–41.

3. Skim one of the following participatory action research studies and comment on the roles of participants and researchers. In what ways would the study have differed if a participatory approach had not been used?
   • Etowa, J., et al., (2007). Depression: The "invisible grey fog" influencing the midlife health of African Canadian women. *International Journal of Mental Health Nursing, 16*, 203–213.
   • Liu, M., et al. (2006). Using participatory action research to provide health promotion for disadvantaged elders in Shaanxi province, China. *Public Health Nursing, 23*, 332–338.
   • Van Loon, A., Koch, T., & Kralik, D. (2004). Care for female survivors of child sexual abuse in emergency departments. *Accident and Emergency Nursing, 12*, 208–214.

4. Read one of the case studies suggested below and evaluate the extent to which the case study approach was appropriate. What were the drawbacks and benefits of using this approach?
   • Pepler, C. J., et al. (2005). Unit culture and research-based nursing practice in acute care. *Canadian Journal of Nursing Research, 37*(3), 66–85.
   • McCurdy, C., et al. (2007). There to here: Young adult patients' perceptions of the process of transition from pediatric to adult transplant care. *Progress in Transplantation, 16*, 309–316.

5. Read one of the studies below, and evaluate the extent to which the problem was amenable to the grounded theory research tradition. Which of the two schools of grounded theory thought was followed in this study? Does the report explicitly discuss how the constant comparative method was used?

   - Brink, E., Karlson, B., & Hallberg, L. (2006). Readjustment 5 months after a first-time myocardial infarction: Reorienting the active self. *Journal of Advanced Nursing, 53*(4), 403–411.
   - Silva-Smith, A. L. (2007). Restructuring life: Preparing for and beginning a new caregiving role. *Journal of Family Nursing, 13,* 99–116.

6. Read one of the studies below, and think about how the researcher could have adopted a critical theory or feminist perspective. In what way would the methods for such a modification differ from the methods used?

   - Forchuk, C., Nelson, G., & Hall, G. (2006). "It's important to be proud of the place you live in": Housing problems and preferences of psychiatric survivors. *Perspectives in Psychiatric Care, 42*(1), 42–52.
   - Oelke, N., & Vollman, A. (2007). "Inside and outside": Sikh women's perspectives on cervical cancer screening. *Canadian Journal of Nursing Research, 39,* 174–189.
   - Price, S., et al. (2007). Women's experience with social presence during childbirth. *MCH: The American Journal of Maternal/Child Nursing, 32,* 184–191.
   - Webb, M., & Gonzalez, L. (2006). The burden of hypertension: Mental representations of African American women. *Issues in Mental Health Nursing, 27*(3), 249–271.

■ D. Application Exercises

EXERCISE 1: STUDY IN APPENDIX B

Read the Design and Methods section of the report by Rasmussen and colleagues ("Young Women with Type 1 Diabetes") in Appendix B. Then answer the following questions:

Questions of Fact

a. In which tradition was this study based?
b. Which specific approach was used—that of Glaser and Strauss, or that of Strauss and Corbin?
c. What is the central phenomenon under study?
d. Was the study longitudinal?
e. What was the setting for this research?
f. Did the report indicate or suggest that constant comparison was used?
g. Was a core variable or basic social process identified? If yes, what was it?
h. Is the research question congruent with a qualitative approach and with the specific research tradition (i.e., is the domain of inquiry for the study congruent with the domain encompassed by the tradition)?

i. Did the researchers use methods that were congruent with the qualitative research tradition?

j. Did this study have an ideological perspective? If so, which one?

Questions for Discussion

a. How well is the research design described in the report? Were design decisions explained and justified?

b. Does it appear that the researchers made all design decisions up-front, or did the design emerge during data collection, allowing them to capitalize on early information?

c. Did any elements of the design or methods appear to be more appropriate for a qualitative tradition other than the one the researchers identified as the underlying tradition?

d. Could this study have been undertaken within an ideological framework? If so, what changes to the research methods would be necessary?

EXERCISE 2: STUDY IN APPENDIX D

Read the method section of the report by Ward-Griffin and colleagues ("Perspectives of Women with Dementia") in Appendix D. Then answer the following questions:

Questions of Fact

a. In which tradition was this study based? Did this study have an ideological perspective?

b. What is the central phenomenon under study?

c. Was the study longitudinal?

d. What was the setting for this research?

e. Is the research question congruent with a qualitative approach and with the specific research tradition (i.e., is the domain of inquiry for the study congruent with the domain encompassed by the tradition)?

f. Did the researchers use methods that were congruent with the qualitative research tradition?

Questions for Discussion

a. How well is the research design described? Were design decisions explained and justified?

b. Does it appear that the researcher made all design decisions up-front, or did the design emerge during data collection, allowing researchers to capitalize on early information?

c. Is there evidence that ideological methods were used and ideological goals were achieved? (e.g., Was there evidence of full collaboration between researchers and participants? Did the research have the power to be transformative, or is there evidence that a transformative process occurred?)

CHAPTER 11

Specific Types
of Research

■ A. Crossword Puzzle

Complete the crossword puzzle below, which uses terms and concepts presented in
Chapter 11.

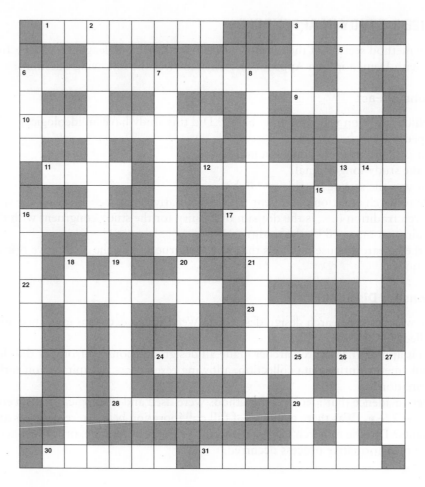

ACROSS

1. Interviews that are done face-to-face
5. Type of trial designed with decision-makers in mind (acronym)
6. A multiphase effort to refine and test the effectiveness of a clinical treatment
9. Another term for interviews done in person is _____ to _____
10. Analysis of data done with an existing data set
11. One method of delivering a survey is through the _____
12. Form used in survey research that participants complete on their own (abbr.)
13. One goal of mixed method research is to generate and then test _____ (abbr.) in a single study.
16. Phase IV clinical trials are sometimes called _____ studies (abbr.).
17. Type of research that focuses on improving research strategies (abbr.)
21. An alternative to in-person interviews is interviews by _____ (abbr.).
22. Method of collecting self-report data
23. Phase II trials often involves a pilot _____ of a new treatment.
24. In evaluations, a(n) _____ analysis describes the extent to which a program is achieving certain goals.
28. A Gallup poll is one of these
29. Paradigm associated with a position emphasizing the "dictatorship of the research question" (abbr.)
30. Type of research that integrates qualitative and quantitative data is mixed _____.
31. An emerging trend is distribution of surveys over the _____.

DOWN

2. Phase III of a clinical trial is a _____ controlled trial.
3. Data collected by asking people questions in a survey is via _____ reports.
4. Type of evaluation that uses an experimental design is a(n) i_ _ _ _ _ analysis.
6. Type of evaluation of the economic effects of an intervention is a(n) _____ analysis.
7. An economic _____ examines the financial costs and benefits of a program or intervention.
8. An evaluation of the process of putting a new intervention into place is a(n) _____ analysis.
14. Nursing intervention research emphasizes the importance of developing an intervention _____ that specifies what must be done to achieve desired outcomes (backwards!).
15. An objective in a phase I clinical trial is to determine the optimal _____ of an intervention.
16. A phase III clinical trial is sometimes called a(n) _____ study.

18. In the Donabedian framework, the three key factors are process, outcomes, and
_____.
19. Another name for an implementation analysis
20. An impact analysis provides information about the _____ effects of a
program.
25. An RCT involves the use of a(n) _____ design (abbr.).
26. In developing a nursing intervention, people who have a _____ in the
intervention should be "brought on board".
27. A mixed method design involving discrete segments of an overall inquiry (abbr.)

■ B. Matching Exercises

Match each feature from Set B with one (or more) of the phrases from Set A that indicates a
type of quantitative research. Indicate the letter(s) corresponding to your response next to
each statement in Set B.

SET A

a. Clinical trial
b. Evaluation research
c. Methodological research
d. Survey research
e. Outcomes research
f. Secondary analysis

SET B   RESPONSES

1. Can involve an experimental design   _____

2. Economic analyses are one type   _____

3. Examines the global effectiveness of nursing services   _____

4. Data are always from self-reports   _____

5. The aim is to develop better instruments and procedures for doing
substantive research   _____

6. Often designed in a series of phases (typically four)   _____

7. Includes process analyses   _____

8. Donabedian's framework is often used in this research   _____

9. The most well-known type is the RCT   _____

10. Avoids time-consuming and costly research steps   _____

■ C. Study Questions

1. Read one of the following studies, in which quantitative data were gathered and analyzed to address a research question. Suggest ways in which the collection of qualitative data might have enriched the study, strengthened its validity, or enhanced its interpretability:

   • Kim, M., Lee, S., Ahn, Y., Bowen, P., & Lee, H. (2007). Dietary acculturation and diet quality of hypertensive Korean Americans. *Journal of Advanced Nursing, 58,* 436–445.

   • Kozachik, S., Wyatt, G., Given, C., & Given, B. (2006). Patterns of use of complementary therapies among cancer patients and their family caregivers. *Cancer Nursing, 29,* 84–94.

   • Moscato, S., Valanis, B., Gullion, C., Tanner, C., Shapiro, S., & Izumi, S. (2007). Predictors of patient satisfaction with telephone nursing services. *Clinical Nursing Research, 16,* 119–137.

2. Read one of the following qualitative studies. Suggest ways that the findings could be validated or the emergent hypotheses could be tested in a quantitative study:

   • Daiski, L. (2007). Perspectives of homeless people on their health and health needs priorities. *Journal of Advanced Nursing, 58,* 273–281.

   • Milne, J., & Moore, K. (2006). Factors impacting self-care for urinary incontinence. *Urologic Nursing, 26,* 41–51.

   • Price, S., Noseworthy, J., & Thornton, J. (2007). Women's experience with social presence during childbirth. *MCN: The American Journal of Maternal/Child Nursing, 32,* 184–191.

3. Suppose you were interested in studying the research questions below by conducting a survey. For each, indicate whether you would recommend using a personal interview, a telephone interview, or a self-administered questionnaire to collect the data. What is your rationale?

   a. What are the coping strategies of newly widowed individuals?

   b. What strategies do emergency department nurses use to identify and correct medical errors?

   c. What type of nursing communications do presurgical patients find most helpful?

   d. What is the relationship between teenagers' health-risk appraisal and their risk-taking behavior (e.g., smoking, unprotected sex, drug use)?

   e. What are the health-promoting activities pursued by inner-city single mothers?

   f. How is employment of parents affected by the health problems or disability of a child?

4. Below is a brief description of a mixed method study, followed by a critique. Do you agree with this critique? Can you add other comments regarding the study design?

Fictitious Study. Garvey conducted a study to examine the emotional well-being of women who had a mastectomy. Garvey wanted to develop an in-depth understanding of the emotional experiences of women as they recovered from their surgery, including the process by which they handled their fears, their concerns about their sexuality, their levels of anxiety and depression, their methods of coping, and their social supports.

Garvey's basic study design was a descriptive qualitative study. She gathered information from a sample of 26 women, primarily by means of in-depth interviews with the women on two occasions. The first interviews were scheduled within 1 month after the surgery. Follow-up interviews were conducted about 12 months later. Several women in the sample participated in a support group, and Garvey attended and made observations at several meetings. Additionally, Garvey decided to interview the "significant other" (usually the husband) of most of the women, when it became clear that the women's emotional well-being was linked to the manner in which the significant other was reacting to the surgery.

In addition to the rich, in-depth information she gathered, Garvey wanted to be able to better interpret the emotional status of the women. Therefore, at both the original and follow-up interview with the women, she administered a psychological scale known as the Center for Epidemiological Studies Depression Scale (CES-D), a quantitative measure that has scores that can range from 0 to 60. This scale has been widely used in community populations, and has cut-off scores designating when a person is at risk of clinical depression (i.e., a score of 16 and above).

Garvey's qualitative analysis showed that the basic process underlying psychological recovery from the mastectomy was something she labeled "Gaining by Losing," a process that involved heightened self-awareness and self-respect after an initial period of despair and self-pity. The process also involved, for some, a strengthening of personal relationships with significant others, whereas for others, it resulted in the birth of awareness of fundamental deficiencies in their relationships. The quantitative findings confirmed that a very high percentage of women were at risk of being depressed at 1 month after the mastectomy, but at 12 months, the average level of depression was actually modestly lower than in the general population of women.

Critique. In her study, Garvey embedded a quantitative measure into her field work in an interesting manner. Most data were qualitative—in-depth interviews and in-depth observations. However, she also opted to include a well-known measure of depression, which provided her with an important context for interpreting her data. A major advantage of using the CES-D is that this scale has known characteristics in the general population and, therefore, provided a built-in "comparison group."

Garvey used a flexible design that allowed her to use her initial data to guide her inquiry. For example, she decided to conduct in-depth interviews with significant others when she learned their importance to the women's process of emotional recovery. Garvey did do some advance planning, however, that provided general guidance. For example, although her questioning undoubtedly evolved while in the field, she had the foresight to realize that to capture a process as it evolved, she would need to collect data longitudinally. She also made the upfront decision to use the CES-D to supplement the in-depth interviews.

In this study, the findings from the qualitative and quantitative portions of the study were complementary. Both portions of the study confirmed that the women initially had emotional "losses," but eventually they recovered and "gained" in terms of their emotional well-being and their self-awareness. This example illustrates how the validity of study findings can be enhanced by the blending of qualitative and quantitative data. If the qualitative data alone had been gathered, Garvey might not have gotten a good handle on the degree to which the women had actually "recovered" (*vis à vis* women who had never had a mastectomy). Conversely, if she had collected only the CES-D data, she would have had no insights into the process by which the recovery occurred.

■ D. Application Exercises

EXERCISE 1: ALL STUDIES IN APPENDICES

Which of the studies in the appendices of this *Study Guide* (if any) could be considered:

a. A clinical trial?
b. An economic analysis?
c. Outcomes research?
d. Survey research?
e. A secondary analysis?
f. Methodological research?

EXERCISE 2: STUDIES IN APPENDICES A TO D

For the quantitative study in either the Appendix A or C, develop a qualitative component that you think would enhance the study. Write one paragraph outlining the design for this component, and indicate how you would sequence the two components (i.e., concurrently or sequentially). Then do the opposite (design a quantitative component) for the qualitative study in either Appendix B or D.

EXERCISE 3: STUDY IN APPENDIX E

Read the article by Tracy and colleagues ("Translating Best Practices") in Appendix E. Then answer the following questions:

Questions of Fact

a. Did this evidence-based practice project use mixed methods? If yes, identify which parts relied on qualitative information and which parts relied on quantitative information.
b. Did this study involve an intervention? If yes, what was it?
c. Did the report note efforts to monitor intervention fidelity?
d. Did this project involve a component that could be described as methodological research?
e. Could any part of this project be considered an *efficacy* study? If yes, what specific research design was involved?
f. Could any part of this project be considered an evaluation? If yes, which specific types of evaluation were undertaken, and which research designs were involved?

Questions for Discussion

a. Comment on the design for the substudy described in this report. Identify possible threats to the internal validity of this design.
b. Defend or refute this statement: "This project provides an example of a practical clinical trial."
c. Comment on the external validity of the overall project. To which types of settings and hospitals do you think the results could be generalized?

CHAPTER 12

Sampling Plans

■ A. Crossword Puzzle

Complete the crossword puzzle below, which uses terms and concepts presented in Chapter 12.

ACROSS

5. Population that is available to a researcher (abbr.)
7. An aggregate set of individuals or objects with specified characteristics
9. Another name for purposive sampling is _____ (abbr.)

Study Guide for Essentials of Nursing Research: Appraising Evidence for Nursing Practice, 7e

10. Cluster sampling is also called _____ stage sampling
11. Type of sampling preferred by grounded theory researchers
13. The most basic unit of a population
18. Sampling approach in which participants are handpicked because of known attributes (abbr.)
20. Ethnographers might begin sampling using a "big _____" approach
21. Qualitative researchers seek opportunities to sample _____-rich data sources (abbr.)
22. Sampling approach in which every *k*th element is selected (abbr.)
23. Type of sampling based on referrals from participants
24. Specific attributes of a population are designated through eligibility _____
25. Qualitative sampling approach in which the most unusual or deviant cases are selected (abbr.)
27. A strong sampling design can enhance the study's value for evidence _____ practice
28. Distortion that arises when a sample is not representative of the population is a sampling _____
30. In quantitative studies, the key criterion for evaluating a sample is whether it is _____ of the population
33. Criteria designating characteristics a population does *not* have (abbr.)
34. A probability sample involves selection at _____

DOWN

1. Term sometimes used in qualitative studies in lieu of "convenience" sample
2. Sampling by convenience, but within specified subgroups of the population
3. Subdivisions of a population
4. Most widely used type of sampling in quantitative research (abbr.)
6. Probability sampling involving successive random selection of smaller units
8. Criteria specifying characteristics that a population must have
12. The rate of participation in a study is the _____ rate
14. Sampling methods in which not every element of a population has an equal chance of being selected (abbr.)
15. Cases selected in a qualitative study to verify preliminary findings
16. Ethnographers rely on a sample of _____ informants
17. Principle used by qualitative researchers to determine when to stop sampling
19. Analysis used by quantitative researchers to estimate the number of subjects needed
22. Number of participants in a study is the sample _____
26. Qualitative sampling approach that yields participants who are "average" (abbr.)
29. Sampling method involving referrals from other people already in the sample (abbr.)
31. Most basic type of probability sampling (acronym)
32. Bias arising when some potential respondents decline is _____ -response bias

■ B. Matching Exercises

1. Match each statement relating to sampling for quantitative studies from Set B with one of the phrases from Set A. Indicate the letter corresponding to your response next to each of the statements in Set B.

SET A

a. Probability sampling

b. Nonprobability sampling

c. Both probability and nonprobability sampling

d. Neither probability nor nonprobability sampling

SET B   **RESPONSES**

1. Includes systematic sampling   _____

2. Allows an estimation of the magnitude of sampling error   _____

3. Guarantees a representative sample   _____

4. Includes quota sampling   _____

5. Requires a sample size of at least 100 subjects   _____

6. Elements are selected by nonrandom methods   _____

7. Can be used with entire populations or with selected strata from the populations   _____

8. Used to select populations   _____

9. Elements have an equal chance of being selected   _____

10. Is required when the population is homogeneous   _____

2. Match each type of sampling approach from Set B with one of the phrases from Set A. Indicate the letter corresponding to your response next to each of the statements in Set B.

SET A

a. Sampling approach for quantitative studies

b. Sampling approach for qualitative studies

c. Sampling approach for either quantitative or qualitative studies

d. Sampling approach for neither quantitative nor qualitative studies

SET B	RESPONSES
1. Typical case sampling	_____
2. Purposive sampling	_____
3. Cluster sampling	_____
4. Weighted sampling	_____
5. Consecutive sampling	_____
6. Snowball sampling	_____
7. Stratified random sampling	_____
8. Quota sampling	_____
9. Power sampling	_____
10. Theoretical sampling	_____

■ C. Study Questions

1. Suppose you have decided to use a systematic sampling design for a study. The known population size is 5,000, and the sample size desired is 250. What is the sampling interval? If the first element selected is 23, what would be the second, third, and fourth elements selected?

2. Suppose you were interested in studying the attitude of clinical specialists toward autonomy in work situations. Suggest a possible target and accessible population. What strata might be identified if quota sampling were used?

3. Identify the type of quantitative sampling design used in the following examples:
    a. One hundred inmates randomly sampled from a random selection of five federal penitentiaries
    b. All the oncology nurses participating in a continuing education seminar
    c. Every 20th patient admitted to the emergency room between January and June
    d. A total of 20 male and 20 female patients admitted to the hospital with hypothermia
    e. A sample of 250 members randomly selected from a roster of American Nurses' Association members
    f. A total of 25 internationally renowned experts in critical care nursing
    g. All patients receiving hospice services from Capital District Hospice in 2009.

4. Nurse A is planning to study the effects of maternal stress, maternal depression, maternal age, and family economic resources on a child's socioemotional development among both intact two-parent and single-parent (mother-headed) families. Nurse B is planning to study body position on patients' respiratory functioning. Describe the kinds of samples that the two nurses would need to use. Which nurse would need the larger sample? Defend your answer.

5. Suppose a qualitative researcher wanted to study the life quality of cancer survivors. Suggest what the researcher might do to obtain a maximum variation sample; a typical case sample; and an extreme case sample.

■ D. Application Exercises

EXERCISE 1: ALL APPENDIX STUDIES

a. Which of the studies in Appendices A through E of this *Study Guide* (if any) used a probability sample?
b. Which of the studies in Appendices A through E of this *Study Guide* (if any) used convenience sampling?
c. Which of the studies in Appendices A through E of this *Study Guide* (if any) used snowball sampling?

EXERCISE 2: STUDY IN APPENDIX C

Read the Methods sections of the report by Vollman and colleagues ("Coping and Depressive Symptoms") in Appendix C. Then answer the following questions:

Questions of Fact

a. What was the target population of this study? How would you describe the accessible population?
b. What were the eligibility criteria for the study?
c. Was the sampling method probability or nonprobability? What specific sampling method was used?
d. How were study participants recruited?
e. What was the response rate in this study?
f. What was the sample size that Vollman and colleagues achieved?
g. Was a power analysis used to determine sample size needs? If yes, what number of subjects did the power analysis estimate as the minimum number needed?
h. Were sample characteristics described? If yes, what were those characteristics?

Questions for Discussion

a. Comment on the adequacy of the researchers' sampling plan and recruitment strategy. What types of sampling biases might be of special concern?
b. Comment on efforts the researchers made (or did not make) to ensure a diverse sample of study participants.
c. Could the researchers have used quota sampling in this study? If so, what stratifying variables do you think they should have used?
d. Assume that you had no resource constraints to address the research questions in this study. What sampling plan would you recommend?

e. Do you think the sample size in this study was adequate? Why or why not?
f. How representative do you think the sample in this study was of the target population? Comment on issues relating to the generalizability of the results.

EXERCISE 3: STUDY IN APPENDIX B

Read the Method section of the report by Rasmussen and colleagues ("Young Women with Type 1 Diabetes") in Appendix B. Then answer the following questions:

Questions of Fact

a. What were the eligibility criteria for this study?
b. How were study participants recruited?
c. What type of sampling approach was used?
d. How many study participants comprised the sample?
e. Was data saturation achieved?
f. Did the sampling strategy include confirming and disconfirming cases?
g. Were sample characteristics described? If yes, what were those characteristics?

Questions for Discussion

a. Comment on the adequacy of the researchers' sampling plan and recruitment strategy for achieving the goals of a grounded theory study.
b. Assume that you had no resource constraints to address the research questions in this study. What sampling plan would you recommend?
c. Do you think the sample size in this study was adequate? Why or why not?
d. Comment on issues relating to the transferability of findings from this study.

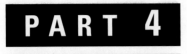

Data Collection

CHAPTER 13

Data Collection Methods

■ A. Crossword Puzzle

Complete the crossword puzzle below, which uses terms and concepts presented in Chapter 13.

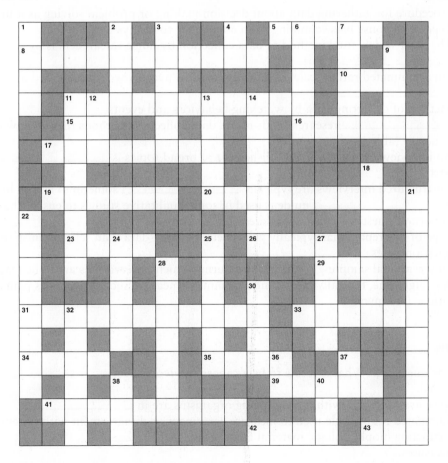

ACROSS

5. A(n) _____ yields a score that places people on a continuum with regard to an attribute.
8. Type of observation used in ethnographies and grounded theory studies
10. In unstructured observation, process questions are "_____" questions (backwards!)
11. Type of question prevalent in mailed questionnaires
15. Type of question that involves having participants put response alternatives in the order of their choice (acronym)
16. Data collection in which specific questions or observations and possible responses or categories are specified in advance (abbr.)
17. Describes a situation or event designed to elicit study participants' reactions
19. Scaling procedure to measure clinical symptoms is a _____ analogue scale.
20. Procedure for gathering data about decision making or problem solving as it unfolds
23. Type of response bias stemming from a tendency to always agree (abbr.)
26. The most widely used method of data collection by nurse researchers is by _____ report.
29. On a summated rating scale, if SD was scored as five, SA would be scored as _____.
31. Method of collecting data by watching behaviors and events
33. _____ research tends to use data collection methods that are low on structure (abbr.).
34. An interview guided by an established list of broad topics is _____ -structured.
35. Unstructured interviews are typically _____, sometimes lasting hours.
39. A(n) _____ guide is used in some qualitative studies to ensure that important question areas are covered.
41. Type of self-report that typically yields better quality data than self-administered questionnaires
42. Observational sampling of the periods during which observations are to be made
43. A straight line, typically measuring 100 mm, to measure such concepts as pain and fatigue (acronym)

DOWN

1. The question, "What is it like to be a cancer survivor?" is _____ ended.
2. Measures obtained within or on living organisms are in _____.
3. Summated rating scale used to measure agreement or disagreement with statements
4. Extracting biophysiologic material from people yields _____ vitro measures.
6. In Q-sorts, the objects being sorted are _____.

7. Mailed questionnaires tend to have _____ response rates than telephone interviews.

9. In structured observation, a(n) _____ list is used with a category system to record frequencies.

11. The _____ incidents technique involves in-depth exploration of specific events or episodes.

12. Participant observers maintain a record of daily events and conversations in a(n) _____.

13. Observational sampling of integral episodes

14. Study participants may be asked to maintain ongoing records of some aspect of their lives in _____.

18. Sometimes observers prefer to _____ themselves to ensure more naturalistic behavior among those being observed.

21. Type of question with only two response options, such as yes or no

22. Two _____ alternatives to "What is your gender?" are "male" and "female"

24. An approach involving the sorting of statements into different piles along a continuum.

25. Bias stemming from people's wanting to "look good" is called a(n) _____ desirability bias.

27. Technique for gathering in-depth information from a group of informants is called a _____ group interview.

28. Bias stemming from distortions of behavior because of the known presence of an observer (abbr.)

30. One advantage of questionnaires is that _____ can be often ensured to protect privacy (abbr.).

32. Respondents rate concepts on a series of bipolar rating scales in a _____ differential (abbr.).

36. Broad opening question in an unstructured interview to gain an overview (acronym)

37. Rating scale along the continuum "exhausted" to "energized" is using _ _polar adjectives

38. Tendency to distort self-report information in characteristic ways is called a response _____ bias.

40. Structured instruments are almost always subjected to a _ _ _test before being used in an actual study.

■ B. Matching Exercises

1. Match each descriptive statement regarding data collection methods from Set B with one (or more) of the statements from Set A. Indicate the letter(s) corresponding to your response next to each item in Set B.

SET A

a. Self-reports

b. Observations

c. Biophysiologic measures

d. None of the above

SET B   **RESPONSES**

  1. Cannot easily be gathered unobtrusively   _____

  2. Can be biased by the subject's desire to "look good"   _____

  3. Can be used to gather data from infants   _____

  4. Is rarely used in qualitative studies   _____

  5. Is a good way to obtain information about human behavior   _____

  6. Can be biased by the researcher's values and beliefs   _____

  7. Can be combined with other data collection methods in a single study   _____

  8. Can range from highly unstructured to highly structured methods   _____

  9. Can yield quantitative information   _____

10. Benefits from pretesting   _____

2. Match each descriptive statement regarding self-report methods from Set B with one of the statements from Set A. Indicate the letter corresponding to your response next to each item in Set B.

SET A

a. Interviews

b. Questionnaires

c. Both interviews and questionnaires

d. Neither interviews nor questionnaires

SET B	RESPONSES

1. Can provide respondents the protection of anonymity   _____

2. Can be used with illiterate respondents   _____

3. Can contain both open- and closed-ended questions   _____

4. Is used in grounded theory studies   _____

5. Is the best way to measure human behavior   _____

6. Generally yields high response rates   _____

7. Can control the order in which questions are asked and answered   _____

8. Is generally an inexpensive method of data collection   _____

9. Requires that the purpose of the study be unknown to the study participants   _____

10. Benefits from pretesting   _____

11. Can be used in longitudinal studies   _____

12. Can be distributed by mail   _____

■ C. Study Questions

1. Below are several research problems. Indicate what methods of data collection (self-report, observation, biophysiologic measures, records) you might recommend using for each. Defend your response.

   a. How does an elderly patient manage the transition from hospital to home?
   b. What are the predictors of intravenous site symptoms?
   c. What are the health and mental health consequences of a sedentary lifestyle among community-dwelling elders?
   d. To what extent and in what manner do nurses interact differently with male and female patients?
   e. What are the coping mechanisms of parents whose infants are hospitalized in neonatal intensive care units for a week or longer?

2. For each of the research problems in Question C.1, indicate where on the four dimensions discussed in this chapter (structure, quantifiability, researcher obtrusiveness, and objectivity) the method of data collection would most likely lie.

3. Below are several research problems. Indicate which type of unstructured self-report approach you might recommend using for each. Defend your response.

   a. How do parents of autistic children manage their frustration and despair?
   b. What are the barriers to preventive health care practices among the urban poor?
   c. What stresses does the spouse of a terminally ill patient experience?
   d. What type of information does a nurse draw on most heavily in formulating pain management decisions?
   e. What are the coping mechanisms and perceived barriers to coping among severely disfigured burn patients?

4. Suppose you were interested in studying the patients' impatience and anxiety waiting for treatment in the waiting area of an emergency department. Develop a topic guide for a semistructured interview on this topic.

5. For the study described in Question C.4, develop five closed-ended questions. Compare the nature of the information you would obtain for the research problem described in Question C.4 using the topic guide versus using the closed-ended questions. Which approach would yield more useful information? Defend your response.

6. Identify five constructs of clinical relevance that would be appropriate for measurement using a visual analogue scale (VAS).

7. Below are several research questions in which the dependent variable is amenable to observation. For each question, specify whether you think a structured or unstructured approach would be preferable. Justify your response.

   a. What is the effect of touch on the crying behavior of hospitalized children?
   b. What is the effect of increased patient-to-staff ratios in psychiatric hospitals on interpersonal conflict among patients?
   c. Are the self-grooming activities of nursing home patients related to the frequency of visits from friends and relatives?
   d. What is the process by which very low-birth-weight infants develop the sucking response?
   e. What types of patient behavior are most likely to elicit empathic behaviors in nurses?
   f. Do nurses reinforce passive behaviors among female patients more than among male patients?

■ D. Application Exercises

EXERCISE 1: VARIOUS APPENDIX STUDIES

Which of the studies in Appendices A (by Hill et al.), B (by Rasmussen et al.), and C (by Vollman et al.) of this *Study Guide* used the following data collection methods:

- Self-reports
- Observational methods
- Biophysiologic measures
- Records

EXERCISE 2: STUDY IN APPENDIX E

Read the Methods sections of the report by Tracy and colleagues ("Translating Best Practices") in Appendix E—specifically the subsections labeled "Instruments" and "Procedures" that described data collection in the pilot substudy. Then answer the following questions:

Questions of Fact

a. How would you describe the data collection methods in the substudy in terms of structure, quantifiability, obtrusiveness, and objectivity?
b. Did the researchers develop their own measures, or did they use instruments or scales that had been developed by others?
c. Did this study use any self-report measures? If no, could they have been used to measure key concepts? If yes, what specific types of self-report were used? How were self-report data recorded? What variables were measured by self-report?
d. Did this study collect any data through observation? If no, could observation have been used to measure key concepts? If yes, what variables were measured through observation and how were data obtained and recorded? What type of observational sampling was used, if any?
e. Did this study collect any biophysiologic measures? If no, could such measures have been used to capture key concepts? If yes, what variables were measured through bio-physiologic methods? How were the measurements made?
f. Were records used in this study? If no, could records have been used to measure key concepts? If yes, what records were used and what variables were captured?
g. Who gathered the data in this study? How were the data collectors trained?
h. Does the report indicate that steps were taken to enhance the quality of the data that were gathered?

Questions for Discussion

a. Comment on the adequacy of the data collection approaches used in this study. Did Tracy and colleagues operationalize their outcome measures in the best possible manner?
b. Comment on factors that could have biased the data in this study.
c. Do you think the researchers should have collected data on any additional outcome variables? Justify your response.

EXERCISE 3: STUDY IN APPENDIX D

Read the Research Design section of the report by Ward-Griffin and colleagues ("Perspectives of Women with Dementia") in Appendix D—specifically the subsections labeled "Data Collection" and "Recruiting and Sampling Method." Then answer the following questions:

Questions of Fact

a. How would you describe the data collection methods of this study in terms of structure, quantifiability, obtrusiveness, and objectivity?
b. Did this study collect any self-report data? If no, could self-reports have been used? If yes, what concepts were captured by self-report? What specific types of qualitative self-report methods were used? How was self-report data recorded?
c. Did this study collect any data through observation? If no, could observation have been used? If yes, what concepts were captured through observation, and how were data obtained and recorded?
d. Did this study collect any biophysiologic measures? If no, could such measures have been used to capture important concepts? If yes, what variables were measured through biophysiologic methods? How were the measurements made?
e. Were records, documents, or artifacts used in this study? If no, could they have been used? If yes, what records were used and what concepts were captured?
f. Who collected the data in this study? How were the data collectors trained?
g. Does the report indicate that steps were taken to enhance the quality of the data that were gathered?

Questions for Discussion

a. Comment on the adequacy of the data collection approaches used in this study. Did Ward-Griffin and colleagues fully capture the concepts of interest in the best possible manner?
b. Comment on factors that could have biased the data in this study.

CHAPTER 14

Measurement and Data Quality

■ A. Crossword Puzzle

Complete the crossword puzzle below, which uses terms and concepts presented in Chapter 14.

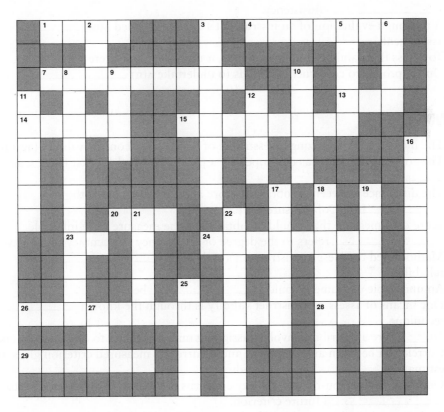

ACROSS

1. Type of validity involving the extent to which a measure "looks" valid
4. Type of validity concerned with adequate representation of all aspects of a concept
7. Predictive validity and concurrent validity are aspects of _____-related validity.
13. An internally consistent scale or subscale measures _____ dimension.
14. Measurement involves assigning numbers according to established _____.
15. Inter-_____ reliability assesses degree of equivalence of categorizations or ratings.
20. Measurement level that ranks or orders objects, but provides no information about distance between objects (abbr.)
23. The ratio of true–positive results to false–positive results is the _ _+
24. The most widely evaluated aspect of reliability is an instrument's _____ consistency.
26. A thorough evaluation of an instrument's quality is called a(n) _____ assessment.
28. To assess the stability of an instrument, it must be administered _____.
29. One approach to construct validity is to undertake a(n) _____ analysis.

DOWN

2. The indicator summarizing assessments of a measure's content validity (acronym)
3. The coefficient alpha was developed by a psychologist whose last name was _____.
5. The difference between an obtained score and the true score is the _____ of measurement.
6. Score on a measure that would be obtained if the measure were infallible
8. _____ refers to the degree of consistency or accuracy of a measure.
9. Method used to assess an instrument's stability is _____-retest reliability.
10. An unreliable instrument could _____ be valid.
11. One means of assessing construct validity is through the known _____ technique.
12. To _ _ _ _ure an attribute involves assigning numeric values to designate its quantity.
16. Correlation between an instrument and a currently measured criterion gives an estimate of _____ validity.
17. One type of criterion-related validity concerns the ability of an instrument to _____ a future criterion.
18. An instrument's ability to identify a case correctly is its _ _ _ _ _ _ _ _ty.

19. The extent to which an instrument actually is measuring what it purports to measure
21. Birth weight is an example of a(n) _____-level measurement.
22. Psychological scales yield _____-level measures.
25. "Nominal" is the lowest _____ of measurement.
27. In screening instruments, "cases" are separated from "noncases" at the _____ off point.

■ B. Matching Exercises

1. Match each variable in Set B with the level of measurement from Set A that captures the highest possible level for that variable. Indicate the letter corresponding to your response next to each variable in Set B.

SET A

a. Nominal scale

b. Ordinal scale

c. Interval scale

d. Ratio scale

SET B   RESPONSES

1. Hours spent in labor before childbirth   _____

2. Religious affiliation   _____

3. Time to first postoperative voiding   _____

4. Responses to a single Likert scale item   _____

5. Temperature on the centigrade scale   _____

6. Nursing specialty area   _____

7. Status on the following scale: in poor health; in fair health; in good health; in excellent health   _____

8. Pulse rate   _____

9. Score on a 25-item Likert scale   _____

10. Highest college degree attained (bachelor's, master's, doctorate)   _____

11. Apgar scores   _____

12. Membership in the American Nurses' Association   _____

2. Match each statement from Set B with one of the phrases from Set A. Indicate the letter corresponding to your response next to each of the statements in Set B.

SET A

a. Reliability

b. Validity

c. Both reliability and validity

d. Neither reliability nor validity

SET B   **RESPONSES**

1. Is concerned with the accuracy of measures   _____

2. The measures must be high on this for the results of a study to be valid   _____

3. If a measure possesses this, then study findings are necessarily sound   _____

4. Can in some cases be estimated by procedures that yield a quantified coefficient _____

5. In some cases, may be assessed by scrutinizing the components (items) of the measure _____

6. Is necessarily high when the measure is high on objectivity   _____

7. Is concerned with whether the researcher has adequately conceptualized the variables under investigation _____

8. Coefficient alpha is an index for this   _____

9. Psychometric assessments evaluate this   _____

10. Is used to establish a cutoff point for screening instruments   _____

■ C. Study Questions

1. The reliability of measures of which of the following attributes would *not* be appropriately assessed using a test–retest procedure with 1 month between administrations. Why?

    a. Attitudes toward abortion
    b. Stress
    c. Achievement motivation
    d. Nursing effectiveness
    e. Depression

Study Guide for Essentials of Nursing Research: Appraising Evidence for Nursing Practice, 7e

2. In the following situation, what might be some of the sources of measurement error?

> One hundred nurses who worked in a large metropolitan hospital were asked to complete a 10-item Likert scale designed to measure job satisfaction. The questionnaires were distributed by nursing supervisors at the end of shifts. The staff nurses were asked to complete the forms and return them immediately to their supervisors.

3. Identify what is incorrect about the following statements:
   a. "My scale is highly reliable, so it must be valid."
   b. "My instrument yielded an internal consistency coefficient of .80, so it must be stable."
   c. "The validity coefficient between my scale and a criterion measure was .40; therefore, my scale must be of low validity."
   d. "My scale had a reliability coefficient of .80. Therefore, an obtained score of 20 is indicative of a true score of 16."
   e. "The validation study proved that my measure has construct validity."
   f. "My advisor examined my new measure of dependence in nursing home residents and, based on its content, assured me the measure was valid."

4. All else equal, in the following situations, for which instrument or situation would reliability be expected to be higher? Why?
   a. An 8-item scale measuring self-efficacy or a 15-item scale of self-efficacy?
   b. A stress scale administered to patients just diagnosed with cancer, or the same stress scale administered to patients just diagnosed with hyperthryroidism?
   c. A test of nursing knowledge administered to freshmen nursing students or senior nursing students?

■ D. Application Exercises

EXERCISE 1: STUDIES IN APPENDICES C AND E

In these two studies (Appendix C, by Vollman et al., and Appendix E, by Tracy et al.), identify which variables were measured on the nominal scale, ordinal scale, interval scale, or ratio scale.

EXERCISE 2: STUDY IN APPENDIX A

Read the Method section of the report by Hill and colleagues ("Chronically Ill Rural Women") in Appendix A—paying special attention to the subsections labeled "Design" and "Measures." Then answer the following questions:

Questions of Fact

a. For the following instruments, did the researchers select measures with previously documented good reliability? Also, describe what methods (if any) were reported as having been used by the researchers themselves to assess the reliability of these instruments—and indicate what the reliability coefficients were in each case.
   - The Personal Resource Questionnaire (PRQ2000)
   - Self-Efficacy Scale
   - Self-Esteem Scale
   - Perceived Stress Scale
   - CES-D Depression Scale
   - UCLA Loneliness Scale

b. Describe what methods (if any) were reported as having been used to assess the validity of the same six instruments.
c. Did Hill and colleagues rely on assessments of quality from other researchers, or did they perform any data quality assessments themselves?
d. Was information about the specificity or sensitivity of any of the instruments provided in the report?
e. What was the level of measurement of variables in this study?

Questions for Discussion

a. Describe what some of the sources of measurement error might have been in this study. Did the researchers take adequate steps to minimize measurement error?
b. Comment on the adequacy of information in the report about efforts to select or develop high-quality instruments.
c. Comment on the quality of the measures that Hill and colleagues used in their study. Do you feel confident that the instruments yielded adequately reliable and valid indicators of the key constructs?

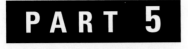

PART 5

Data Analysis and Interpretation

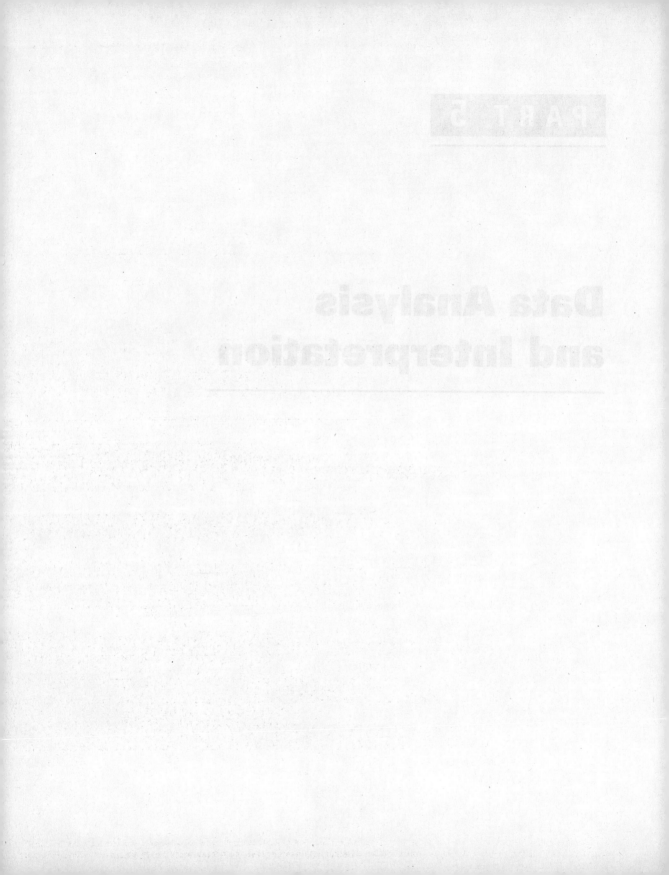

CHAPTER 15

Statistical Analysis of Quantitative Data

■ A. Crossword Puzzle

Complete the crossword puzzle below, which uses terms and concepts presented in Chapter 15.

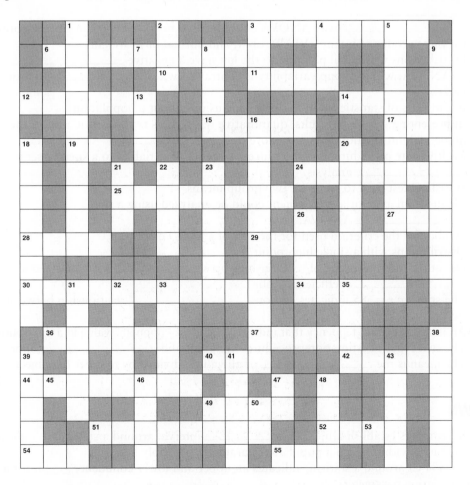

ACROSS

3. Most common index of variability, the _____ deviation
6. ANCOVA is an acronym for analysis of _____.
10. Symbol sometimes used in reports to designate a mean
11. Most stable, and most frequently used, index of central tendency
12. A(n) _____ size index summarizes the magnitude of an impact of the independent variable on the dependent variable.
14. Risk index summarizing a comparison of two risks (acronym)
15. Risk of making a Type I error is the _____ of significance
17. One approach to inferential statistics involves parameter _____ (abbr.)
19. Number of observations free to vary about a parameter (acronym)
24. Another name for the product-moment correlation coefficient is _____'s r.
25. Quantitative researchers make sense of their data through statistical _____.
27. A _____-way ANOVA could be used to compare mean Apgar scores for three groups of infants (VBLW, LBW, and normal birth weight)
28. Distributions with a tail pointing to the left have a negative _____.
29. In ANOVA, within-group variability is contrasted with _____-group variability
30. Broad class of statistics used to draw conclusions about a population
34. In presenting statistical results, quantitative researchers typically put a lot of their numerical information in one or more _____.
36. Multivariate procedure used to reduce a large set of variables to a smaller set is _____ analysis.
37. Statistical test used to compare two group means
40. Means from a factorial experiment could be analyzed using a two-_____ ANOVA.
42. Symbol for the criterion used for the risk of a Type I error
44. Distributions with a single high point
49. Direction and magnitude of relationships between variables are summarized in _____ coefficients (abbr.).
51. The statistic $r = .85$ indicates a strong, _____ relationship between two variables.
52. An index of central tendency that indicates the most "popular" value in a distribution
54. The two types of estimation procedures are point and _____ (abbr.).
55. The mean is the _____ of all values, divided by number of subjects.

DOWN

1. Researchers establish a(n) _____ interval around a statistic to indicate the range within which a population parameter probably lies.
2. A 95% CI around a statistic indicates an upper and lower confidence _ _ _it for a population parameter.

3. Standard deviation in a sampling distribution of means (acronym)
4. Inferential statistics without rigorous assumptions about distributional properties of variables are _____-parametric.
5. Multiple _____ analysis could be used to predict body weight, based on multiple predictors.
7. Statistical symbol for the index summarizing the direction and strength of a correlation
8. A Type I error involves the incorrect rejection of a true _____ hypothesis.
9. A two-dimensional frequency distribution for nominal-level variables is called a(n) _____ table.
13. Distributions for two nominal-level variables can be displayed in a cross_ _ _ .
16. Range and SD are two indexes for describing a distribution's _____
18. Type of regression used to predict a nominal-level dependent variable from multiple predictors
20. Index indicating the highest score value minus the lowest score value in a distribution
21. Acronym for a multivariate analysis of variance: _ _ _OVA (abbr.)
22. A(n) _____ analysis is an approach to causal modeling.
23. Error committed when a false null hypothesis is accepted
26. Descriptive index (e.g., a mean, percentage) to describe a *sample* value (abbr.)
31. Statistic computed in analysis of variance
32. Highest level of measurement, appropriate for the dependent variables in ANOVAs and *t*-tests
33. A bell-shaped curve is a popular name for a _ _ _ _ _l distribution.
35. Risk of making a Type II error, i.e., 1-Beta
38. A two-dimensional display of *r* values is a correlation _____ .
39. Distribution with two or more peaks is _____ modal.
41. Statistical test used to compare three or more group means (acronym)
43. A Type II error can occur when the analysis has insufficient _____, usually reflecting too small a sample.
45. Symbol used to designate total sample size
46. Class of statistics used to summarize data, not to estimate population parameters (abbr.)
47. A widely used risk index that summarizes the ratio of two probabilities—the likelihood of occurrence versus nonoccurrence (acronym)
48. A distribution without a skew is a _____ distribution (abbr.).
49. The precision of a point estimate can be expressed with a 95% or 99% _____ (acronym).
50. A _ _peated measures ANOVA can be used to test the comparability of means measured 3+ times.
51. The probability that obtained results are owing to chance is expressed by a(n) _____ value.
53. An effect size indicator that captures the magnitude of difference between two group means

■ B. Matching Exercises

Match each statement or phrase from Set B with one of the phrases from Set A. Indicate the letter corresponding to your response next to each of the statements in Set B.

SET A

a. Index(es) of central tendency

b. Index(es) of variability

c. Index(es) of neither central tendency nor variability

d. Index(es) of both central tendency and variability

SET B   **RESPONSES**

  1. The range   _____

  2. In lay terms, an average   _____

  3. A percentage   _____

  4. Descriptor(s) of a distribution of scores   _____

  5. Descriptor(s) of how heterogeneous a set of values is   _____

  6. The standard deviation   _____

  7. The mode   _____

  8. The median   _____

  9. A normal distribution   _____

10. The mean   _____

■ C. Study Questions

1. Prepare a frequency distribution and frequency polygon for the set of scores below, which represent the ages of 30 women receiving hormone replacement therapy (HRT).

   47 50 51 50 48 51 50 51 49 51

   54 49 49 53 51 52 51 52 50 53

   49 51 52 51 50 55 48 54 53 52

Describe the resulting distribution in terms of its symmetry and modality (i.e., whether it is unimodal or multimodal).

2. Calculate the mean, median, and mode for the following pulse rates:

78 84 69 98 102 72 87 75 79 84 88 84 83 71 73

Mean:_____   Median:_____   Mode:_____

3. Suppose a researcher has conducted a study concerning lactose intolerance in children. Of a sample of 60 children of each gender, the data reveal that 12 boys and 16 girls have lactose intolerance. Construct a contingency table and calculate the row, column, and total percentages for each cell in the table. Discuss the meaning of these statistics.

4. Suppose that 400 subjects (200 per group) were in the intervention study described in connection with Table 15.7 in the textbook, and that 60% of those in the experimental group and 90% of those in the control group continued smoking. Compute the absolute risk reduction (ARR) and the odds ratio in this scenario.

5. A group of nurse researchers measured the amount of time (in minutes per week) spent in recreational activities by a sample of 200 hospitalized paraplegic patients. They compared male and female patients as well as those aged 50 and younger versus those 50 years of age and older. The four group means (50 subjects per group) were as follows:

Age	Male	Female
≤50 years	98.2	70.1
>50	50.8	68.3

A two-way ANOVA yielded the following results

	F	df	p
Sex	3.61	1,196	ns
Age group	5.87	1,196	<.05
Gender × age group	6.96	1,196	<.01

Interpret the meaning of these results.

6. The correlation between the number of days absent per year and annual salary in a sample of 100 nurses was found to be −.23, $p < 0.05$. What does this result mean?

7. Indicate which statistical tests you would use to analyze data for the following variables:

a. Variable 1 is a psychiatric patient's gender; variable 2 is whether or not the patient has attempted suicide in the past 6 months.

b. Variable 1 is the participation versus nonparticipation of patients with a pulmonary embolus in a special treatment group; variable 2 is the pH of the patients' arterial blood gases.

c. Variable 1 is serum creatinine concentration levels; variable 2 is daily urine output.

d. Variable 1 is patient's marital status (married versus divorced, separated, or widowed versus never married); variable 2 is the patient's degree of self-reported depression (measured on a 30-item depression scale).

8. In the following examples, which multivariate procedure is most appropriate for analyzing the data?

a. A researcher is testing the effect of verbal expressiveness, self-esteem, age, and the availability of family supports among a group of recently discharged psychiatric patients on recidivism (i.e., whether they will be readmitted within 12 months after discharge).

b. A researcher is comparing the bereavement and coping processes of recently widowed and divorced individuals, controlling for their age.

c. A researcher wants to test the effects of two drug treatments and two dosages of each drug on blood pressure, and the pH and Po_2 levels of arterial blood gases.

d. A researcher wants to predict hospital staff absentee rates (number of days absent) based on staff rank, shift, number of years with the hospital, and marital status.

9. Below is a list of variables. Assume that you have data from 500 nurses on these variables. Develop two or three hypotheses regarding the relationships among these variables, and indicate what statistical tests you would use to test your hypotheses.

- Number of years of nursing experience
- Type of employment setting (hospital, nursing home, public school system, other)
- Annual salary
- Marital status (single, married, other)
- Job satisfaction (as measured on a 10-item Likert-type scale)
- Number of children under 18 years of age
- Gender
- Type of nursing preparation (diploma, Associate, Bachelor)

■ D. Application Exercises

EXERCISE 1: STUDY IN APPENDIX A

Read the Results section of the report by Hill and colleagues ("Chronically Ill Rural Women") in Appendix A. Then answer the following questions:

Questions of Fact

a. Which descriptive statistics did Hill and colleagues use to describe their sample (Table 1 and associated text)? Could they have used other descriptive statistics to summarize sample characteristics?

b. Did Hill and colleagues analyze the comparability of their experimental and control group subjects to assess potential selection biases? If yes, what statistical tests did they perform? If not, what statistical tests could they have used?

c. Was there any attrition in this study (i.e., did some participants drop out of the study)? Did Hill and colleagues analyze the comparability of subjects who remained and those who dropped out to assess potential attrition biases?

d. Which bivariate statistical tests discussed in Chapter 15 did Hill and colleagues use to address their research questions or test their hypotheses?

e. Did Hill and colleagues present information about hypothesis tests? About parameter estimation? About effect sizes?

f. Referring to Table 3, answer the following questions:
   - What was the correlation between the women's Depression and Self-Efficacy scores?
   - Which variables were negatively correlated with Loneliness scores?
   - Scores on the Stress scale were significantly correlated with which other variables?
   - What is the strongest correlation in this matrix?
   - What is the weakest correlation in this matrix?
   - How many correlations were statistically significant at or beyond the .05 level? How many were *not* statistically significant?
   - What is the name of the test statistic presented in this table?

g. Referring to Table 5 and the accompanying text, answer the following questions:
   - What is the independent variable in the analyses presented in this table?
   - Explain what the results for the Empowerment scale scores mean.
   - Explain what the results for the Self-Efficacy scores mean.
   - For how many dependent variables were there significant (at the .05 level) experimental–control group differences over time?
   - For how many dependent variables were there significant changes over time for the sample as a whole at the .05 level?
   - What statistical test was used in the analyses presented in this table?

h. Did the report indicate that a power analysis was done while planning the study to estimate sample size needs?

Questions for Discussion

a. Discuss the effectiveness of the presentation of information in the tables. What, if anything, could be done to make the tables more informative, more comprehensible, or more efficient? Should there have been other tables? Create one such table, using information summarized in the text of the article.

b. Did Hill and colleagues use the appropriate statistical tests to analyze their data? If not, what tests should have been performed?

c. Did the researchers present a sufficient amount of information about their statistical tests? What additional information would have been helpful?

d. Discuss the possibility of selection and attrition biases in this study.

e. Discuss the possibility of Type I and Type II errors.

EXERCISE 2: STUDY IN APPENDIX C

Read the Results section of the report by Vollman and colleagues ("Coping and Depressive Symptoms") in Appendix C. Then answer the following questions:

Questions of Fact

a. Which descriptive statistics did the researchers use to describe the characteristics of their study participants? Were sample characteristics described in a table?

b. Which bivariate statistical tests discussed in Chapter 15 did Vollman and colleagues use?

c. Did the researchers present information about hypothesis tests? About parameter estimation? About effect sizes?

d. Did the researchers undertake any multivariate analyses? If yes, which one(s)?

e. Referring to Table 2 and the accompanying text, answer the following questions:

- What is the dependent variable in this analysis? What is the measurement level of this variable?
- How many predictor variables did the researchers use *initially* in their effort to predict the dependent variable? Why were some predictor variables removed from the analysis?
- How many predictor variables were significantly related to the dependent variable, according to the results shown in the table?
- What are the measurement levels of all predictor variables in the final analysis?
- Interpret the signs associated with all of the beta coefficients in Table 2.
- Which predictor was most strongly associated with the dependent variable in this analysis, with other predictors controlled?
- What is the name of the test statistic presented in this table? What was its value? What percentage of variability in the dependent variable was explained by the predictors?

f. Did the report indicate that a power analysis was done while planning the study to estimate sample size needs?

Questions for Discussion

a. Discuss the effectiveness of the presentation of information in the tables. What, if anything, could be done to make the tables more informative, more comprehensible, or more efficient? Should there have been other tables?

b. Did Vollman and colleagues use the appropriate statistical tests to analyze their data? If not, what tests should have been performed?

c. Did Vollman and colleagues present a sufficient amount of information about their statistical tests? What additional information would have been helpful?

d. Discuss the possibility of Type I and Type II errors.

CHAPTER 16

Rigor and Interpretation in Quantitative Research

■ A. Crossword Puzzle

Complete the crossword puzzle below, which uses terms and concepts presented in Chapter 16.

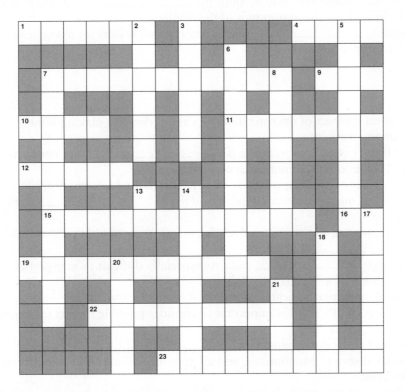

ACROSS

1. Both researchers and consumers of quantitative research must develop a(n) _____ of the accuracy, meaning, and importance of the results (abbr.).
4. A significant result is not necessarily of any _ _ _ _ical importance to practicing nurses.

Study Guide for Essentials of Nursing Research: Appraising Evidence for Nursing Practice, 7e

7. A famous research precept is that _____ does not prove that one variable caused another.
9. _ _ _ect size estimates help to understand the importance of the results better.
10. After assessing the accuracy of their results, researchers must interpret what they _____.
11. Reporting guidelines that include a flow chart documenting participant flow in a study
12. When some hypotheses are supported and others are not, the results are _____.
15. One interpretive task is to suggest _____ of the findings for practice, theory, or future research.
16. Hospital unit acronym and name of long-running TV program
19. Researchers should take the _____ of their study into account when interpreting their findings.
22. Researchers should take into account the _____ of effects in coming to conclusions about the importance of the results.
23. A research _____ that is actually null is difficult to evaluate through standard statistical methods.

DOWN

2. An important aspect of interpretation for clinical decision-making is the _ _ _ _ _ _ion of estimates of effects.
3. One difficulty with interpretation is that _____ are pervasive, despite researchers' efforts to minimize or control them.
5. Process or act of drawing conclusions based on limited information
6. Researchers' interpretations are presented in the _____ section of a report.
7. Before evaluating the meaning of results, researchers should evaluate their accuracy and _____.
8. Results that are _____ are especially difficult to interpret because of the possibility of a Type II error (abbr.).
13. Statistical index that indicates precision of results (acronym)
14. In assessing credibility, it is important to consider possible threats to various aspects of _____.
17. Analysis of study data yields the _____.
18. A famous slogan of Missourians, and an appropriate mindset for interpreting results (backwards!)
20. The flow chart recommended in the widely used clinical trial reporting guidelines helps to _____ participants from recruitment to study completion.
21. An assessment of whether results are "real" and accurate involves a careful scrutiny of the researcher's _____ decisions (abbr.).

■ B. Matching Exercises

Match each statement or phrase from Set B with one or more of the phrases from Set A. Indicate the letter(s) corresponding to your response next to each of the statements in Set B.

SET A

a. Credibility of results

b. Precision of results

c. Magnitude of effects and importance

d. Generalizability of results

e. Implications of results

SET B   **RESPONSES**

1. Confidence intervals provide information about this   _____

2. An analysis of threats to study validity is a way to address this   _____

3. A consideration of how study limitations could be corrected in
   subsequent research is part of this   _____

4. In addressing this, consideration is given to the characteristics of
   the study sample and the research setting   _____

5. Effect size information can be especially useful for considering this   _____

6. An analysis of the success of the researcher's "proxies" is an
   approach to this   _____

7. Biases can reduce this   _____

8. Statements about the utility of findings for clinical practice are
   part of this   _____

■ C. Study Questions

1. Read one of the following studies, and evaluate the extent to which the researchers assessed possible biases. Can you think of analyses that could have been performed to strengthen the credibility of the results?
   - Doorenbos, A., Given, B., Given, C., & Verbitsky, N. (2006). Physical functioning: Effect of a behavioral intervention for symptoms among individuals with cancer. *Nursing Research, 55*(3), 161–171.
   - Mantler, J., Armstrong-Stassen, M., Horsburgh, M., & Cameron, S. (2006). Reactions of hospital staff nurses to recruitment incentives. *Western Journal of Nursing Research, 28*(1), 70–84.

2. In the following research article, a team of researchers reported that they obtained nonsignificant results that were not consistent with expectations. Review and critique the researchers' interpretation of the findings and suggest some possible alternatives.

   • Holzemer, W., Bakken, S., Portillo, C., Grimes, R., Welch, J., Wantland, D., & Mullan, J. (2006). Testing a nurse-tailored HIV medication adherence intervention. *Nursing Research, 55,* 189–197.

3. In the following report, the researchers did not present a flow chart to track participant flow, as recommended in the CONSORT guidelines. Use information in the report to create one, to the extent possible.

   • Gill, S., Reifsnider, E., & Lucke, J. (2007). Effects of support on initiation of breastfeeding. *Western Journal of Nursing Research, 29,* 708–723.

4. Skim one of the following articles, the titles for which imply a causal connection between phenomena. Do you think a causal inference is warranted? Why or why not?

   • Laschinger, H., Purdy, N., & Almost, J. (2007). The impact of leader-member exchange quality, empowerment, and core self-evaluation on nurse manager's job satisfaction. *Journal of Nursing Administration, 37,* 221–229.
   • Barakzai, M., Gregory, J., & Fraser, D. (2007). The effect of culture on symptom reporting: Hispanics and irritable bowel syndrome. *Journal of the American Academy of Nurse Practitioners, 19,* 261–267.

5. Below is a fictitious research report with a critique of various aspects of it. This example is designed to highlight features about the form and content of both a written report and a written evaluation of the study's worth. To economize on space, the report is brief, but it incorporates essential elements for a meaningful appraisal.

   Read the report and critique, and then determine whether you agree with the critique. Can you add other comments relevant to a critical appraisal of the study?

The Report: The Role of Health Care Providers in Teenage Pregnancy

by Phyllis Clinton

Background. Of the 20 million teenagers living in the United States, about one in four is sexually active by age 14; more than half have had sexual intercourse by age 17 (Kelman & Saner, 1998).[1] Despite increased availability of contraceptives, the number of teenage pregnancies has remained fairly stable over the past two decades. About 1 million girls under age 20 become pregnant each year and, of these, about 500,000 become teenaged mothers (U.S. Bureau of the Census, 1998).

---

[1]All references in this example are fictitious, although most of the information in this fictitious literature review is based on real research.

Public concern regarding teenage pregnancy stems not only from the high rates, but also from the extensive research that has documented the adverse consequences of early parenthood in the health arena. Pregnant teenagers have been found to receive less prenatal care (Tremain, 2000), to be more likely to develop toxemia (Schendley, 1991; Waters, 2001), to be more likely to experience prolonged labor (Curran, 1999), to be more likely to have low-birth-weight babies (Tremain, 2000; Beach, 1999), and to be more likely to have babies with low Apgar scores (Beach, 1995) than older mothers. The long-term consequences to the teenaged mothers themselves are also extremely bleak: Teenaged mothers get less schooling; they are more likely to be on public assistance, to earn lower wages, and to get divorced if they marry than their peers who postpone parenthood (Jamail, 1999; North, 1992; Smithfield, 2001).

The 1 million teenagers who become pregnant each year are caught up in a tough emotional decision—to carry the pregnancy to term and keep the baby, to have an abortion, or to deliver the baby and surrender it for adoption. Despite the widely reported adverse consequences of young parenthood cited above, most young women today are opting for delivery and child-rearing, often out of wedlock (Jaffrey, 2002; Henderson, 2001). Relatively few young mothers in recent years have been relinquishing their babies for adoption, forcing many couples with fertility problems to seek adoption options overseas (Smith, 1998).

This study was conducted to test the effect of a special intervention based in an outpatient clinic of a Chicago hospital on improving the health outcomes of a group of pregnant teenagers. Specifically, it was hypothesized that pregnant teenagers who were in the special program would (a) receive more prenatal care, (b) be less likely to develop toxemia, (c) be less likely to have a low-birth-weight baby, (d) spend fewer hours in labor, (e) have babies with higher Apgar scores, and (f) be more likely to use a contraceptive at 6 months postpartum than pregnant teenagers not enrolled in the program.

The theoretical model on which this research was based is an ecologic model of personal behavior (Brandenburg, 1984). A schematic diagram of the ecologic model is presented in Figure A. In this framework, the actions of the person are the focus of attention, but those actions are believed to be a function not only of the person's own characteristics, attitudes, and abilities but also of other influences in their environment. Environmental influences can be differentiated according to their proximal relationship with the target person. According to the model, health care workers and institutions are more distant influences than family, peers, and boyfriends. Yet it is assumed that these less immediate forces are real and can intervene to change the behaviors of the target person. Thus, it is hypothesized that pregnant teenagers can be influenced by increased exposure to a health care team providing a structured program of services designed to promote improved health outcomes.

Method. A special program of services for pregnant teenagers was implemented in the outpatient clinic of an inner-city public hospital in Chicago. The intervention involved 8 weeks of nutrition education and counseling, parenting education, instruction on prenatal health care, preparation for childbirth, and contraceptive counseling.

All teenagers with a confirmed pregnancy attending the clinic were asked if they wanted to participate in the special program. The goal was to enroll 150 pregnant

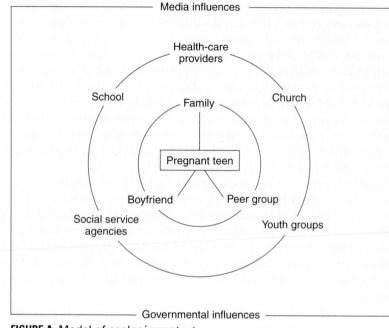

FIGURE A Model of ecologic contexts

teenagers during the program's first year of operation. A total of 276 teenagers attending the clinic were invited to participate; of these, 59 had an abortion or miscarriage, and 108 declined to participate, yielding an experimental group sample of 109 girls.

To test the effectiveness of the special program, a comparison group of pregnant teenagers was needed. Another inner-city hospital agreed to cooperate in the study. Staff obtained information on the labor and delivery outcomes of the 120 teenagers who delivered at the comparison hospital, where no special teen-parent program was available. For both experimental group and comparison group subjects, a follow-up telephone interview was conducted 6 months postpartum to determine if the teenagers were using birth control.

The outcome variables in this study were the teenagers' labor and delivery and postpartum outcomes and their contraceptive behavior. Operational definitions of these variables were as follows:

Prenatal care: Number of visits made to a physician or nurse during the pregnancy, exclusive of the visit for the pregnancy test

Toxemia: Presence versus absence of preeclamptic toxemia as diagnosed by a physician

Labor time: Number of hours elapsed from the first contractions until delivery of the baby, to the nearest half hour

Low infant birth weight: Infant birth weights of less than 2,500 g versus those of 2,500 g or greater

Apgar score: Infant Apgar score (from 0 to 10) taken at 3 minutes after birth
Contraceptive use postpartum: Self-reported use of any form of birth control 6 months postpartum versus self-reported nonuse

The two groups were compared on these six outcome measures using *t*-tests and chi-squared tests.

Results. The teenagers in the sample were, on average, 17.6 years of age at the time of delivery. The mean age was 17.0 in the experimental group and 18.1 in the comparison group (*p* <.05).

By definition, all the teenagers in the experimental group had received prenatal care. Two of the teenagers in the comparison group had no health care treatment before delivery. The distribution of visits for the two groups is presented in Figure B. The experimental group had a higher mean number of prenatal visits than the comparison group, as shown in Table A, but the difference was not statistically significant at the .05 level, using a *t*-test for independent groups.

In the sample as a whole, about 1 girl in 10 was diagnosed as having preeclamptic toxemia. The difference between the two groups was in the hypothesized direction, with 1.6% more of the comparison group teenagers developing this complication, but the difference was not significant using a chi-squared test.

The hours spent in labor ranged from 3.5 to 29.0 in the experimental group and from 4.5 to 33.5 in the comparison group. On average, teenagers in the experimental group spent 14.3 hours in labor, compared with 15.2 for the comparison group teenagers. The difference was not statistically significant.

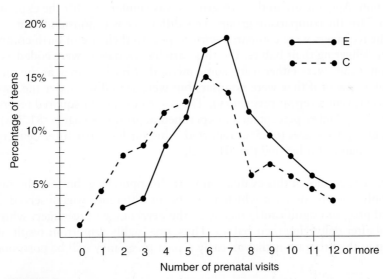

FIGURE B Frequency distribution of prenatal visits, by experimental versus comparison group. (*E*, experimental group; *C*, comparison group)

TABLE A Summary of Experimental and Comparison Group Differences

Outcome Variable	Group Experimental ($n = 109$)	Comparison ($n = 120$)	Difference	Test Statistic
Mean number of prenatal visits	7.1	5.9	1.2	$t = 1.83$, $df = 227$, NS
Percentage with toxemia	10.1%	11.7%	−1.6%	$\chi^2 = 0.15$, $df = 1$, NS
Mean hours spent in labor	14.3	15.2	−.09	$t = 1.01$, $df = 227$, NS
Percentage with low-birth-weight baby	16.5%	20.9%	−4.4%	$\chi^2 = 0.71$, $df = 1$, NS
Mean Apgar score	7.3	6.7	.6	$t = 0.98$, $df = 227$, NS
Percentage adopting contraception post-partum	81.7%	62.5%	19.2%	$\chi^2 = 10.22$, $df = 1$, $p < .01$

With regard to low-birth-weight babies, a total of 43 of 229 girls in the sample gave birth to babies who weighed under 2,500 g (5.5 pounds).[2] More of the comparison group teenagers (20.9%) than experimental group teenagers (16.5%) had low-birth-weight babies, but, once again, the group difference was not significant.

The 3-minute Apgar score in the two groups was similar: 7.3 for the experimental group and 6.7 for the comparison group. This difference was nonsignificant.

Finally, the teenagers were compared with respect to their use of birth control 6 months after delivering their babies. For this variable, teenagers were coded as users of contraception if they were either using some method of birth control at the time of the follow-up interview or if they were nonusers but were sexually inactive (i.e., were using abstinence to prevent a repeat pregnancy). The results of the chi-squared test revealed that a significantly higher percentage of experimental group teenagers (81.7%) than comparison group teenagers (62.5%) reported using birth control after delivery. This difference was significant beyond the .01 level.

Discussions. The results of this evaluation were disappointing, but not discouraging. There was only one outcome for which a significant difference was observed. The experimental program significantly increased the percentage of teenagers who used birth control after delivering their babies. Thus, one highly important result of participating in the program is that an early repeat pregnancy will be postponed.

---

[2]All mothers gave birth to live infants; however, there were two neonatal deaths within 24 hours of birth in the comparison group.

Abundant research has shown that repeat pregnancy among teenagers is especially damaging to their educational and occupational attainment and leads to particularly adverse labor and delivery outcomes in the higher-order births (Klugman, 1985; Jackson, 1997).

The experimental group had more prenatal care, but not significantly more. Perhaps part of the difficulty is that the program can only begin to deliver services once pregnancy has been diagnosed. If a teenager does not come in for a pregnancy test until her fourth or fifth month, this obviously puts an upper limit on the number of visits she will have; it also gives less time for her to eat properly, avoid smoking and drinking, and take other steps to enhance her health during pregnancy. Thus, one implication of this finding is that the program needs to do more to encourage early pregnancy screening. Perhaps a joint effort between the clinic personnel and school nurses in neighboring middle schools and high schools could be launched to publicize the need for a timely pregnancy test and to inform teenagers where such a test could be obtained. The two groups performed similarly with respect to the various labor and delivery outcomes chosen to evaluate the effectiveness of the new program. The issue of timeliness is again relevant here. The program may have been delivering services too late in the pregnancy for the instruction to have made much of an impact on the health of the mother and her child. This interpretation is supported, in part, by the one variable for which timeliness was *not* an issue—postpartum contraception—which, indeed, was positively affected by program participation. Another possible implication is that the program itself should be made more powerful, for example, by lengthening or adding to instructional sessions.

Given that the experimental and comparison group differences were all in the hypothesized direction, it is also tempting to criticize the study's sample size. A larger sample (which was originally planned) might have yielded some significant differences.

In summary, the experimental intervention is not without promise. A particularly exciting finding is that participation in the program resulted in better contraceptive use, which will presumably lower the incidence of repeat pregnancy. It would be interesting to follow these teenagers 2 years after delivery to see if the groups differ in the rates of repeat pregnancy. It appears that more needs to be done to get these teenagers into the program early in their pregnancies. Perhaps then the true effectiveness of the program would be demonstrated.

Critique of the Research Report

In the following critique, we present some comments on various aspects of this research report. You are urged to read the report and formulate your own opinion about its strengths and weaknesses before reading our critique. An evaluation of a study is necessarily partly subjective. Therefore, you might disagree with some of the points that follow, and you might have additional criticisms and comments. We believe, however, that most of the serious methodological flaws of the study are highlighted in our critique.

Title. The title for the study is misleading. The research does *not* investigate the role of health care professionals in serving the needs of pregnant teenagers. A more appropriate title would be "Health-Related Outcomes of an Intervention for Pregnant Teenagers."

Background. The background section of this report consists of three distinct elements that can be analyzed separately: a literature review, statement of the problem, and a theoretical framework.

The literature review is relatively clearly written and well organized. It serves the important function of establishing a need for the experimental program by documenting the prevalence of teenage pregnancy and some of its adverse consequences. However, the literature review could be improved. First, an inspection of the citations suggests that the author is not as up-to-date on research relating to teenage pregnancy as she might have been. Most of the references are from the 1990s, meaning that this literature review is about a decade old. Second, some material in the literature review section is not relevant and should be removed. For example, the paragraph on the options with which a pregnant teenager is faced (paragraph 3) is not germane to the research problem. A third and more critical flaw is what the review does *not* cover. Given the research problem, there are probably four main points that should be addressed in the review:

1. How widespread is teenage pregnancy and parenthood?
2. What are the social and health consequences of early child-bearing?
3. What has been done (especially by nurses) to address the problems associated with teenage parenthood?
4. How successful have other interventions been?

The review adequately handles the first question: the need for concern is established. The second question is covered in the review, but perhaps more depth and more recent research is needed here. The new study is based on an assumption of negative health outcomes in teenaged mothers. The author has strung together a series of references without giving the reader any clues about the reliability of the information. The author would have made her point more convincingly if she had added a sentence such as, "For example, in a carefully executed prospective study involving nearly 8,000 pregnant women, Beach (1995) found that young maternal age was significantly associated with higher rates of prematurity and other negative neonatal outcomes." The third and fourth points that should have been covered are totally absent from the review. Surely the author's experimental program does not represent the first attempt to address the needs of pregnant teenagers. How is Clinton's intervention different from or better than other interventions? What reason does she have to believe that such an intervention might be successful? Clinton has provided a rationale for addressing the problem but no rationale for the manner in which she has addressed it. If, in fact, little information about other interventions and their effectiveness in improving health outcomes exists, then the review should say so.

The problem statement and hypothesis were stated succinctly and clearly. The hypothesis is complex (there are multiple dependent variables) and directional (it predicts better outcomes among teenagers participating in the special program).

The third component of the background section of the report is the theoretical framework. In our opinion, the theoretical framework chosen does little to enhance the research. The hypothesis is not generated on the basis of the model, nor does the intervention itself grow out of the model. One gets the feeling that the model was slapped on as an afterthought to try to make the study seem more sophisticated or theoretical. Actually, if more thought had been given to this conceptual framework, it might have proved useful. According to this model, the most immediate and direct influences on a pregnant teenager are her family, friends, and sexual partner. One programmatic implication of this is that the intervention should involve one or more of these influences. For example, a workshop for the teenagers' parents could have been developed to reinforce the teenagers' need for adequate nutrition and prenatal care. A research hypothesis that could have been tested in the context of the model is that teenagers who are missing one of the direct influences would be especially susceptible to the influence of less proximal health care providers (i.e., the program). For example, it might be hypothesized that pregnant teenagers who do not live with both parents have to depend on alternative sources of social support (e.g., health care personnel) during the pregnancy. Thus, it is not that the theoretical context selected is far-fetched, but rather that it was not convincingly linked to the actual research problem. Perhaps an alternative theoretical context would have been better. Or perhaps the researcher simply should have been honest and admitted that her research was practical, not theoretical.

Method. The design used to test the research hypothesis was a widely used quasi-experimental design. Two groups, whose equivalence is assumed but not established, were compared on several outcome measures. The design is one that has serious problems because the preintervention comparability of the groups is unknown.

The most serious threat to the internal validity of the study is selection bias. Selection bias can work both ways—either to mask true treatment effects or to create the illusion of a program effect when none exists. This is because selection bias can be either positive (i.e., the experimental group can be initially advantaged in relation to the comparison group) or negative (i.e., the experimental group can have pretreatment disadvantages). In the present study, it is possible that the two hospitals served clients of different economic circumstances, for example. If the average income of the families of the experimental group teenagers was higher, then these teenagers would probably have a better opportunity for adequate prenatal nutrition than the comparison group teenagers. Or the comparison hospital might serve older teens, a higher percentage of married teens, or a higher percentage of teens attending a special school-based program for pregnant students. None of these confounding variables, which could affect the mother's health, has been controlled.

Another way in which the design was vulnerable to selection bias is the high refusal rate in the experimental group. Of the 217 eligible teenagers, half declined to participate in the special program. We cannot assume that the 109 girls who participated were a random sample of the eligible girls. Again, biases could be either positive or negative. A positive selection bias would be created if, for example, the teenagers who were the most motivated to have a healthy pregnancy selected themselves into the experimental group. A negative selection bias would result if the teenagers from the most disadvantaged households or from families offering little support elected to participate in the program. In the comparison group, hospital records were used primarily to collect the data, so this self-selection problem could not occur (except for refusals to answer the contraceptive questions 6 months postpartum).

The researcher could have taken a number of steps either to control selection biases or, at the least, to estimate their direction and magnitude. The following are among the most critical confounding variables: social class and family income; age; race and ethnicity; parity; participation in another pregnant teenager program; marital status; and prepregnancy experience with contraception (for the postpartum contraception outcome). The researcher should have attempted to gather information on these variables from experimental group and comparison group teenagers *and* from eligible teenagers in the experimental hospital who declined to participate in the program. To the extent that these groups were similar on these variables, credibility in the internal validity of the study would be enhanced. If sizable differences were observed, the researcher would at least know or suspect the direction of the biases and could factor that information into her interpretation and conclusions.

Had the researcher gathered information on the confounding variables, another possibility would have been to match experimental and comparison group subjects on one or two variables, such as family income and age. Matching is not an ideal method of controlling extraneous variables; for one thing, matching on two variables would not equate the two groups in terms of the other confounding variables. However, matching is preferable to doing nothing to control extraneous variation.

So far we have focused our attention on the research design, but other aspects of the study are also problematic. Consider the decision the researcher made about the population. The target population is not explicitly defined by the researcher, but we can perhaps infer that the target population is pregnant young women under age 20 who carry their infants to delivery. The accessible population is pregnant teenagers from one area in Chicago. Is it reasonable to assume that the accessible population is representative of the target population? No, it is not. It is likely that the accessible population is quite different with regard to health care, family intactness, and many other characteristics. The researcher should have more clearly discussed exactly who was the target population of this research.

Clinton would have done well, in fact, to delimit the target population; had she done so, it might have been possible to control some of the confounding variables discussed previously. For example, Clinton could have established eligibility criteria that excluded multigravidas, very young teenagers (e.g., under age 15), or married teenagers. Such a specification would have limited the generalizability of the findings, but it would have enhanced the internal validity of the study because it probably would have increased the comparability of the experimental and comparison groups.

The sample was one of convenience, the least effective sampling design for a quantitative study. There is no way of knowing whether the sample represents the accessible and target populations. Although probability sampling likely was not feasible, the researcher might have improved her sampling design by using a quota sampling plan. For example, if the researcher knew that in the accessible population, half of the families received public assistance, then it might have been possible to enhance the representativeness of the samples by using a quota system to ensure that half of the research subjects came from welfare-dependent families.

Sample size is a difficult issue. Many of the reported results were in the hypothesized direction but were nonsignificant. When this is the case, the adequacy of the sample size is always suspect, as Clinton pointed out. Each group had about 100 subjects. In many cases, this sample size would be considered adequate, but in the present case, it is not. One of the difficulties in testing the effectiveness of new interventions is that, generally, the experimental group is not being compared with a no-treatment group. Although the comparison group in this example was not getting the special program services, it cannot be assumed that this group was getting no services at all. Some comparison group members may have had ample prenatal care during which the health care staff may have provided much of the same information as was taught in the special program. The point is not that the new program was not needed, but rather that unless an intervention is extremely powerful and innovative, the incremental improvement will typically be rather small. When relatively small effects are anticipated, the sample must be very large for differences to be statistically significant. Indeed, power analysis can be performed using the study findings. For example, a power analysis indicates that to detect a significant difference between the two groups with respect to one outcome—the incidence of toxemia—a sample of more than 5,000 pregnant teenagers would have been needed. Had the researcher done a power analysis before conducting the study, she might have realized the insufficiency of her sample for some of the outcomes and might have developed a different sampling plan or identified different outcome variables.

The third major methodological decision concerns the measurement of the research variables. For the most part, the researcher did a good job in selecting objective, reliable, and valid outcome measures. Also, her operational definitions were clearly worded and unambiguous. Two comments are in order, however. First, it might have been better to operationalize two of the variables differently. Infant birth weight might have been more sensitively measured as actual weight (a ratio-level measurement) or as a three-level ordinal variable ($<1,500$ g; $>1,500$ g, but $<2,500$ g; and $>2,500$ g) instead of as a dichotomous variable. The contraceptive variable could also have been operationalized to yield a more sensitive (i.e., more discriminating) measure. For example, rather than measuring contraceptive use as a dichotomy, Clinton could have measured frequency of using contraception (e.g., never, sometimes, usually, or always), effectiveness of the *type* of birth control used, or a combination of these two.

A second consideration is whether the outcome variables adequately captured the effects of program activities. It would have been more directly relevant to the intervention to capture group differences, for instance, in dietary practices during pregnancy than in infant birth weight. None of the outcome variables measured the effects of parenting education. In other words, Clinton could have added additional and more direct measures of the effectiveness of the intervention.

One other point about the methods relates to ethical considerations. The article does not specifically say that subjects were asked for their informed consent, but that does not necessarily mean that no written consent was obtained. It is quite likely that the experimental group subjects, when asked to volunteer for the special program, were advised about their participation in the study and asked to sign a consent form. But what about the control group subjects? The article implies that comparison group members were given no opportunity to decline participation and were not aware of having their birth outcomes used as data in the research. In some cases, this procedure is acceptable. For example, a hospital or clinic might agree to release patient information without the patients' consent if the release of such information is done anonymously—that is, if it can be provided in such a way that even the researcher does not know the identity of the patients. In the present study, however, it is clear that the names of the comparison subjects *were* given to the researcher because she had to contact the comparison group at 6 months postpartum to determine their contraceptive practices. Thus, this study does not appear to have adequately safeguarded the rights of the comparison group subjects.

In summary, the researcher appears not to have given the new program a particularly fair test. Clinton should have taken a number of steps to control confounding variables and should have attempted to get a larger sample (even if this meant waiting for additional subjects to enroll in the program). In addition to concerns about the internal validity of the study, its generalizability is also questionable.

Results. Clinton did an adequate job of presenting the results of the study. The presentation was straightforward and succinct and was enhanced by the inclusion of a good table and figures. The style of this section was also appropriate: It was written objectively and was well organized.

The statistical analyses were also reasonably well done. The descriptive statistics (means and percentages) were appropriate for the level of measurement of the variables. The two types of inferential statistics used (the *t*-test and chi-squared test) were also appropriate, given the levels of measurement of the outcome variables. The results of these tests were efficiently presented in a single table. Of course, more powerful statistics could have been used to control extraneous variables (e.g., analysis of covariance). It appears, however, that the only extraneous variable that could have been controlled statistically was the subjects' ages; no data were apparently collected on other confounding variables (social class, ethnicity, parity, and so on).

Discussion. Clinton's discussion section fails almost entirely to take the study's limitations into account in interpreting the data. The one exception is her acknowledgment that the sample size was too small. She seems unconcerned about the many threats to the internal or external validity of her research.

Clinton lays almost all the blame for the nonsignificant findings on the program rather than on the research methods. She feels that two aspects of the program should be changed: (*a*) recruitment of teenagers into the program earlier in their pregnancies and (*b*) strengthening program services. Both recommendations might be worth pursuing, but little in the data suggests these modifications. With nonsignificant results such as those that predominated in this study, there are two possibilities to consider: (*a*) the results are accurate—that is, the program is not effective for those outcomes examined (although it might be effective for other measures), and (*b*) the results are false—that is, the existing program is effective for the outcomes examined, but the tests failed to demonstrate it. Clinton concluded that the first possibility was correct and, therefore, recommended that the program be changed. Equally plausible is the possibility that the study methods were too weak to demonstrate the program's true effects.

We do not have sufficient information about the characteristics of the sample to conclude with certainty that substantial selection biases existed. We do, however, have a clue that selection biases were operative in a direction that would make the program look less effective than it actually is. Clinton noted in the beginning of the results section that the average age of the teenagers in the experimental group was 17.0, compared with 18.1 in the comparison group—a difference that was significant. Age is inversely related to positive labor and delivery outcomes; indeed, that is the basis for having a special program for teenaged mothers. Therefore, the experimental group's performance on the outcome measures was possibly depressed by the youth of that group. Had the two groups been equivalent in terms of age, the group differences might have been larger and could have reached levels of statistical significance. Other uncontrolled pretreatment differences could also have masked true treatment effects.

For the one significant outcome, we cannot rule out the possibility that a Type I error was made—that is, that the null hypothesis was in fact true. Again, selection biases could have been operative. The experimental group might have contained many more girls who had preprogram experience with contraception; it might have contained more highly motivated teenagers, or more single teenagers, or more teenagers who had already had multiple pregnancies than the comparison group. There simply is no way of knowing whether the significant outcome reflects true program effects or merely initial group differences.

Aside from Clinton's disregard for the problems of internal validity, she overstepped the bounds of scholarly speculation. She assumed that the program *caused* contraceptive improvements: "the experimental program significantly increased the percentage of teenagers who used birth control. . . ." Worse yet, she went on to conclude that repeat pregnancies will be postponed in the experimental group, although she does not know whether the teenagers used an effective contraception, whether they used it all the time, or whether they used it correctly.

As another example of going beyond the data, Clinton became overly invested in the notion that teenagers need greater and earlier exposure to the program. It is not that her hypothesis has no merit; the problem is that she builds an elaborate rationale for program changes with no apparent empiric support. She probably had information on when in the pregnancy the teenagers entered the program, but that information was not shared with readers. Her argument about the need for more publicity on early screening would have been stronger if she had reported that most teenagers entered the program during the fourth month of their pregnancies or later. Additionally, she could have marshaled more evidence in support of her proposal if she had been able to show that earlier entry into the program was associated with better health outcomes. For example, she could have compared the outcomes of teenagers entering the program in the first, second, and third trimesters of their pregnancies.

In conclusion, the study has several positive features. As Clinton noted, some reason exists to be cautiously optimistic that the program *could* have some beneficial effects. However, the existing study is too seriously flawed to reach any conclusion. A replication with improved research methods is needed to solve the research problem.

■ D. Application Exercises

EXERCISE 1: STUDY IN APPENDIX A

Read the Method, Results, and Discussion sections of the report by Hill and colleagues ("Chronically Ill Rural Women") in Appendix A. Then answer the following questions:

Study Guide for Essentials of Nursing Research: Appraising Evidence for Nursing Practice, 7e

Questions of Fact

a. Did the researchers provide evidence about the success of randomization (i.e., whether experimentals and controls were equivalent at the outset) and, thus, selection biases were absent?

b. Did any study participants withdraw from the study? What was the rate of attrition in the two groups? Did the researchers report an analysis of attrition biases?

c. With regard to Aim 1 (intercorrelations among psychosocial variables), were hypotheses supported, nonsupported, or mixed?

d. With regard to Aim 2 (experimental-control group differences on psychosocial variables), were hypotheses supported, nonsupported, or mixed?

e. Did the report provide information about the precision of results via confidence intervals?

f. Did the report provide information about magnitude of effects via calculation of effect sizes?

g. In the Discussion section, was there any explicit discussion about the study's internal validity?

h. In the Discussion section, was there any explicit discussion about the study's external validity?

i. In the Discussion section, was there any explicit discussion about the study's statistical conclusion validity?

j. Did the Discussion section link study findings to findings from prior research (i.e., did the authors place their findings into a broader context)?

k. Did the Discussion section explicitly mention any study limitations?

Questions for Discussion

a. Critique the analysis of biases in this report and possible resulting effects on the interpretation of the findings.

b. Do you agree with the researchers' interpretations of their results? Why or why not?

c. Discuss the extent to which the Discussion included all important results.

d. Compare your assessment about the internal and external validity of the study with that of the researchers.

e. To what extent do you think the researchers' adequately described the study's limitations and strengths?

EXERCISE 2: STUDY IN APPENDIX C

Read the Methods, Results, and Discussion sections of the report by Vollman and colleagues ("Coping and Depressive Symptoms") in Appendix C. Then answer the following questions:

Questions of Fact

a. Did any study participants withdraw from the study? Did the researchers report an analysis of attrition biases?

b. Were any other biases analyzed in this study? If yes, what was the analysis and what type of bias was addressed?

c. Did the researchers state or imply any hypotheses? With regard to any hypotheses, were they supported, nonsupported, or mixed?

d. Did the report provide information about the precision of results via confidence intervals?

e. Did the report provide information about magnitude of effects via calculation of effect sizes?

f. In the Discussion section, was there any explicit discussion about the study's internal validity?

g. In the Discussion section, was there any explicit discussion about the study's external validity?

h. In the Discussion section, was there any explicit discussion about the study's statistical conclusion validity?

i. Did the Discussion section link study findings to findings from prior research (i.e., did the authors place their findings into a broader context)?

j. Did the Discussion section explicitly mention any study limitations?

Questions for Discussion

a. Do you agree with the researchers' interpretations of their results? Why or why not?

b. Discuss the extent to which the Discussion included all important results.

c. To what extent do you think the researchers adequately described the study's limitations and strengths?

CHAPTER 17

Analysis of Qualitative Data

■ A. Crossword Puzzle

Complete the crossword puzzle below, which uses terms and concepts presented in Chapter 17.

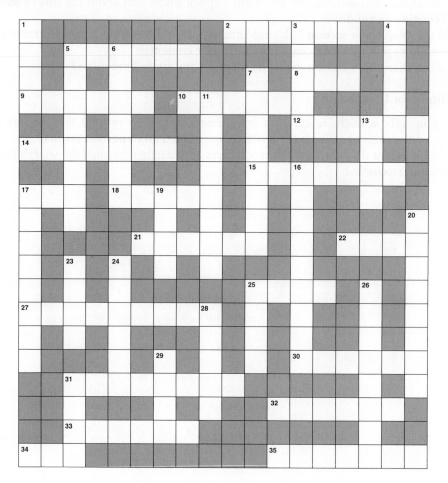

ACROSS

2. Nurse researcher who helped develop an alternative approach to grounded theory
5. Phenomenologic analysis involves the identification of essential _____.
8. In Glaser & Strauss' method, there are theoretical codes and _ _ _stantive codes.
9. In ethnographies, a broad unit of cultural knowledge
10. In vivo codes
12. The hermeneutic _____ involves movement between parts and whole of a text being analyzed.
14. _ _ _ _ _ _ _i was a prominent analyst and writer in the Duquesne school of phenomenology.
15. In Diekelmann's analytic approach, the discovery of a constitutive _____ forms the highest level of analysis.
17. In grounded theory, _____ has to do with how closely concepts map onto incidents they represent.
18. Phenomenologist _ _ _ _ _i was one of the writers in the Duquesne school who proposed an approach to the collection and analysis of data.
21. Hermeneutic approach developed by _____ includes an analysis of exemplars.
22. _____ from a descriptive qualitative study are sometimes analyzed through a process called content analysis.
25. Timelines and _____ charts are devices that can be used to highlight time sequences in qualitative analysis.
27. Most interpretive and subjective of three prototypical qualitative analysis styles
30. After a category system is developed, the main task involves _____ the data.
31. Dutch phenomenologist who encouraged the use of artistic data sources
32. Basic analytic strategy in grounded theory research is _ _ _ _ _ _nt comparison.
33. Qualitative researchers often begin analysis by developing a category _____.
34. All of a phenomenologist's transcribed interviews would comprise a qualitative data _____.
35. In grounded theory, the type of coding focused on the core variable is _ _ _ _ _ _ _ve coding.

DOWN

1. A recurring _____ in a set of interviews can sometimes be the basis for an emerging theme.
3. One type of core variable in grounded theory is a(n) _____ social process that evolves over time.
4. Type of coding in Strauss and Corbin's approach wherein the analyst links subcategories

5. Guide for sorting narrative data that may be developed before data collection
6. Grounded theorists and phenomenologists typically use this broad type of qualitative analysis style.
7. Literary device sometimes used as part of an analytic strategy, especially by interpretive phenomenologists
11. Concept of _____ fit in grounded theory involves comparing emerging concepts with similar concepts from previous studies.
13. In grounded theory, the _____ category is a central pattern that is relevant to participants.
16. Second level of analysis in Spradley's ethnographic method, yielding an organizational structure for the data
17. Glaser proposed 18 _____ of theoretical codes to help grounded theorists conceptualize relationships.
19. First stage of constant comparison involves _____ coding
20. _____ cases are strong examples of ways of being in the world.
23. Grounded theorists document an idea in an analytic_____.
24. Gadamer is associated with interpretive phenomenology or _ _ _ _ _ _eutics.
25. In manual organization of qualitative data, excerpts are cut up and inserted into a conceptual _____.
26. In Van Manen's most global (_____) approach, the analyst sees the text as a whole and tries to capture its meaning.
28. The field _____ of an ethnographer are an important source of data for analysis.
29. Van _____ was a phenomenologist from the Duquesne school.
31. The amount of data collected in a typical qualitative study typically is

_____.

■ B. Matching Exercises

Match each descriptive statement from Set B with one or more types of qualitative analyses from Set A. Indicate the letter(s) corresponding to your response next to each item in Set B.

SET A

a. Grounded theory analysis
b. Phenomenologic/hermeneutic analysis
c. Ethnographic analysis
d. None of the above

SET B	RESPONSES
1. Involves the development of coding categories	_____
2. Begins with "open coding"	_____
3. One method of analysis was developed by Colaizzi	_____
4. Data can be organized using computer software	_____
5. One method of analysis was developed by Glaser & Strauss	_____
6. May involve the development of a taxonomy	_____
7. One analytic approach involves identifying paradigm cases	_____
8. Requires the use of quasi-statistics	_____

■ C. Study Questions

1. What is wrong with the following statements?
   a. Lopez conducted a grounded theory study about coping with a miscarriage in which she was able to identify four major themes.
   b. Schwartz's ethnographic analysis of Haitian clinics involved gleaning related thematic material from French poetry.
   c. Allen's phenomenologic study of the lived experience of Parkinson's disease focused on the domain of fatigue.
   d. Denny's grounded theory study of widowhood yielded a taxonomy of coping strategies.
   e. In her ethnographic study of the culture of a nursing home, Tower used a rural nursing home as a paradigm case.

2. Use the category scheme presented in Box 17.1 of the textbook to code the following segments from actual interviews:

   "Birthdays—what do they mean to me? For me, a birthday prior to the start of the new millennium meant joy, presents, relaxation, and celebration. Now it has a darker side to it, a profound depth that I never could have imagined was possible. As the birthday nears, I find I question my own abilities much more than usual and I am aware that I experience high levels of anxiety and fear. On the day before his birthday I watch the clock continually and plot what was happening at minute by minute. I find it very difficult to sleep for several weeks before the birthday and usually cannot sleep at all the night before his birthday. He was born at 6:15 AM so labor was overnight. I get very angry with myself for not being more assertive and taking more control of the situation.
   The first birth anniversary was particularly difficult. I had very mixed feelings about celebrating Jon's birth—for me what was there to celebrate? What became important to me (indeed all consuming) was that the birthday should be a technical

success (i.e., the food should be good, the guests right, and the weather fine). It, however, was not an enjoyable event and I was very emotional. It did bring the whole experience flooding back, the sense of extreme violation by a rough, arrogant, male doctor who invaded my space and made me feel disgusting and ruined my inner self. For me, when people ask what it was like, I say it was as close to a sense of rape without being physically raped. These feelings were vividly present both before and then subsequently. Although they are heightened around the time of the anniversary, they are often with me. The birthday is no longer the celebration of the child but the anniversary of a wrong.

Jon's second birthday was a children's party and again I focused heavily on getting it right—of being successful. I do feel so ambivalent about the whole thing—yes, I want to celebrate the fact he is a gorgeous little boy, who survived a particularly horrible birth without any apparent long-term damage. But on the other hand, each birthday brings back memories of the wrong.

Although this is getting better year by year, I am not sure it will ever really disappear. The reawakening of the birth each birthday does mean I think again about what happened, my role in it, what I could have done to prevent it from happening and my sadness at what was taken away from me. The feelings of having let myself down and allowed this to happen remain with me. The decisions I made that led down the path which led to birth trauma haunt me."

3. Suppose a researcher was studying people with hypertension who were struggling unsuccessfully for months to manage their weight. The researcher planned to interview 10 to 20 people for this study. Answer the following questions:

a. What might be the research question that a phenomenologist would ask relating to this situation? And what might the research question be for a grounded theory researcher?

b. Which do you think would take longer to do—the analysis of data for the phenomenologic or the grounded theory? Why?

c. What would the final "product" of the analyses be for the two different studies?

d. Which study would have more appeal to you? Why?

■ D. Application Exercises

EXERCISE 1: STUDY IN APPENDIX B

Read the "Design and Methods" and "Findings" sections of the report by Rasmussen and colleagues ("Young Women with Type 1 Diabetes") in Appendix B. Then answer the following questions:

Questions of Fact

a. Did the researchers audiotape and transcribe the interviews? If yes, who did the transcription? Did the report state how many pages of data comprised the data set?

b. Was constant comparison used in analyzing the data?

c. Did Rasmussen and colleagues create conceptual files? Was a computer used to analyze the data? If yes, what software was used?

d. Did the researchers calculate any quasi-statistics?

e. Which grounded theory analytic approach was adopted in this study?

f. Did the researchers prepare any analytic memos?

g. Did the authors describe the open coding process? If so, what did they say?

h. Did the authors describe the process of theoretical coding? If so, what did they say? Did they offer any examples of their theoretical codes?

i. How many categories emerged in the analysis? How many major categories were ultimately developed and refined? What were they?

j. What was the BSP? What does the BSP entail?

k. Did the report include a figure that represented the grounded theory?

Questions for Discussion

a. Discuss the thoroughness of Rasmussen and colleagues' description of their data analysis efforts. Did the report present adequate information about the data coding and the steps taken to analyze the data?

b. Was there any evidence of "method slurring"—that is, did Rasmussen and colleagues apply any analytic procedures that are inappropriate for a grounded theory approach?

c. Discuss the effectiveness of the researchers' presentation of results. Does the analysis seem sensible, thoughtful, and thorough?

d. Were data presented in a manner that allows you to be confident about the researchers' conclusions? Comment on the inclusion or noninclusion of figures that graphically represent the grounded theory.

EXERCISE 2: STUDY IN APPENDIX D

Read the "Data Analysis" and "Findings" sections of the report by Ward-Griffin and colleagues ("Perspectives of Women with Dementia") in Appendix D. Then answer the following questions:

Questions of Fact

a. Did the researchers audiotape and transcribe the interviews? If yes, who did the transcription? Did the report state how many pages of data comprised the data set?

b. Did Ward-Griffin and colleagues create conceptual files? Was a computer used to analyze the data? If yes, what software was used?

c. Did the researchers describe the coding process? If so, what did they say?

d. Did the researchers calculate any quasi-statistics?

e. Did the researchers prepare any analytic memos?

f. Which analytic approach was adopted in this study?

g. How many themes emerged in analysis? What were they?

h. Did Ward-Griffin and colleagues provide supporting evidence for their themes, in the form of excerpts from the data?

i. Did the report include a figure that summarized the findings?

Questions for Discussion

a. Discuss the thoroughness of Ward-Griffin and colleagues' description of their data analysis efforts. Did the report present adequate information about the data coding and the steps taken to analyze the data?

b. Discuss the effectiveness of the researchers' presentation of results. Does the analysis seem sensible, thoughtful, and thorough?

c. Were data presented in a manner that allows you to be confident about the researchers' conclusions? Comment on the inclusion or noninclusion of figures that graphically represent the conceptualization of the findings.

CHAPTER 18

Trustworthiness and Integrity in Qualitative Research

■ A. Crossword Puzzle

Complete the crossword puzzle below, which uses terms and concepts presented in Chapter 18.

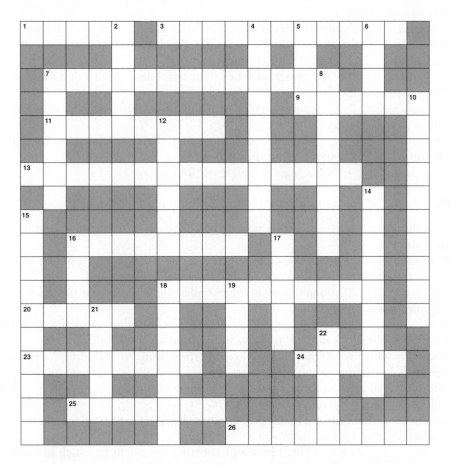

ACROSS

1. Confirmability can be addressed through a scrutiny of documents and procedures in an inquiry _____.
3. A key criterion for assessing quality in qualitative studies, in both frameworks described in the textbook
7. Use of multiple means of converging on the truth
9. The stability of data over time and conditions, analogous to reliability, is called _ _ _ _ _ _ability.
11. A secondary criterion in the Whittemore et al. framework, referring to the ability to follow researchers' decisions and interpretations, is _ _ _ _ _ _ _ness.
13. Extent to which qualitative findings can be applied to other settings
16. Auditability can be enhanced by a(n) _____ trail that documents judgments and choices.
18. A secondary criterion in the Whittemore et al. framework, referring to interconnectedness
20. Collecting data in multiple sites is a form of _____ triangulation.
23. Credibility in qualitative inquiry has been described as analogous to _____ validity in quantitative inquiry.
24. _ _ _ _ _ness involves the presentation of rich, artful descriptions that highlight salient themes in the data.
25. A(n) _____ audit involves scrutiny of data and supporting documents by an external reviewer.
26. Persistent _ _ _ _ _ _ _ _ _on refers to a focus on the aspects of a situation that are relevant to the phenomena being studied.

DOWN

2. An audit _____ is a systematic collection of materials for an independent auditor.
4. Word used by some as an overarching goal for qualitative inquiry, in lieu of validity
5. An electronic music device (brand name—unrelated to research!)
6. _____ triangulation involves collecting data about a phenomenon at multiple points.
7. With _____ triangulation, researchers examine competing hypotheses or conceptualizations in their analysis and interpretation of data.
8. Process by which researchers revise their interpretations by including cases that appear to disconfirm earlier hypotheses is a _____ case analysis.
10. Credibility can be enhanced through a thorough search for _ _ _ _ _ _ _ _ _ing evidence.
12. One method of addressing credibility involves going back to participants to do member _____.
14. _ _ _ _ _ _ _ _ _ity is a quality criterion indicating the extent to which the researchers fairly and faithfully portray a range of different realities.

15. _ _ _ _ _ _ _ _ _ _or triangulation is achieved by having two or more researchers make key decisions and interpretations.
16. Interviewing patients *and* family members about a phenomenon is an example of _____ source triangulation.
17. Qualitative researchers strive for the _____worthiness of their data and their methods.
18. _ _ _ _ _ _ity is a secondary criterion in the Whittemore et al. framework, reflecting challenges to traditional ways of thinking.
19. Lincoln and _____ proposed criteria for evaluating the trustworthiness of qualitative inquiries.
21. Researchers typically "_____" transcribe data by comparing transcriptions with recordings and making necessary corrections.
22. Term that is hotly debated in terms of appropriateness for evaluating quality in qualitative inquiry

▪ B. Matching Exercises

Match each statement from Set B with one of the phrases from Set A. Indicate the letter corresponding to your response next to each of the statements in Set B.

SET A

a. Data source triangulation
b. Investigator triangulation
c. Theory triangulation
d. Method triangulation

SET B   **RESPONSES**

1. A researcher studying health beliefs of the rural elderly interviews old people and health care providers in the area   _____

2. A researcher tests narrative data, collected in interviews with people who attempted suicide, against two alternative explanations of stress and coping   _____

3. Two researchers independently interview 10 informants in a study of adjustment to a cancer diagnosis, and debrief with each other to review what they have learned   _____

4. A researcher studying school-based clinics observes interactions in the clinics and also conducts in-depth interviews with students   _____

5. A researcher studying the process of resolving an infertility problem interviews husbands and wives separately   _____

6. Themes emerging in the field notes of an observer on a psychiatric ward are categorized and labeled independently by the researcher and an assistant   _____

■ C. Study Questions

1. Suppose you were conducting a grounded theory study of couples' coming to terms with infertility. What might you do to incorporate various types of triangulation into your study?

2. In the previous chapter, one of the study questions involved an exercise to elicit descriptions of the unsuccessful efforts of people with hypertension to manage their weight (Study question C.3 in Chapter 17). Describe efforts you could take to enhance the integrity of this inquiry.

3. What is your opinion about the value of member checking as a strategy to enhance credibility? Defend your position.

4. Read a research report in a recent issue of the journal *Qualitative Health Research*. Identify several examples of "thick description." Also, identify areas of the report in which you feel additional thick description would have enhanced the inquiry.

■ D. Application Exercises

EXERCISE 1: STUDY IN APPENDIX B

Read the report by Rasmussen ("Young Women with Type I Diabetes") in Appendix B. Then answer the following questions:

Questions of Fact

a. Did the researchers devote a section of their report to describing their quality-enhancement strategies? If so, what was it labeled? If not, where was information about such strategies located?

b. What types of triangulation, if any, were used in this study?

c. Were any of the following methods used to enhance the credibility of the study and its data:
   - Prolonged engagement, persistent observation, or both
   - Peer review and debriefing
   - Member checks
   - Search for disconfirming evidence
   - Researcher credibility

d. Describe what methods (if any) were used to enhance the following aspects of the study:
   - Dependability
   - Confirmability
   - Transferability
   - Authenticity
   - Explicitness

Questions for Discussion

a. Discuss the thoroughness with which Rasmussen and colleagues described their efforts to enhance and evaluate the quality and integrity of their study.
b. In the section titled "Rigor and Credibility," the authors state that their strategies "were all very important assuring credibility." Comment on this statement.
c. How would you characterize the integrity and trustworthiness of this study, based on the researchers' documentation?

EXERCISE 2: STUDY IN APPENDIX D

Read the report by Ward-Griffin and colleagues ("Perspectives of Women with Dementia") in Appendix D. Then answer the following questions:

Questions of Fact

a. Did the researchers devote a section of their report to describing their quality-enhancement strategies? If so, what was it labeled? If not, where was information about such strategies located?
b. What types of triangulation, if any, were used in this study?
c. Were any of the following methods used to enhance the credibility of the study and its data:
   - Prolonged engagement, persistent observation, or both
   - Peer review and debriefing
   - Member checks
   - Search for disconfirming evidence
   - Researcher credibility
d. Describe what methods (if any) were used to enhance the following aspects of the study:
   - Dependability
   - Confirmability
   - Transferability
   - Authenticity
   - Sensitivity

Questions for Discussion

a. Discuss the thoroughness with which Ward-Griffin and colleagues described their efforts to enhance and evaluate the quality and integrity of their study.

b. How would you characterize the integrity and trustworthiness of this study, based on the researchers' documentation?

c. Do you think that the researchers' maintenance of "an extensive audit trail" contributed to the integrity and trustworthiness of this study? Why or why not?

CHAPTER 19

Systematic Reviews: Meta-Analysis and Metasynthesis

■ A. Crossword Puzzle

Complete the crossword puzzle below, which uses terms and concepts presented in Chapter 19.

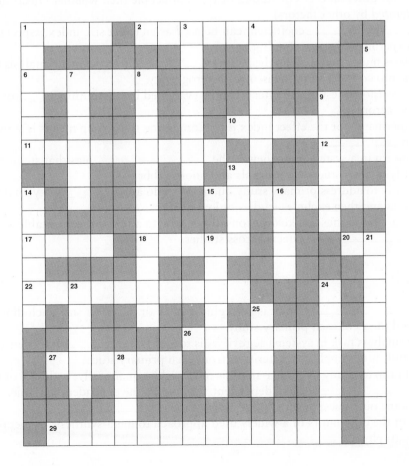

ACROSS

1. A(n) _____-safe number estimates the number of studies with zero effect that would be needed to reverse the conclusion of a significant effect.
2. A(n) _____ effect size is the ratio of reports with a particular thematic finding, divided by all reports describing qualitative study results on a phenomenon.
6. The type of meta-analytic model that is preferred with heterogeneity is called a(n) _____ effects model.
10. Study quality can be assessed using a formal rating _____ and many such multicomponent instruments have been developed.
11. The _____ level ($5k + 10$) is the number against which a fail-safe number is compared.
12. In extracting and coding data for meta-analysis, it is preferable to have _____ or more people so that intercoder reliability can be assessed.
15. A(n) _____ analysis involves examining the extent to which effects differ for different types of studies or types of people (i.e., whether effects are *moderated* by other factors).
17. A _____ coefficient can be used as an effect size index, especially for nonexperimental research (abbr.).
18. Analysts must choose an analysis _____ for the meta-analysis that takes into consideration the issue of heterogeneity.
20. The precision of estimated effects can be evaluated by computing a _ _ around each index (acronym).
22. Another name for the effect index *d* for comparing two group means is standardized mean _____.
26. A concern in a systematic review is the _____ bias that stems from identifying only studies in journals and books (abbr).
27. One way to address primary study quality is to do a(n) _ _ _ _ _ _ivity analysis that includes and then excludes studies of low quality.
29. A meta-analyst must make decisions about how to address the inevitable _____ of effects across studies.

DOWN

1. A(n)_____ plot is a graphic display of the effect size (including CIs around them) of each primary study.
3. A preanalysis task in systematic reviews is to _____ information about the study and sample characteristics from each primary study.
4. Each primary study in a meta-analysis must yield a quantitative estimate of the _____ of the independent variable on the dependent variable.
5. For some outcomes, the effect size index is the odds _____.
7. One of the originators of a widely used approach to meta-synthesis or meta-ethnography

8. A(n) _____, which involves calculating manifest effect sizes, can lay the foundation for a meta-synthesis.

9. In Paterson and colleagues' scheme, the three aspects of a meta-synthesis are meta-data analysis, meta-theory, and meta-_____.

13. There is evidence of a bias against the _____ hypothesis in published studies.

14. In a meta-analysis, after extracting information from primary studies it is necessary to _____ it so that it can be included in the analysis.

16. The body of unpublished studies is sometimes referred to as _____ literature.

19. In a meta-analysis, researchers sometimes must opt to _____ primary studies written in a language other than English.

21. A(n) _____ effect size is the ratio of the number of themes represented in one report, divided by all relevant themes relating to a phenomenon across all reports.

23. To use a(n) _____ effects model to analyze aggregate effects, heterogeneity should be low.

24. _____ appraisal is undertaken in most meta-analyses, although approaches to using the information vary.

25. A funnel _____ is often used to detect publication biases.

28. The index *d* provides an estimate of effect _____ for comparing means.

■ B. Matching Exercises

Match each of the statements in Set B with the appropriate phrase in Set A. Indicate the letter(s) corresponding to your response next to each of the statements in Set B.

SET A

a. Meta-analysis

b. Meta-synthesis

c. Neither meta-analysis nor meta-synthesis

d. Both meta-analysis and meta-synthesis

SET B   **RESPONSES**

1. Involves gathering data from human participants   _____

2. Focuses on synthesizing information from prior studies   _____

3. Relies on findings from qualitative studies   _____

4. Almost always involves an assessment of study quality   _____

5. Sandelowski developed important approaches for this   _____

6. Often involves calculating d or OR statistics   _____

7. CINAHL would be used for this   _____

8. Can involve the calculation of a frequency effect size   _____

■ C. Study Questions

1. Read one of the following meta-analysis reports:
   - Beck, C. T. (2001). Predictors of postpartum depression: An update. *Nursing Research, 50,* 275–285.
   - Floyd, J., Medler, S., Ager, J., & Janisse, J. (2000). Age-related changes in initiation and maintenance of sleep: A meta-analysis. *Research in Nursing & Health, 23,* 106–117.
   - Peters, R. (1999). The effectiveness of therapeutic touch: A meta-analytic review. *Nursing Science Quarterly, 12,* 52–61.

   Then, search the literature for related quantitative primary studies published *after* this meta-analysis. Are new study results consistent with the conclusions drawn in the meta-analytic report? Are there enough new studies to warrant a new meta-analysis?

2. Read one of the following meta-synthesis reports:
   - Beck, C. T. (2002). Postpartum depression: A metasynthesis. *Qualitative Health Research, 12,* 453–472.
   - Burke, S., Kauffmann, E., Costello, E., Wiskin, N., & Harrison, M. (1998). Stressors in families with a child with a chronic illness: An analysis of qualitative studies and a framework. *Canadian Journal of Nursing Research, 30,* 71–95.
   - Russell, C., Bunting, S., & Gregory, S. (1997). Protective care-receiving: The active role of care recipients. *Journal of Advanced Nursing, 25,* 532–540.

   Then, search the literature for related qualitative primary studies published *after* this meta-synthesis. Are new study results consistent with the conclusions drawn in the meta-synthesis report? Are there enough new studies to warrant a new meta-synthesis?

3. Read the following report, which involved a systematic review without a meta-analysis. Did the authors adequately justify their decision not to conduct a meta-analysis?
   - McGillion, M., Watt-Watson, J., Kim, J., & Yamada, J. (2004). A systematic review of psychoeducational intervention trials for the management of stable angina. *Journal of Nursing Management, 12*(3), 174–182.

■ D. Application Exercises

EXERCISE 1: STUDY IN APPENDIX F

Read the report on the meta-analysis by Lee, Soeken, and Picot ("Interventions for Informal Stroke Caregivers") in Appendix F. Then answer the following questions:

Questions of Fact

a. What was the stated purpose of this review? What were the independent and dependent variables in this review?

b. Which bibliographic databases were searched? What key words were used? Was there an effort to identify and locate "grey literature"?

c. Were non-English language primary study reports excluded from the review?

d. How many initial citations were obtained? What inclusion criteria were stipulated? How many studies met all inclusion criteria? Were studies omitted for other reasons? If yes, how many were in the actual analysis?

e. If a primary study was an RCT that examined the effect of an intervention on caregivers' mental health using the CES-D depression scale as the outcome variable, would it have been included in the meta-analysis?

f. How many of the studies included in this meta-analysis used an experimental design? How many were nonexperimental?

g. Did the researchers rate each study in the data set for its quality? If yes, what aspects of the study were appraised? What was the highest possible quality score? How many people scored the studies for quality? Was inter-rater agreement assessed?

h. What was the cutoff score for high versus low quality? How many studies were rated low quality and how many were high quality? Did the researchers set a threshold for study quality as part of their inclusion criteria? If yes, what was it? Were any studies excluded because of a low quality rating?

i. What effect size measure was used in the analysis? By what were the effect sizes weighted?

j. Did the researchers perform any tests for statistical heterogeneity? If yes, what were the findings?

k. Was a fixed effects or random effects model used?

l. How many subjects were there in total, in all studies combined?

m. Answer the following questions regarding information in Table 2 or Figure 1:
   • In which study was the effect size the largest? Was this effect size statistically significant?
   • In which study was the effect size the smallest? Was this effect size statistically significant?
   • Were effect sizes nonsignificant in any studies? If yes, which one(s)?
   • For all four studies combined, what was the mean weighted effect size and was it statistically significant? What does the effect size mean?

n. Were subgroup analyses undertaken? If yes, what subgroups were examined?

o. Were sensitivity analyses undertaken? If yes, what was done and what were the findings?

p. Did this meta-analysis address the issue of publication bias? What did the researchers conclude?

Questions for Discussion

a. Was the size of the sample (studies and subjects) sufficiently large to draw conclusions about the overall effect of caregiver interventions and about subgroup effects?

b. What other subgroups might have been interesting to examine (assume there was sufficient information in the original studies)?

c. Did the researchers draw reasonable conclusions about the quality, quantity, and consistency of evidence?

d. How would you assess the overall rigor of this meta-analysis? What would you recommend to improve the quality of this systematic review?

e. Based on this review, what is the evidence regarding interventions for caregivers of patients with stroke? What are the implications for nursing practice?

EXERCISE 2: STUDY IN APPENDIX G

Read the report on the meta-synthesis by Xu ("Strangers in Strange Lands") in Appendix G. Then answer the following questions:

Questions of Fact

a. What was the stated purpose of this meta-synthesis? What was the central phenomenon and how was it defined?

b. Which bibliographic databases were searched? What key words were used? Was there an effort to identify and locate "grey literature"? In addition to electronic database searches, what did Xu do to locate relevant studies?

c. What was Xu's position in the controversy regarding integration across research traditions?

d. How many primary studies were included in the integration? Were the primary studies described?

e. Were primary studies appraised for quality? Were any studies excluded because of poor quality?

f. Were the data in the primary studies derived from interviews, observations, or both?

g. What approach was used to conduct this meta-synthesis? Was the analytic process described?

h. Was a meta-summary performed?

i. How many study participants were there in all of the studies combined?

j. How many shared themes were identified in this meta-synthesis? What were those themes?

k. Was Xu's analysis supported through the inclusion of raw data from the primary studies?

l. Did the report discuss the meta-synthesis findings? Did Xu present possible implications?

Questions for Discussion

a. Was the size of the sample (studies and subjects) sufficiently large to conduct a meaningful meta-synthesis? Did the diversity of the sample (in terms of participant characteristics, timing of data collection, or research tradition) enhance the study or weaken it?

b. Did the analysis and integration appear reasonable and thorough?

c. Were primary studies adequately described?

d. Did Xu draw reasonable conclusions about the quality and consistency of evidence?

e. How would you assess the overall rigor of this meta-synthesis? What would you recommend to improve its quality?

f. Based on this meta-synthesis, what is the evidence regarding the experiences of immigrant Asian nurses working in Western countries? What are the implications for nursing practice, nursing administration, or health care policy?

INFLUENCE OF A COMPUTER INTERVENTION ON THE PSYCHOLOGICAL STATUS OF CHRONICALLY ILL RURAL WOMEN

Preliminary Results

Wade Hill • Clarann Weinert • Shirley Cudneyc

■ **Background:** Adaptation to chronic illness is a lifelong process presenting numerous psychological challenges. It has been shown to be influenced by participating in support groups. Rural women with chronic illness face additional burdens as access to information, healthcare resources, and sources of support are often limited. Developing virtual support groups and testing the effects on psychosocial indicators associated with adaptation to chronic illness may help remove barriers to adaptation.

■ **Objective:** To examine the effects of a computer-delivered intervention on measures of psychosocial health in chronically ill rural women including social support, self-esteem, empowerment, self-efficacy, depression, loneliness, and stress.

■ **Methods:** An experimental design was used to test a computer-delivered intervention and examine differences in psychosocial health between women who participated in the intervention ($n = 44$) and women in a control group ($n = 56$).

■ **Results:** Differences between women who participated in the intervention and controls were found for self-esteem, $F(1,98) = 5.97$, $p = .016$; social support, $F(1,98) = 4.43$, $p = .038$; and empowerment, $F(1,98) = 6.06$, $p = .016$. A comparison of means for depression, loneliness, self-efficacy, and stress suggests that differences for other psychosocial variables are possible.

■ **Discussion:** The computer-based intervention tested appears to result in improved self-esteem, social support, and empowerment among rural women with chronic illness. Descriptive but non-significant differences were found for other psychosocial variables (depression, loneliness, self-efficacy, and stress); women who participated in the intervention appeared to improve more than women in the control group.

■ **Key Words:** chronic illness • computer-based intervention • psychosocial outcomes • rural

Adaptation to chronic disease is a lifelong challenge to persons with long-term health problems. Being diagnosed with a chronic illness, unlike an acute illness, is a profound and life-altering event that can result in alterations in physical functioning, loss of control over life circumstances, and subsequently emotional strain (Emery, 2003). The psychological task imposed on these individuals is that of maintaining an acceptable quality of life while living with the changes in lifestyle that long-term illness imposes. For chronically ill, middle-aged, rural women who live where there are relatively few healthcare resources and limited access to those that do exist, it is

Reprinted with permission from *Nursing Research* 2006; 55(1):34–42.

particularly difficult to maintain a semblance of normalcy and balance in their lives. They often must struggle in isolation to meet the psychological challenges of adapting to their chronic illnesses.

Emotional distress often accompanies these challenges, yet not all experience significant emotional problems (Earll, Johnson, & Mitchell, 1993), particularly if they have adequate social support and access to quality health information. Social support has been demonstrated to be a constructive influence on the experience of dealing with illness (Finfgeld-Connett, 2005; Hegyvary, 2004) and positively affects psychosocial adjustment, enhances quality of life, and reduces the incidence of depression. Those with intact psychosocial health can live healthier lives and better manage living with long-term illness (Stuifbergen, Seraphine, & Roberts, 2000). Historically, traditional support groups where participants interact in person are known to influence psychosocial health (Hunter & Hall, 1989; Lin, Simeone, Ensel, & Kuo, 1979; Williams, 1990), although little is known about the effects of virtual support groups.

■ Background

Social support, based on the work of Weiss (1969), includes the provision of attachment or intimacy, facilitation of social integration, opportunity for nurturant behavior, reassurance of self-worth, and availability of informational and material assistance. Social support can buffer the negative effects of life events on health (Paykel, 1994; Pollachek, 2001; Thomas, 1995) and positively influence psychosocial adjustment and self-management of the chronic illness experience (Gallant, 2003; Symister & Friend, 2003). Inadequate social support can contribute to increased levels of depression and stress (Connell, Davis, Gallant, & Sharpe, 1994; Gray & Cason, 2002). Not all persons with chronic illness suffer from significant emotional problems (Earll et al., 1993), particularly if they have adequate social support and access to quality

health information that enable them to live healthy and productive lives while successfully adapting to and managing the many challenges of chronic illness. Social support resources may buffer the consequences of a chronic disease by enhancing recovery, increasing adherence to treatment recommendations, and promoting overall psychological adaptation (Wallston, Alagna, DeVellis, & DeVellis, 1983; Wortman & Conway, 1985). An effective and efficient means of providing support and facilitating the mobilization of support is through self-help groups (Schaefer, 1995). For those who live in geographically isolated areas, distance, travel time, weather, and road conditions often prohibit contact with others like themselves who are attempting to maintain psychosocial health (Sullivan, Weinert, & Cudney, 2003).

Computer-based support systems can be one solution to the problem of isolation. It has been shown that ill individuals using a computer-based health support system had better health outcomes, exerted greater efforts to improve functioning, and demonstrated greater resistance to psychological dysfunction (Gustafson et al., 1999).

The diagnosis of a chronic illness sets in motion a complex process of adaptation that requires balancing the demands of the situation and the individual's ability to respond (Pollock, Christian, & Sands, 1990). Adaptation has been a major theoretical concept guiding nursing practice over the past 20 years as delineated in the Roy Adaptation Model (RAM; Roy & Andrews, 1999). Pollock et al. (Pollock, 1986, 1993; Pollock et al., 1990) used the RAM as the theoretical framework for integrating the major variables of chronicity, stress, hardiness, and adaptive behavior. Their investigation identified and measured selected intervening variables that influenced adaptation. These variables included the ability to tolerate stress, presence of the hardiness characteristic, demographic characteristics, involvement in health promotion activities, and participation in health education programs (which enhance optimal self-management). The end result or level of adaptation was the individual's functioning as measured in the psychological and physiologic domains (Pollock, 1986). Chen (2005) tested the fit of the RAM as a framework for studying the nutritional health of community-dwelling elders using a conceptual–theoretical–empirical approach for examining factors that influence adaptation level. Stuifbergen et al. (2000) developed a model of health promotion and quality of life (QOL) in chronic disabling conditions that has implications for associating optimal self-management with QOL. The central concept for management of chronic illness throughout the literature has been psychosocial health and represents the key component of interest in this study.

One example of a computer-based intervention designed to support adaptation for chronically ill rural women was the Women to Women Project (WTW; Cudney & Weinert, 2000; Cudney, Winters, Weinert, & Anderson, 2005; Weinert, 2000; Weinert, Cudney, & Winters, 2005). The WTW was an online self-help support group designed to enhance social support and teach women the computer literacy skills necessary to find and evaluate health information available on the World Wide Web (WWW). Indicators of the potential for adaptation used in this project were social support, self-esteem, empowerment, self-efficacy, stress, depression, and loneliness. The purposes of this article are: to (a) examine the relationships among the psychosocial indicators and (b) determine the effect of the intervention on social support, self-esteem, empowerment, self-efficacy, stress, depression, and loneliness.

■ Method

DESIGN

This research was approved and monitored through the university's institutional review board for protection of human subjects. Women for this study were recruited ($N = 125$) from the Intermountain West using a variety of techniques including mass media, agency and service organization newsletters, and word of mouth (see Figure 1). After eliminating the names of five women who lived in urbanized areas, 120 women were randomized into intervention and control groups (intervention = 61; control = 59). At the completion of the intervention, 17 women from the intervention group dropped out due to declining health, inadequate time for participation, or moving to urban areas. Only two women from the control group dropped from the study due to failing to return the questionnaires. Data analyzed here are based on 43 women that completed the intervention and 57 women in the control group. One woman from the intervention group was dropped due to missing data.

To determine the impact of the intervention on the women's psychological status, measures were administered via a mail questionnaire composed of psychosocial health indicators: social support, self-esteem, empowerment, self-efficacy, stress, depression, and loneliness. *Illustrative comments from the women's online conversations were added to illuminate the data related to emotional and informational support.* A detailed description of the intervention is provided elsewhere (Weinert et al., 2005); thus, only a limited description of WTW will be repeated here.

The intervention included 22 weeks of participation in an online, asynchronous, peer-led support group and health teaching units. The WebCT (2005) platform was used to deliver the intervention and was available 24 hours a day, 7 days a week, thus allowing women to participate at any convenient time. Women in the intervention group had access to "Koffee Klatch," an asynchronous chat room in which they exchanged feelings, expressed concerns, provided support, and shared life experiences. The e-mail function ("Mailbox") gave the women private access to each other and to the research team. Women also engaged in health teaching unit activities independently, which included accessing health information on the WWW and participating in expert-facilitated chat room ("Health Roundtable") discussions related to the health teaching unit activities.

SAMPLE

The sample consisted of 100 chronically ill rural women. Participants were required to be 35–65 years of age and have a chronic illness

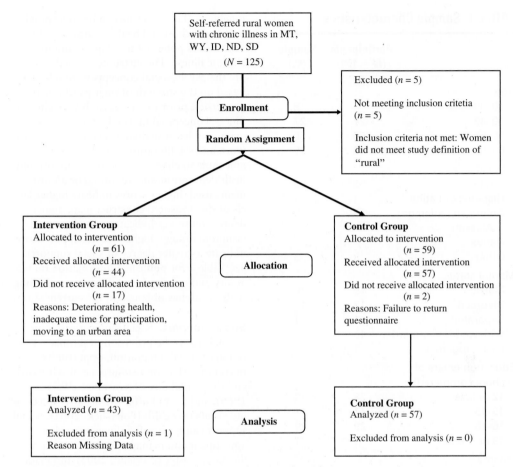

FIGURE 1 Participant progression.

such as diabetes, rheumatoid condition, heart disease, cancer, or multiple sclerosis. They lived at least 25 miles outside an urbanized area (a city of 12,500 or more) on a ranch, farm, or small town in Montana, Idaho, North Dakota, South Dakota, or Wyoming. On average, women in the sample traveled almost 57 (SD = 74.2) miles one-way for routine healthcare. The women were primarily older than 40 years of age (92%), were married or living with someone (80%), and had 13 or more years of education (77%). A majority of the sample were not employed outside of the home (64%) and household income varied from less than $15,000 (21%) to $55,000 or greater (16%). The length of

chronic illness (time since diagnosis) was 1–51 years with a mean of 13.0 years (SD = 11.1). Additional demographic details are presented in Table 1.

MEASURES

Disease may coexist with health in the same person at any point in the life span; thus, health maintenance is an important part of the quality of life equation for people with chronic illness. Promoting health, even in the presence of chronic illness, includes activities that educate, guide, and motivate the individual to take personal actions which improve

TABLE 1 Sample Characteristics

	Participants (*N* = 100)	Sample (%)
Age		
30–39	8	8
40–49	27	27
50–59	50	50
60–69	15	15
Ethnicity		
White	93	93
Hispanic or Latina	1	1
American Indian or Alaskan Native	3	3
Other	3	3
Marital status		
Married	79	79
Divorced	13	13
Separated	1	1
Widowed/Never married	15	15
Living together	1	1
Education (years of school completed)		
12 or less	23	23
13–15	47	47
16–18	29	29
19 or greater	1	1
Income		
Less than $15,000	21	21
$15,000–24,999	14	14
$25,000–34,999	16	16
$35,000–44,999	16	16
$45,000–54,999	17	17
$55,000–64,999	8	8
$65,000–74,999	4	4
$75,000–84,999	4	4
Employment (outside home)		
Yes	36	36
No	64	64

the likelihood of sustained good health (Fries, 1997). Factors considered to influence the success of these activities in promoting good health are social support, self-esteem, empowerment, self-efficacy, stress, depression, and loneliness. These factors can be conceptualized as psychosocial health indicators of the individual's potential to adapt to and manage chronic illness. The instruments used to measure the psychosocial concepts were selected based on the strength of their psychometric properties, prior use in research with chronic illness, conceptual fit, use by the research team, and because there is evidence in earlier work and the literature that they are amenable to change, based on a support and health education intervention. For all instruments used, higher scores indicate higher levels of the measured construct (e.g., higher depression scores indicate more depression symptomatology; higher social support scores indicate a greater degree of social support). See Table 2 for published information on reliability and validity for each instrument along with the alphas obtained in the current study.

Social Support. Social support can be conceptualized as the provision of intimacy, facilitation of social integration, opportunity for nurturant behavior, reassurance of self-worth, and the availability of assistance (Weiss, 1969), and it can buffer the negative effects of life events on health (Pollachek, 2001). Social support can positively influence psychosocial adjustment and management of the chronic illness (Symister & Friend, 2003) and inadequate support can increase depression and stress (Gray & Cason, 2002). Interventions designed to enhance social support can facilitate coping and problem solving (Spiegel, 1993) and encourage the reciprocal aspects of providing comfort and support to others, which is critical to many women's sense of worth and well-being. The Personal Resource Questionnaire (PRQ) was developed to measure situational support and perceived support (Brandt & Weinert, 1981) and has systematically and consistently undergone psychometric evaluation over the past 20 years resulting in the current 15-item version, the PRQ2000 (Weinert, 2003).

Self-Esteem. Self-esteem is the extent to which people value, approve, or like themselves (Baumeister, Campbell, Krueger, &

TABLE 2 Psychological Concepts, Indicators, Items, Reliability, Validity

Concepts	Indicators	No. of Items	Reported α	Study α	Validity
Self-efficacy	Self-Efficacy Scale (Sherer et al., 1982)	23	.71–.86	.88	Construct criterion
Self-esteem	Self-Esteem Scale (Rosenberg, 1965)	10	.77–.88	.87	Convergent discriminant
Empowerment	Diabetes Empowerment Scale (Anderson et al., 2000)	10	.91	.96	Concurrent
Social support	PRQ2000 (Weinert, 2003)	15	.87–.92	.90	Construct divergent
Stress	Perceived Stress Scale (Cohen et al., 1983)	14	.84–.86	.90	Convergent discriminant
Depression	CES-D (Devine & Orme, 1985)	20	.84–.90	.90	Convergent discriminant
Loneliness	UCLA Loneliness Scale (Rosenberg, 1965)	20	.94	.94	Convergent discriminant

Vohs, 2003). Self-esteem is considered an indicator, among others, of psychological well-being and can be thought of as one dimension of the potential to manage chronic illness. People who have a positive sense of self-worth, believe in their own control, and are optimistic about the future may be more likely to exhibit better health behaviors (Taylor, Kemeny, Reed, Bower, & Gruenewald, 2000). The Rosenberg Self-Esteem Scale (SES) was designed originally to measure global feelings of self-worth or self-acceptance for ease of administration, economy of time, and unidimensionality. The 10 items are a self-report of feelings about the self (Robinson, Shaver, & Wrightsman, 1991).

Empowerment. In its most general sense, empowerment refers to the ability of people to gain understanding and control over personal, social, economic, and political forces to take action to improve their life situations. Control over destiny emerges as a disease risk factor and a strategy for health promotion (Wallerstein, 2002); lack of control of destiny enhances susceptibility to illness. These

deficits can be overcome through the use of computer-based support systems that have been shown to be extremely valuable in helping participants understand their illness and as a result became a source of empowerment (Gustafson et al., 1993). For this study, the Diabetes Empowerment Scale (Anderson, Funnell, Fitzgerald, & Marrero, 2000) was modified with the permission of the author of the tool. The 10-item Setting and Achieving Goals subscale was used after changing the word "diabetes" in the stem to "chronic illness."

Self-Efficacy. Self-efficacy is the belief that by personal behavior one may be able to affect health or other futures and is an essential key to subsequent changes in health risk behavior (Fries, Koop, Sokolov, Beadle, & Wright, 1998). One hallmark of a successful information and support program is its power to develop individuals' skills and confidence in their ability to take responsibility for managing their healthcare and provide access to social support to foster self-efficacy (Gustafson et al., 1999). The Self-Efficacy

Scale (Sherer et al., 1982) was designed to measure generalized self-efficacy expectations dependent on past experiences and on tendencies to attribute success to skill as opposed to chance. The items were written to measure general self-efficacy expectancies in areas such as social skills or vocational competence (17 items) and social self-efficacy (6 items).

Stress. Chronic illness and stress are closely aligned. The diagnosis and treatment of a chronic illness affects an individual's physical, psychological, and social self, and it affects sense of stress and well-being (Pollachek, 2001). Developing the capacity to manage stress is often helpful in managing the additional problems of a chronic illness (Cagle, 2004). The Perceived Stress Scale (PSS; Cohen, Kamarck, & Mermelstein, 1983) measures the degree to which situations in one's life are perceived as stressful. The PSS is based on the argument that the causal event is the cognitively mediated response to the objective event, not the objective event itself.

Depression. Depression is very common among people who have chronic illness and can impair their ability to cope with their diseases and detract from their quality of life (Davis & Gershtein, 2003). Chronic physical conditions affect depression directly and indirectly by affecting domestic relationships, reducing occupational performance, imposing economic strains, and undermining personal resources (e.g., self-esteem and empowerment; Vilhjalmsson, 1998). The Center for Epidemiological Studies Depression Scale (CES-D) is a 20-item self-report measure of depressive symptomatology that was initially developed for use in epidemiology surveys of depression within the general population (Devine & Orme, 1985). The CES-D assesses the frequency and duration of cognitive, affective, behavioral, and somatic symptoms associated with depression in the preceding week. Positive affect is also assessed by the instrument.

Loneliness. Loneliness can be defined as a deficit in human intimacy and negative feelings about being alone (Hall & Havens, 1999). The significance of loneliness is that it often results in human suffering, whereas freedom from loneliness contributes to a feeling of well-being and a positive mental health outlook (Perlman, Gerson, & Spinner, 1977). For chronically ill rural women, the risk for loneliness is compounded by their geographic isolation. The UCLA Loneliness Scale (Version 3), a widely used measure of loneliness, was used in this study (Robinson et al., 1991). It is a Likert-type measure focusing on the quality of a respondent's relationships with others. Advantages of the scale are that the word "loneliness" does not appear in any of the items, which helps reduce response bias, and loneliness is conceptualized as a unidimensional affective state.

▪ Results

For the first aim, bivariate correlations were produced to examine the relationships among the psychosocial variables of interest from data collected at baseline. On Table 3, the correlations among self-efficacy, self-esteem, empowerment, social support, stress, depression, and loneliness are shown. All correlations were statistically significant ($p = .01$, two-tailed) and in the anticipated direction. For example, self-esteem is positively associated with social support ($r = .414$), empowerment ($r = .354$), and self-efficacy ($r = .566$). Alternatively, psychosocial outcomes such as stress, loneliness, and depression were negatively associated with positive outcomes such as self-esteem, social support, empowerment, and self-efficacy. The highest absolute correlations are found between loneliness and stress ($r = .716$), depression and stress ($r = .708$), depression and loneliness ($r = .701$), and social support and loneliness ($r = -.646$).

For the second aim, repeated-measures analysis of variance was conducted to evaluate the effects of the computerized intervention on changes in the seven psychosocial outcomes of interest. The models tested included the dependent variable of scale scores for the SES (self-esteem), the PRQ (social support), Chronic Illness Empowerment Scale (CIES;

TABLE 3 Correlations Among Psychosocial Measures

	Self-esteem	Social Support	Empowerment	Self-efficacy	Depression	Loneliness
Social support	.414					
Empowerment	.354	.488				
Self-efficacy	.566	.546	.564			
Depression	−.599	−.447	−.487	−.586		
Loneliness	−.686	−.646	−.390	−.549	.701	
Stress	−.600	−.413	−.380	−.454	.708	.716

Note. Correlation is significant at the .01 level (two-tailed).

empowerment), Self-Efficacy Scale (Sherer et al., 1982), CES-D (depression), University of California, Los Angeles (UCLA) Loneliness Scale (version 3), and PSS (stress) (Cohen et al.) scales, one within-subjects factor of time (i.e., baseline measurement to the 3-month measurement, at the conclusion of the computer intervention) and one between-subjects factor of membership in the intervention or control groups. The means and standard deviations for all scale scores found for both time periods are presented in Table 4.

TABLE 4 Baseline and 3-month Means for Psychosocial Measures (N = 100)

	Baseline Mean (*SD*)	3-Month Mean (*SD*)
Self-esteem		
Intervention	29.57 (5.83)	30.83 (5.17)
Control	31.82 (4.82)	31.21 (5.32)
Social support		
Intervention	79.05 (13.40)	83.46 (12.42)
Control	79.91 (14.86)	78.96 (17.15)
Empowerment		
Intervention	36.79 (7.15)	40.30 (4.83)
Control	35.73 (7.24)	36.14 (6.48)
Self-efficacy		
Intervention	110.33 (21.08)	111.26 (18.86)
Control	109.61 (17.32)	106.09 (19.82)
Depression		
Intervention	18.52 (11.64)	15.50 (11.90)
Control	18.13 (10.34)	16.91 (11.82)
Loneliness		
Intervention	45.73 (9.99)	43.15 (8.69)
Control	43.97 (10.53)	43.11 (10.94)
Stress		
Intervention	28.49 (7.51)	26.15 (7.83)
Control	28.46 (7.32)	27.28 (8.80)

TABLE 5 ANOVA Results for Effect of Intervention on Psychosocial Measures

	Sum of Squares	df	Mean Square	F	p
Self-esteem					
Time	5.15	1	5.15	0.733	.394
Time × Treatment	41.92	1	41.92	5.973	.016
Social support					
Time	142.38	1	142.38	1.855	.176
Time × Treatment	340.15	1	340.15	4.432	.038
Empowerment					
Time	187.10	1	187.10	9.699	.002
Time × Treatment	116.94	1	116.94	6.062	.016
Self-efficacy					
Time	81.43	1	81.43	0.90	.346
Time × Treatment	240.62	1	240.62	2.65	.107
Depression					
Time	215.54	1	215.54	5.00	.028
Time × Treatment	39.29	1	39.29	0.91	.342
Loneliness					
Time	141.94	1	141.94	6.51	.012
Time × Treatment	35.29	1	35.29	1.62	.206
Stress					
Time	144.931	1	144.93	8.44	.005
Time × Treatment	15.58	1	15.58	0.91	.343

After assurance that ANOVA assumptions were met (e.g., normality, homogeneity of variance), the results for the ANOVAs indicate that significant Time × Treatment interactions exist for self-esteem, $F(1,98) = 5.97$, $p = .016$, social support, $F(1,98) = 4.43$, $p = .038$, and empowerment, $F(1,98) = 6.06$, $p = .016$, thereby suggesting that the group's scores changed differently across time. An examination of the means and standard deviations in Table 4 shows that for all three psychosocial outcomes the intervention group improved across time; for example, social support increased from 79.05 at baseline to 83.46 at 3 months, whereas the control groups either improved very little or decreased. These results suggest that the intervention had an appreciable effect on self-esteem, social support, and empowerment within the sample.

The results for the other psychosocial outcomes of interest are less clear (see Table 5). ANOVA results for depression, loneliness, and stress show that significant main effects for time only are evident, suggesting that the groups together changed significantly across time, but did not differ statistically. For depression, $F(1,98) = 5.00$, $p = .028$, results of the ANOVA and descriptive statistics indicate that both groups became less depressed over time, although subjects in the treatment group showed a much greater change (i.e., treatment group declined by 3.02; control declined by 1.22). Likewise, both loneliness, $F(1,98) = 6.51$, $p = .012$, and stress, $F(1,98) = 8.44$, $p = .005$, yield main effects for time, but do not indicate statistical differences between groups despite greater improvements made among the participants of the intervention when examining descriptive statistics. These findings suggest that cautious optimism is warranted in conclusions that the computer intervention had effects on depression, loneliness, and stress.

■ Discussion

The purpose of this study was to examine the impact of a computer-delivered intervention on measures of psychosocial health (social support, self-esteem, empowerment, self-efficacy, depression, loneliness, and stress) in chronically ill rural women. Although statistically significant differences between intervention and control groups were found only for social support, self-esteem, and empowerment, all psychosocial indicators improved in the intervention group and declined or remained stable among controls.

SOCIAL SUPPORT

Although the nature and function of social support on various states of health is debated, agreement exists that social support and social networks have important causal influences on health (Finfgeld-Connett, 2005). As expected, the intervention had appreciable effects on social support because women in the intervention group were provided access to others with similar conditions and the means, via computers, to access an asynchronous support environment. Essentially, women created new social networks and provided and received support at will, without regard to time of day or distance between participants.

Self-esteem is thought to mediate the relationships between social support and variables such as depression that have been used to define psychological adjustment to chronic illness (Druley & Townsend, 1998). Although it is unknown whether manipulating self-esteem regulates the relationship between social support and psychological adjustment, or alternatively if persons with high or low self-esteem receive differential support or per-

ceive support differently, recent research supports the idea that social support operates through self-esteem and can influence both optimism and depression (Symister & Friend, 2003). Bivariate relationships from previous studies compare favorably with the findings here, providing further evidence about the connectedness of self-esteem, social support, and depression. Symister and Friend (2003) used a sample of 86 people with end-stage renal disease to study psychosocial response to chronic illness and found correlations of .47 ($p < .001$) between social support and self-esteem, $-.51$ ($p < .001$) between social support and depression, and $-.62$ ($p < .001$) between self-esteem and depression. Our findings for the relationships between social support and self-esteem, social support and depression, and self-esteem and depression were .41 ($p < .01$), $-.45$ ($p < .01$), and $-.60$ ($p < .01$), respectively. Our ability to demonstrate positive effects on self-esteem and social support suggests that Web-based interventions may be an effective tool to assist persons with adjusting to chronic illness.

Paterson (2001) noted that discussions about patient participation in healthcare decisions and self-care are based on a model of empowerment. Findings from the current study suggest that women participating in the intervention improved in their ratings of empowerment more significantly than women in the control group. Professional dominance may delegitimize knowledge and experience of people with chronic illness (Paterson, 2001) and understanding where power resides becomes central to the idea of empowerment (Wallerstein, 2002). In this study, we suggest that the mechanism for empowering women who participated in the intervention includes learning and practicing with a new set of skills that guide them in the use of the WWW to find information and subsequently evaluate that information for credibility and usefulness. As rural residents, many of these women relied solely on healthcare providers and informal networks for health information. By having access to the WWW and the experience provided through participation in the intervention (Hill & Weinert, 2004), the women had a new and valuable source of information with which to make self-care decisions or lessen the maldistribution of power between themselves and their health-care providers.

LIMITATIONS

Despite favorable initial findings from this ongoing study, several limitations are important to note. First, the total anticipated sample was not available for analysis and this decreased our statistical power and may have led to nonsignificant findings for changes in self-efficacy, depression, loneliness, and stress. Further analysis of these data will be necessary in the future as sample size increases and the program continues to evolve. Second, it is unknown whether effects resulting from the intervention will be sustained over time. The posttest measurements on which the analysis was based were performed immediately after participants concluded the intervention when anticipated effects were thought to be greatest. Because psychosocial adjustment to chronic illness is thought to be a dynamic process where individuals must respond to daily challenges, it will be important to examine effects over time to determine whether this intervention provides lasting benefits. Third, because this intervention was tested with rural chronically ill women who were predominantly white, generalization to urban dwellers, men, and communities of color is not possible. Fourth, statistically significant results presented here indicate apparently small differences between the groups on self-esteem and empowerment and moderate differences in social support. For individual psychosocial factors, caution is warranted in interpreting these findings as clinically significant. However, taken together, small changes in many of the psychosocial factors representing adaptation may have a compounding effect on the ability of women to adapt to their chronic illnesses. Future research should examine the effects of similar interventions among more heterogeneous populations.

STRENGTHS

Despite these limitations, this study has a number of strengths. Much of the previous research on adaptation to chronic illness generally uses homogenous samples where single illnesses are selected (Stuifbergen, Seraphine, Harrison, & Adachi, 2005; Symister & Friend, 2003). A particular strength of this study is that psychosocial benefits of participation in a Web-based intervention were tested among women with a variety of chronic illnesses. Thus, external validity is somewhat improved. Second, rural populations that have limited access to health information and resources were targeted. An efficient way to meet the needs of geographically isolated populations was demonstrated through the efficacy of this intervention.

As technology becomes increasingly available among rural populations, strategies for using computers and the WWW to improve health need to be developed and tested. The success of the WTW project in making a difference in women's psychosocial outcomes provides impetus to researchers and clinicians interested in harnessing technology to assist people in adapting to chronic illness.

Wade Hill, PhD, RN, is Assistant Professor; Clarann Weinert, SC, PhD, RN, FAAN, is Professor; and Shirley Cudney, MA, RN, GNP, is Retired Associate Professor, College of Nursing, Montana State University.

Accepted for publication August 7, 2005.
Funded by The NIH/National Institute of Nursing Research (1RO1NR07908-01), SC Ministry Foundation, Arthritis Foundation.
Correspondence: Wade Hill, PhD, RN, College of Nursing, Montana State University, MT 59717 (e-mail: whill@montana.edu).

REFERENCES

Anderson, R. M., Funnell, M. M., Fitzgerald, J. T., & Marrero, D. G. (2000). The Diabetes Empowerment Scale: A measure of psychosocial self-efficacy. *Diabetes Care, 23*(6), 739–743.

Baumeister, R. F., Campbell, J. D., Krueger, J. I., & Vohs, K. D. (2003). Does high self-esteem cause better performance, interpersonal success, happiness, or healthier lifestyles? *Psychological Science in the Public Interest, 4*(1), 1–44.

Brandt, P. A., & Weinert, C. (1981). The PRQ—A social support measure. *Nursing Research, 30*(5), 277–280.

Cagle, C. S. (2004). 3 themes described how self care management was learned and experienced by patients with chronic illness. *Evidence-Based Nursing, 7*(3), 94.

Chen, C. C. (2005). A framework for studying the nutritional health of community-dwelling elders. *Nursing Research, 54*(1), 13–21.

Cohen, S., Kamarck, T., & Mermclstein, R. (1983). A global measure of perceived stress. *Journal of Health and Social Behavior, 24*(4), 385–396.

Connell, C. M., Davis, W. K., Gallant, M. P., & Sharpe, P. A. (1994). Impact of social support, social cognitive variables, and perceived threat on depression among adults with diabetes. *Health Psychology, 13*(3), 263–273.

Cudney, S., Winters, C., Weinert, C., & Anderson, K. (2005). Social support in cyberspace: Lessons learned. *Rehabilitation Nursing, 30*(1), 25–29.

Cudney, S. A., & Weinert, C. (2000). Computer-based support groups. Nursing in cyberspace. *Computers in Nursing, 18*(1), 35–43.

Davis, J. M., & Gershtein, C. M. (2003). Screening for depression in patients with chronic illness: Why and how? *Disease Management & Health Outcomes, 11*(6), 375–378.

Devine, G., & Orme, C. (1985). Center for epidemiologic studies depression scale. In D. J. Keyser & R. C. Sweetland (Eds.), *Test critiques* (Vol. I, pp. 144–160).

Druley, J. A., & Townsend, A. L. (1998). Self-esteem as a mediator between spousal support and depressive symptoms: A comparison of healthy individuals and individuals coping with arthritis. *Health Psychology, 17*(3), 255–261.

Earll, L., Johnson, M., & Mitchell, E. (1993). Coping with motor neuron disease—An analysis using self-regulation theory. *Palliative Medicine, 7*(4 Suppl.), 21–30.

Emery, C. (2003). Women living with chronic illness experienced transition that involved stages of distress and a quest for ordinariness. *Evidence-Based Nursing, 6*(2), 63.

Finfgeld-Connett, D. (2005). Clarification of social support. *Journal of Nursing Scholarship, 37*(1), 4–9.

Fries, J. F. (1997). Reducing the need and demand for medical care: Implications for quality management and outcome improvement. *Quality Management in Health Care, 6*(1), 34–44.

Fries, J. F., Koop, C. E., Sokolov, J., Beadle, C. E., & Wright, D. (1998). Beyond health promotion: Reducing need and demand for medical care. *Health Affairs, 17*(2), 70–84.

Gallant, M. P. (2003). The influence of social support on chronic illness self-management: A review and directions for research. *Health Education & Behavior, 30*(2), 170–195.

Gray, J., & Cason, C. L. (2002). Mastery over stress among women with HIV/AIDS. *Journal of the Association of Nurses in AIDS Care, 13*(4), 43–51.

Gustafson, D., Wise, M., McTavish, F., Taylor, J. O., Wolberg, W., Stewart, J., et al. (1993). Development and pilot evaluation of a computer based support system for women with breast cancer. *Journal of Psychosocial Oncology, 11*(4), 69–93.

Gustafson, D. H., McTavish, F. M., Boberg, E., Owens, B. H., Sherbeck, C., Wise, M., et al. (1999). Empowering patients using computer based health support systems. *Quality in Health Care, 8*(1), 49–56.

Hall, M., & Havens, B. (1999). *The effects of social isolation and loneliness on the health of older women.* Winnipeg, Manitoba: Prairie Women's Health Center of Excellence.

Hegyvary, S. T. (2004). Clarifying social support. *Journal of Nursing Scholarship, 36*(4), 287.

Hill, W., & Weinert, C. (2004). An evaluation of an online intervention to provide social support and health education. *CIN: Computers, Informatics, Nursing, 22*(5), 282–288.

Hunter, S. M., & Hall, S. S. (1989). The effect of an educational support program on dyspnea and the emotional status of COPD clients. *Rehabilitation Nursing, 14*(4), 200–202.

Israel, B. A., Checkoway, B., Schulz, A., & Zimmerman, M. (1994). Health education and community empowerment: Conceptualizing and measuring perceptions of individual, organizational, and community control. *Health Education Quarterly, 21*(2), 149–170.

Lin, N., Simeone, R. S., Ensel, W. M., & Kuo, W. (1979). Social support, stressful life events, and illness: A model and an empirical test. *Journal of Health and Social Behavior, 20*(2), 108–119.

Paterson, B. (2001). Myth of empowerment in chronic illness. *Journal of Advanced Nursing, 34*(5), 574–581.

Paykel, E. S. (1994). Life events, social support and depression. *Acta Psychiatrica Scandinavica Supplementum, 377*, 50–58.

Perlman, D., Gerson, A., & Spinner, B. (1977). Loneliness among senior citizens: A report. *Essence, 6*, 3–17.

Pollachek, J. B. (2001). *The relationship of hardiness, social support, and health promoting behaviors to well-being in chronic illness.* Newark, NJ: Rutgers, The State University of New Jersey.

Pollock, S. E. (1986). Human responses to chronic illness: Physiologic and psychosocial adaptation. *Nursing Research, 35*(2), 90–95.

Pollock, S. E. (1993). Adaptation to chronic illness: A program of research for testing nursing theory. *Nursing Science Quarterly, 6*(2), 86–92.

Pollock, S. E., Christian, B. J., & Sands, D. (1990). Responses to chronic illness: Analysis of psychological and physiological adaptation. *Nursing Research, 39*(5), 300–304.

Robinson, J., Shaver, P., & Wrightsman, L. (1991). *Measures of personality and social psychological attitudes.* New York: Academic Press.

Rosenberg, M. (1965). *Society and the adolescent self image.* Princeton, NJ: University Press.

Roy, C., & Andrews, H. A. (1999). *The Roy Adaptation Model* (2nd ed.). Stamford, CT: Appleton & Lange.

Schaefer, K. M. (1995). Women living in paradox: Loss and discovery in chronic illness. *Holistic Nursing Practice, 9*(3), 63–74.

Sherer, M., Maddix, J., Mercandante, B., Prentice-Dunn, S., Jacobs, B., & Rogers, R. (1982). The Self-Efficacy Scale: Construction and validation. *Psychological Reports, 51,* 663–671.

Spiegel, D. (1993). Psychosocial intervention in cancer. *Journal of the National Cancer Institute, 85*(15), 1198–1205.

Stuifbergen, A. K., Seraphine, A., Harrison, T., & Adachi, E. (2005). An explanatory model of health promotion and quality of life for persons with post-polio syndrome. *Social Science and Medicine, 60*(2), 383–393.

Stuifbergen, A. K., Seraphine, A., & Roberts, G. (2000). An explanatory model of health promotion and quality of life in chronic disabling conditions. *Nursing Research, 49*(3), 122–129.

Sullivan, T., Weinert, C., & Cudney, S. (2003). Management of chronic illness: Voices of rural women. *Journal of Advanced Nursing, 44*(6), 566–574.

Symister, P., & Friend, R. (2003). The influence of social support and problematic support on optimism and depression in chronic illness: A prospective study evaluating self-esteem as a mediator. *Health Psychology, 22*(2), 123–129.

Taylor, S. E., Kemeny, M. E., Reed, G. M., Bower, J. E., & Gruenewald, T. L. (2000). Psychological resources, positive illusions, and health. *American Psychologist, 55*(1), 99–109.

Thomas, S. P. (1995). Psychosocial correlates of women's health in middle adulthood. *Issues in Mental Health Nursing, 16*(4), 285–314.

Vilhjalmsson, R. (1998). Direct and indirect effects of chronic physical conditions on depression: A preliminary investigation. *Social Science and Medicine, 47*(5), 603–611.

Wallerstein, N. (2002). Empowerment to reduce health disparities. *Scandinavian Journal of Public Health Supplement, 59,* 72–77.

Wallston, B. S., Alagna, S. W., DeVellis, B. M., & DeVellis, R. F. (1983). Social support and physical health. *Health Psychology, 2,* 367–391.

WebCT campus edition. (2005). Retrieved July 5, 2005, from http://www.webct.com/software/viewpage?name=software_campus_edition.

Weinert, C. (2000). Social support in cyberspace for women with chronic illness. *Rehabilitation Nursing, 25*(4), 129–135.

Weinert, C. (2003). Measuring social support: PRQ2000. In O. Strickland & C. Dilorio (Eds.), *Measurement of nursing outcomes: Self care and coping* (Vol. 3, pp. 161–172). New York: Springer.

Weinert, C., Cudney, S., & Winters, C. (2005). Social support in cyberspace: The next generation. *CIN: Computers, Informatics, Nursing, 23*(1), 7–15.

Weiss, R. (1969). The fund of sociability. *Transaction, 6,* 36–43.

Williams, M. H. (1990). The self-help movement in head injury. *Rehabilitation Nursing, 15*(6), 311–315.

Wortman, C. B., & Conway, T. L. (1985). The role of social support in adaptation and recovery from physical illness. In S. Cohen & S. L. Syme (Eds.), *Social support and health* (pp. 281–302). Orlando, FL: Academic Press.

Qualitative Health Research
Volume 17 Number 3
March 2007 300-310
© 2007 Sage Publications
10.1177/1049732306298631
http://qhr.sagepub.com
hosted at
http://online.sagepub.com

Young Women With Type 1 Diabetes' Management of Turning Points and Transitions

Bodil Rasmussen
Beverly O'Connell
Patricia Dunning
Helen Cox
Deakin University, Burwood, Victoria, Australia

The authors used grounded theory to explore and develop a substantive theory to explain how 20 young women with type 1 diabetes managed their lives when facing turning points and undergoing transitions. The women experienced a basic social problem: being in the grip of blood glucose levels (BGLs), which consisted of three categories: (a) the impact of being susceptible to fluctuating BGLs, (b) the responses of other people to the individual woman's diabetes, and (c) the impact of the individual women's diabetes on other people's lives. The women used a basic social process to overcome the basic social problem by creating stability, which involved using three interconnected subprocesses: forming meaningful relationships, enhancing attentiveness to blood glucose levels, and putting things in perspective. Insights into the processes and strategies used by the women have important implications for provision of care and service delivery.

Keywords: *type 1 diabetes; women; transitions; turning points; grounded theory.*

Diabetes is a significant chronic illness and a growing global public health problem. It represents a considerable personal and public burden (Commonwealth of Australia, 1999). In Australia, diabetes was nominated as the fifth National Health Priority in 1998. Diabetes affects more than 940,000 Australians over the age of 25 years, and it is estimated that there will be 1.23 million Australians with diabetes by the year 2010 (Dunstan et. al., 2001). Diabetes is the seventh leading cause of death in Australia and contributes significantly to morbidity, disability, poor quality of life, and loss of potential years of life (Australian Institute of Health and Welfare, 2004).

Individuals living with diabetes and their families and friends face many challenges. Researchers have argued that people with chronic illness handle their conditions in individual ways, often in isolation and with little information (Glasgow, Fisher, Anderson, & La Greca, 1999). Likewise, ill people adopt innovative ways of managing their lives, which are often unnoticed by health professionals and relatives and friends (Paterson, 2001; Paterson, Thorne, Crawford, & Tarko, 1999; Rayman & Ellison, 2000). Learning to help people with a chronic illness is challenging for health professionals as more people develop chronic illnesses (Glasgow, Hiss, Anderson, & Friedman, 2001).

Life transitional processes have been a research focus for some years; however, more clarity about the concept is needed (Anderson & Wolpert, 2004; Liddle, Carlson, & McKenna, 2003). Although the literature from different disciplines raises germane questions about life course perspectives, there is limited information linking people's experiences of chronic illness to their life trajectory, or to identify what signifies a turning point for individuals (Charmaz, 1991; Moen, 1997). A turning point is defined as an event that results in a fundamental shift in the meaning, purpose, or direction of a person's life and must include a self-reflective awareness of or insight into the significance of the change (Clausen, 1995). Turning points can sometimes be predictable, but are often unpredictable, uncontrollable, and linked to a specific context (Gotlib & Wheaton, 1997). They can

Authors' Note: This research was supported by a scholarship provided by Deakin University, Victoria, Australia. The research team thanks the participants for their time and willingness to share their experiences and Reality Check, a support group for young people with diabetes.

Reprinted with permission from *Qualitative Health Research* 2007; 17:300–310.

165

provoke transitions and change people's life courses in positive and negative directions. Transitions accommodate both the continuities and discontinuities in the life processes of humans and are invariably related to change and development (Chick & Meleis, 1986). Transitions have many characteristics, including how they are experienced, their developmental and growth value, and their function in linking people to their social context (Wheaton, 1990).

The current study was based on the findings from a pilot study that explored the experiences of young adults with type 1 diabetes when they accessed health services in Victoria, Australia (Rasmussen, Wellard, & Nankervis, 2001). In Rasmussen et al.'s study, the participants recounted that the transition from adolescence into young adulthood was difficult and complex. Female participants identified the transition into motherhood as being particularly difficult and stressful. They described lack of services to support decision making in family planning and perinatal care as well as the ongoing difficulties associated with being a parent with diabetes. However, there is a paucity of evidence to verify and describe the strategies young women with type 1 diabetes use to address issues related to transition into motherhood. The findings of the pilot study were the basis for focusing exclusively on women in the current study.

The aim of the current study was to develop a substantive theory of how women with type 1 diabetes managed turning points and transitions in their lives.

Design and Methods

Grounded theory was used to address the study objectives. This involves seeking social processes within a given phenomenon about which little is known (Charmaz, 1995).

Setting and Sample

The study was conducted in Victoria, Australia. Participants were women who volunteered for the study in response to an advertisement in Diabetes Australia newsletters and local diabetes support group Web sites. Ethics approval was obtained from Deakin University.

The initial sample comprised 20 women, age range 20 to 36 years, mean 28 years, who volunteered and consented to participate in the study. They had lived with diabetes for between 4 and 28 years, mean 17 years. Twelve women had no family history of type 1

diabetes. Five women had immediate family members with diabetes, and 3 had remote family members with diabetes. All of the women spoke English but came from Indian, Italian, and Greek backgrounds.

Sampling Procedure

Both purposeful and theoretical sampling procedures were used. Initially, as a part of the purposeful sampling procedure, women who had diabetes since childhood (between 5 and 11 years) were invited to participate. This age group was selected because they had more opportunities to experience transitions while living with diabetes. A total of 20 initial interviews were conducted.

Data analysis revealed a need for further theoretical sampling to assist with the development of the theory (Charmaz, 2000). Therefore, individual interviews were conducted with women who had experienced childbirth, relatives of young women with type 1 diabetes, and health professionals involved in managing diabetes of women with type 1 diabetes. Ten interviews were conducted in the theoretical sampling phase of the study.

Data Collection

The main source of data was formal interviews with 20 women; however, other sources were used such as informal interviews, relevant documents, newspapers, and nonverbal communication.

The interviews lasted between 30 and 140 minutes and were conducted over a period of 1½ years. These interviews were audiotaped. Immediately after each interview, the researcher recorded her observations and thoughts in a nonprioritized manner.

Data Analysis

The recorded interviews were transcribed verbatim by the first author, examined line by line, and coded using open coding techniques, which is the first stage of developing a theory (Glaser & Strauss, 1967). Theoretical coding was applied simultaneously and involved connecting the developing categories through open coding with emerging relationships between categories and their properties (Glaser, 1992). Constant comparative analysis was used throughout the study.

In the current study, the core category was the main problem experienced by the women and was identified as being in the grip of blood glucose levels (BGLs). The core category was identified as the basic social problem, because it accounted for the greatest variation in the data, was related to all of the other categories in the data, and accurately described the problem the women experienced during transitional periods. The basic social process the women used to overcome the basic social problem was labeled "creating stability".

Throughout the study, memos were written by the first author to guide her in identifying links between categories, compare and identify differences in the data, develop new questions, and test assumptions. O'Connell and Irurita (2000) described a visual data analysis procedure, which was used to schematize the linkages between categories and the developing theory.

Rigor and Credibility

It has been argued that grounded theory involves methodological procedures that promote rigor and credibility (Silverman, 2001). Constant comparative analysis presented the first author with opportunities to confirm or deny her interpretation of data. Applying theoretical sampling also provided a flexible mode to verify information from multiple sources. Credibility was enhanced in the study by lengthy contact with the women, which Lincoln and Guba (1985) referred to as prolonged engagement, and Charmaz (2000) described as "sustained involvement with research participants" (p. 519).

The substantive theory in the study was validated through peer review throughout the research process. For example, national and international conference presentations where abstracts were peer reviewed, and the findings were evaluated by clinical and academic colleagues. In addition, the women in the study checked the researcher's interpretation of the data. These strategies were all very important assuring credibility (Glaser & Strauss, 1967).

Findings

Core Problem: Being in the Grip of Blood Glucose Levels (BGLs)

The findings revealed that the women experienced a basic social problem, which emerged from the understandings and meanings the women made of their transitional experiences. Although the experiences were based on individual perceptions, and the individual woman managed and responded differently to these experiences, it was possible to explicate a story line

about a central phenomenon around which other categories were integrated with linked strategies. The basic social problem was identified and described as being in the grip of blood glucose levels (BGLs). Three subcategories emerged from the data as having the most impact on the women's experiences of turning points and transitions: (a) the impact of being susceptible to fluctuating BGLs, (b) the responses of other people to the woman's diabetes, and (c) the impact of the woman's diabetes on other people's lives.

Impact of Being Susceptible to Fluctuating BGLs

Fluctuating BGLs profoundly affected the women's daily activities, their emotional responses to diabetes, and their responses to other people in their social networks and health professionals. The women were aware of the potential impact of hypo- and hyperglycemia on their physical, psychological, and social health. The long-term impact of diabetes was the major concern for the women, who stated that the "forever" aspect made it very difficult for them to acknowledge and accept that they had diabetes. There was an important distinction between acknowledging having diabetes and accepting it. However, acknowledgment was the beginning of the journey of transition toward acceptance, which started at the time of diagnosis, which was a turning point. Some women acknowledged that diabetes was present, but integrating it into their self-perception and identity was a complex and often long process. The women developed many ways of coping with diabetes shortly after being diagnosed, but the transition to accepting diabetes as a part of their identity took years for some women.

The transition from perceiving themselves to be a "healthy person" to "a person with diabetes" was a major one with complex and long-term implications.

The fear of developing diabetes complications greatly affected their lives and made the women feel vulnerable, and intensified the grip of BGLs. The women described their fear of diabetes complications, in particular when circumstances in their lives changed and when they went through life transitions, such as leaving home or becoming a student, worker, partner, or mother.

Fearing complications. In general, the women did not discuss long-term complications, such as developing renal, cardiovascular, or other comorbidities. Their primary fears related to four areas: (a) having an acute episode of ketoacidosis, (b) having a hypoglycemic episode, (c) developing eye complications, (d) and having complications during pregnancy.

Of the four areas, hypoglycemic episodes, or fear of developing hypoglycemia, had the most significant impact on the women's daily lives, in particular when imbalances in their blood glucose levels required acute hospitalization. The experience of being unconscious and waking up in a hospital, sometimes in intensive units, was referred to as a "wake-up call" or turning point, because it made the women realize they had sole responsibility for their diabetes management. These experiences made some women reconsider their diabetes management; for other women, it was the beginning of a transition in their lives. The women found it was extremely difficult to balance their social needs with the demands of their diabetes regimens during transitions.

> I felt scared, because I normally have good control, but during the first year of University, I just wanted to have fun. I'm not saying it is right to live badly with that sort of behaviours, but I think that has to be factored in [when considering transition and diabetes].

Fluctuating BGLs and entering the workforce. The transition into the workforce raised other prominent issues for the women in terms of adjusting fluctuating BGLs. The women experienced difficulties trying to adjust their insulin requirements to accommodate their new lifestyles, as they were often unable to eat or inject when necessary because of unpredictable work schedules, not knowing how long a meeting would take, or not knowing when they would be able to take a break and eat.

> It was the first job interview I had ever gone for, and thank goodness, I came straight out and said that I had type 1[diabetes] and no, no that will not a problem. They wanted 9-to-9 shifts and I actually ended up having a hypo. I ended up passing out behind the counter and knocking my head on the glass counter.

The women acted differently in each work situation, but the decision whether to disclose their diabetes was difficult for all of the women. The underlying factor that influenced disclosure was fear of unpredictable hypoglycemia, which often triggered the decision to disclose diabetes to help them feel safe at work.

Fluctuating BGLs during pregnancy and in transition to motherhood. Planning and going through pregnancy made the grip of BGLs particularly tight. The

women had to be more vigilant in their diabetes management. They attempted to keep their BGLs within the recommended level, which was lower than their usual blood glucose level and increased the potential for hypoglycemia. The women were anxious about the impact diabetes could have on their and their babies' health. The women often felt their previous knowledge of and skills in managing diabetes were inadequate to cope with "hypos" during pregnancy.

The women who had experienced the transition into motherhood found it was particularly complex because of the impact of diabetes on their bodies and their lives in general. The women's fear of hypos increased dramatically because of the hormonal changes associated with pregnancy and lactation. Their fears became reality when they had hypos, some for the first time in their lives. Often these hypos occurred at unusual times, for example, overnight or when they least expected it. The women struggled to balance diabetes management, their own needs, and the needs of their babies. The feeling of being in the grip of BGLs was particularly tight during this transition.

Responses of Other People to the Individual Woman's Diabetes

The responses and reactions of other people to the woman's diabetes had a profound impact on their sense of being in control of their lives at the time of diagnosis, and had an ongoing and long-lasting effect on their lives. The responses and reactions from people in the women's social networks and health professionals affected how tightly or loosely the women felt the grip of BGLs. When the women felt the responses and reactions were negative, the grip was tight and exacerbated their sense of losing control of their diabetes and their lives in general.

Social network. The women were not able to control the negative or unexpected responses of other people to their diabetes, which made them feel emotionally vulnerable, especially in the context of family and school communities and when people exhibited misconceptions and lack of understanding diabetes, especially differences between type 1 and type 2 diabetes.

Lack of knowledge and understanding about diabetes was consistently displayed in the wider community, particularly when people confused type 1 and type 2 diabetes. The confusion between the two types of diabetes had a major impact on the women and caused frustration, anger, and feelings of not being understood or of being judged by other people.

They say diabetes and there are such misconceptions of the two types of diabetes. People often do not even realise that type 2 is a completely different thing or how you get type 1 or how you get type 2 and why you get it. It is very frustrating.

Health professionals. The women realized the importance of having a good relationship with health professionals, especially during transitional periods, and tried to maintain good relationships. One of the most prominent issues the women raised was that health professionals tended to focus on their BGLs rather than on their personal issues. This exacerbated the women's sense of being in the grip of BGLs, especially when blood glucose monitoring dominated their interactions with health professional, and sometimes made them reluctant to continue consulting health professionals.

> I don't see a dietitian or anyone like that anymore. It was just always pointless. They did not really seem to be that concerned about how I was. They just wanted to look at my HbA1c. They just wanted to see the test result. If I was in what was considered as good control [blood glucose result], which is under nine, then "Good, see you later."

The women felt they were being judged on the basis of their blood glucose results. Indeed, a "bad girl" or "good girl" dichotomy emerged from the data. As one woman said, "There is definitely a good-bad girl association, you know, if your blood glucoses are good you are good, and if your glucoses are bad, you are bad. There is kind of stigma attached to people [with diabetes]."

Health professionals' comments about and constant gaze on the BGLs became deeply embedded in the women's mind-set and contributed to their perception of themselves as being either a "bad" girl or "good" girl. There was a shift from being "seen" as a bad girl by others "to feeling" they "were" bad girls, which exacerbated feelings of guilt if the women did not comply with their diabetes regimen.

Impact of the Individual Woman's Diabetes on Other People's Lives

Diabetes affected other people's lives when the women went through transitions, because the changes occurring at these times also affected people in their social networks. The level of dependency had to be renegotiated with their social support people, in particular mothers, husbands, or partners. The women felt they were a burden to their families, which exacerbated the grip of BGLs. As one woman said, "I felt I was just being a burden to my husband and to my family and everybody else. That was really difficult for me to overcome."

Generally, the women perceived coping with diabetes was "a big ask" and identified a lack of support from health services for their partners. The women indicated their partners needed opportunities to share their experiences with other partners in similar situations. They said diabetes highlighted their dependence on their partners when they became mothers, and they found this dependency burdensome and frustrating.

The data analysis confirmed family members also felt they were in the grip of BGLs because of the impact diabetes had on their lives, and transitional times were particularly difficult for them too.

Creating Stability: A Basic Social Process

The consequences of being in the grip of BGLs were complex, and the women applied interrelated processes to overcome the grip of BGLs. Certain patterns could be discerned in the processes and were identified as the basic social and psychological process labeled Creating Stability, which involved three interconnected subprocesses that tended to occur simultaneously: forming meaningful relationships; enhancing attentiveness to blood glucose levels (BGLs); and putting things in perspective.

Forming meaningful relationships. All of the women described personal interactions and social support as important factors that influenced how they stabilized their lives with diabetes. They reassessed their personal relationships with people in their social networks during transitional periods to overcome their sense of isolation, low self-esteem, and uncertainty.

Achieving a sense of belonging was a major aspect of creating stability. Being with other people with diabetes enhanced the women's self-confidence and was a major factor in their ability to achieve a sense of belonging, especially when the group consisted of people of their own age. Some of the women explained how, when they were young, they met other children at diabetes camps, which they felt contributed to their having a sense of belonging.

> I participated in camps as a child, which was a great way of growing up with peers and knowing that I wasn't all alone, because today when I mix with diabetes support people, some people say, oh, look I

haven't known one other person with diabetes in my whole life.

One consistent source of frustration, and a dimension of being in the grip of BGLs, was other people's ignorance about diabetes. The women usually responded by "cutting them out" of their networks, for example, when people became "food" police: "I can say, 'Look, I can have it [chocolate cake], leave me alone'. I can do this, leave me alone, and I will cut them out. I tend to do it that way." By selectively drawing on supportive people, the women felt they had a higher degree of control, which enhanced stability in their lives.

The women needed to trust other people and sometimes to maintain anonymity to manage transitions well. Using Web sites and e-mails was a way of obtaining information anonymously and forming new, meaningful relationships when appropriate during transitions. The women's need for information constantly changed, and Web sites and e-mails were able to accommodate these changing needs quickly. The women indicated that sensitive issues, such as discriminatory behaviors in workplaces due to diabetes, stigma, contraception, and sexual issues, were easier to discuss anonymously.

Enhancing attentiveness to blood glucose levels. The women said they needed to feel prepared for unexpected events and situations by knowing how to manage their diabetes and recognize and respond to their body reactions quickly. For example, one woman said, "I guess relating it [uncertainty] to the diabetes thing, what do I know, do I need to take insulin with me, so I need to take it with me. Do I need to carry food?"

Learning to read body clues was generally the first measure the women took when taking control of their BGLs.

> You have got to know your own body and how different things affect it and how, you know, what to do to prevent the high sugar levels. Yes, vigilance, you got to, because some people when they exercise they go hypo, some people go high because of the adrenalin, you know.

The women experienced increased well-being when they had good blood glucose control. Improved well-being was important to their ongoing motivation and made them feel more assertive in getting what they needed to stay in control. One assertive action

was to apply up-to-date medical technology to their diabetes management, for example, by using insulin pumps. The pumps made the women's day-to-day lives easier, reduced their fear of fluctuating BGLs, and increased their sense of control. The women said that reaching a stage where they were in full control was very difficult. Nevertheless, they explained, they could achieve a sense of balance and tried to create stability by putting things in perspective.

Putting things in perspective. The main difficulties the women experienced during transitions were associated with the demands of their new social roles that were often imposed by changes and the demands of diabetes management. Putting things in perspective helped the women achieve balance in their lives.

> Just do not let things stress you out too much. Try to keep it in perspective and try to maintain balance. You might be having a real bad day with your diabetes, but you sort of learn to keep it in perspective. It is only a day and the next day will be a different day.

The women explained that putting things in perspective helped them accept life with diabetes. Accepting diabetes was a difficult journey for some women because it involved changing their self-perception, which became a part of the strategy of accepting diabetes and moving on. For example, one woman said, "That is the thing, it is when I decide and not when someone else, parents or friends or doctors, tell me to do something. It is when I decide for myself, that it is time for change."

The importance of having role models who managed diabetes very well, for example by not letting diabetes get in the way of their aspirations and goals in life, was a repeated theme raised by the women. The women said role models influenced how they perceived their opportunities and achievements, and helped them to put their difficulties into perspective.

> I guess, the other people who had a big impact were the diabetic leaders on the camps—I looked up to them. I think, camp leaders are real positive role models. It is good to look up to someone who says, "I turned out all right," and this person, who could be a doctor, a nurse or a scientist or recreation team leader, and then say, "I can do that as well."

The women regarded their transitions as evaluation processes that enabled them to reevaluate their lives, including their life aims, goals, priorities, and perspectives. Diabetes affected the women's quality of life in different ways. The basic social problem described how some women felt diabetes reduced their quality of life. However, this study clearly indicates that the women's perceived quality of life was strongly associated with their sense of being in control of diabetes. The higher the women's perception of control was, the higher they rated their quality of life. According to one woman, "The pump definitely increased my quality of life. I have not had complications, but psychologically the pump is what has truly affected and changed my life for the better." Viewing diabetes in a more positive light was clearly connected to hope of a cure and better treatment. The majority of the women placed great hope in stem cell and islet cell transplantations. One women moved interstate to be closer to " 'where things happen' in diabetes research."

> Melbourne is probably a good place to be when looking for cures and things. They are doing a lot of research and stem cell stuff. You feel, when you are in a country town and certainly when I was in [name of small town in NSW], I felt much, much further away from any talk about cures.

Hoping for a cure affected how the women created stability by applying other strategies to help them on a day-to-day basis, for example comparing diabetes to other illnesses and people they considered to be "worse off" than they, such as those with asthma, other chronic illnesses, or terminal illnesses. The women used the comparative strategy as a general coping mechanism that helped them put things in perspective and create stability.

Consequences of Being in the Grip of Blood Glucose Levels

There were many consequences of being in the grip of diabetes. The worst of these was when the women felt stuck or unable to adapt to changes associated with transitions. Despite the women's ability to identify opportunities to change their behavior, they still found it difficult. One woman said, "I could do things differently but for some reasons I just feel stuck."

Feeling stuck or unable to adapt to transitional changes was not always the outcome of being in the grip of BGLs. In general, the women said that they experienced different levels of control, which affected their emotions, their lives, their and health. When the women felt they had little control, they also felt a high level of vulnerability, uncertainty, and guilt.

The women explained that transitions caused instability in their lives. The women's sense of being unstable deeply affected other people in their social networks. Family members also experienced high levels of guilt, uncertainty, and the grip of BGLs. They could not escape diabetes either and also focused on the women's BGLs, particularly strongly during transitions.

The women explained that being in the grip of BGLs was reduced when they felt supported by people in their social networks. Turning points and transitions made the women appreciate and make better use of the resources and support around them. When social support was perceived to be good, the women experienced growing confidence and self-worth, which helped them to develop new skills and knowledge.

Discussion

In this study, transition represented a passage from one life phase to another, which embraced the elements of a process that consisted of change, perception, passage of time, and outcomes of transitions. The women referred to turning points, such as losing a job or getting divorced, as life events that caused instability in their lives. Some of the women's definitions concur in the literature, which describe life events in terms of crises (Erikson, 1968). Specifically related to women with chronic illnesses, some researchers have described transitions as processes or movements that occur in a non-linear, cyclical way and potentially recur throughout the course of life (Ellison & Rayman, 1998; Kralik, 2002; Rayman & Ellison, 2004). The women in the current study also identified transition (e.g., becoming an adult or a mother) from a life course perspective.

The substantive theory provides unique insight into how the ever-present grip of BGLs made the management of turning points and transitions a complex social and psychological process in which the women constantly tried to stabilize their lives. The metaphor of being in the grip of BGLs illustrates the physical, psychological, and social impact of type 1 diabetes on young women. As a consequence of experiencing transitions, the women felt their lives were unbalanced, which made them feel vulnerable. Other researchers have established that people with diabetes have a high sense of vulnerability (Weiss & Hutchinson, 2000), particularly during life course transitions (Seiffge-Krenke, 2001). In the current study, "stability" during transitions meant taking control and maintaining stable

BGLs in changing social and psychological environments. However, to achieve stability, it was necessary for the women to enhance attention to BGLs, because stable BGLs allow them to feel more positive about their diabetes management. Paterson (2001) referred to this situation as one of the paradoxes in diabetes management, because "illnesses require attention in order not to have to pay attention to it" (p. 24) and fostering a shift in people's perception of a threat to control. The individual's perception of reality, not the reality itself, is the essence of how people respond (Paterson, 2001). As the personal and social context changes, people's perspectives shift in the degree to which illness is in the foreground or background of their reality. It is an ongoing, continuously shifting process in which people experience a complex dialectic between themselves and their world that contains elements of both illness and wellness. People's experience is depicted as an ever-changing perspective about illness that enables them to make sense of their experiences (Paterson, 2003).

During transitions, women with type 1 diabetes felt there was a constant gaze on their BGLs, which they found oppressive. It both helped and hindered successful transitions. The constant gaze was hindering when the women felt people's attention to their BGLs was judgmental, disrespectful, and ignorant. In contrast, when the women felt valued and involved in decisions about their care and treatment, they felt encouraged to disclose their concerns. The findings challenge health professionals to review their attitudes toward patients. Health professionals can help by paying attending to attributes of expertise in everyday diabetes management (Paterson & Thorne, 2000a; Thorne, Nyhlin, & Paterson, 2000), in particular, how people negotiate their assessment of risks, make comparative analysis of their previous experiences, seek explanations for changing in their BGLs, make choice of actions, and evaluate their decisions (Paterson & Thorne, 2000b).

The women found that disclosing their diabetes was particularly difficult in their work environment. They feared stigmatization and discrimination if they disclosed. If they did not disclose, on the other hand, they feared they would be blamed for "telling a lie" should their diabetes become apparent. They felt more at risk by nondisclosure, because their colleagues might not be able to assist them should they need it: for example, if they developed a "hypo."

The decision to disclose diabetes was a major source of internal conflict, which sometimes took years for people with diabetes to resolve (Hernandez, 1996).

Charmaz (1991) noted that individuals with chronic illness attempt to control stigma by being highly selective about the individuals to whom they reveal their condition and rely on them to withhold the information from others. These measures also emerged in the current study. In some circumstances, disclosure increased support from selected individuals or groups (Charmaz, 1991; Joachim & Acorn, 2000). However, trying to pass as "normal" caused stress, because the individual worried about being found out as "calculated cheating" or "caught in a lie" (Thorne, Paterson, & Russell, 2003, p. 1345). There is a risk of being rejected and stigmatized, of having difficulty handling the responses of others, and of losing control (Charmaz, 1991). The current study further highlighted the importance of maintaining autonomy and staying anonymous about diabetes until the women chose to disclose it.

The concept of autonomy has been widely explored and is an important aspect of coping with diabetes. However, the association between autonomy and anonymity in the process of how young people with type 1 diabetes establish their networks has not been extensively explored, and neither has young people's perceptions of the impact of the responses of health professionals. Health professionals need to consider the triad between autonomy, anonymity, and how their actions and responses affect young people with diabetes.

Forming meaningful relationships with people in their social networks, including health professionals, was essential to the women's management of transitions. Certain qualities were vital to forming meaningful relationships, especially with health professionals. The women sought health professionals who showed respect, empathy, recognition, autonomy, and, an important point, nonjudgmental attitudes. The study demonstrates that when the women felt supported and engaged in meaningful relationships, they were capable of and resourceful in managing diabetes during transitions. The values of honesty, trust, and openness were an integral part of useful communication with health professionals. When the women perceived health professional's attitudes to be judgmental, lacking in genuine concern for their well-being, and focused only on the BGLs rather than on the women's concerns, they chose not to listen to their health professional's advice or consult them again.

The current study indicates that health professionals need a higher degree of awareness of the impact their attitudes have on young adults with diabetes. Health professionals must be sensitive to the powerful influences their values and attitudes have on the self-management decisions their patients make (Thorne, Nyhlin, et al., 2000). The current study also illuminated that during transitions, young women feel it is important to involve family members in management, particularly during pregnancy and early motherhood, when the women felt torn in two directions between their babies' needs and the requirement of their diabetes regimens. Managing motherhood and diabetes is a balancing act (Poirier-Solomon, 2002) and increased the women's dependence on their partners and mothers.

It was critical to the management of transitions that simultaneous to forming meaningful relationships, the women had to take control of their fluctuating BGLs. Unpredictable experiences, such as hypo- or hyperglycemia, called forth unknown and unused resources essential for generating positive ways of responding and adapting to new situations (Antonovsky, 1987). Responding to new situations in positive ways depends on the resources under direct individual control and the resources accessible from family, friends, or the community (Rayman & Ellison, 2004; Schlossberg, Waters, & Goodman, 1995). Manageability largely depends on people's experiencing a practical and physical sense of self-empowerment in coping with their biology and threats to their health (Sanden-Eriksson, 2000). Manageability and self-empowerment also emerged in the current study, evidenced by the women's enhanced attentiveness to body clues and controlling their BGLs by using medical technology, such as modern blood glucose meters and insulin pumps.

In Ellison and Rayman's (1998) study among women with type 2 diabetes, engagement and ability to adjust diabetes management helped the participants to move on in the process where the diabetes was just a part of the life, not the whole life. Furthermore, the ability to reframe problems with a positive perspective required transformation (Paterson, 2001) and integration (Hernandez, 1996) of oneself in relation to diabetes management.

In this study, the women tried to remain positive and indicated that "things could have been worse." Comparative strategies helped the women put things in perspective and sustain or gain stability in their lives after turning points and during transitions. Comparing their situation with others was part of the normalization process the women used to help them to accept diabetes and move on. Making comparisons is a way of positioning oneself in terms of time, space, and relationship

to others, and helps the individual adjust to his or her chronic illness (Dewar & Lee, 2000; Meleis, Sawyer, Im, Messias, & Schumacher, 2000). To feel integrated into the world again and included, and to reduce feelings of isolation, individuals must learn to live with new limits and find new ways to accommodate the transitional changes. In addition, the women in the current study indicated that positive role models gave them hope and were integral to the adjustment process.

Practice Implications and Further Research

The substantive theory developed in this study has the potential to be used in future studies considering life transitions and decision-making situations that chronically ill people encounter, including people with asthma and epilepsy.

There is a need to explore further how health professionals can evaluate their communication strategies and be flexible in their communication with young people with type 1 diabetes. A shared decision making and understanding of attributes of expertise in everyday diabetes management process that develops an equal, respectful, and productive relationship between health professionals and women with diabetes needs to be adopted. Particular attention needs to be paid to the good girl–bad girl association. The study indicates that diabetes camps helped the women and their families cope with diabetes, and so health professionals need to support and encourage families to attend diabetes camps.

Health professionals and health policy makers need to take up the challenge to put more emphasis on the social and psychological issues associated with disclosing diabetes, especially in the context of stigma and discrimination in workplaces. The differences between type 1 and type 2 diabetes, and the impact the lack of understanding about the differences can have on young women with type 1 diabetes and their families, is also important and worth exploring in more depth. It is particularly important to support current and potential employers of young people with diabetes to enhance employers' understanding of diabetes and reduce discrimination in workplaces.

It is necessary to involve individuals with diabetes, and people in their social networks, in health service planning and resource allocation so their experiences and specific needs can be utilized to benefit young women with diabetes and to guide health professionals.

References

Anderson, B. J., & Wolpert, H. A. (2004) A developmental perspective on the challenge of diabetes education and care during the young adult period. *Patient Education and Counseling, 53*, 347-352.

Antonovsky, A. (1987). *Unraveling the mystery of health: How people manage to stay well*. San Francisco: Jossey-Bass.

Australian Institute of Health and Welfare. (2004). *Australia's health 2004*. Canberra, Australia: Author.

Charmaz, K. (1991). *Good days, bad days: The self in chronic illness and time*. New Brunswick, NJ: Rutgers University Press.

Charmaz, K. (1995). Grounded theory. In J. A. Smith, R. Harré, & L. Van Langenhove (Eds.), *Rethinking methods in psychology* (pp. 27-49). London: Sage.

Charmaz, K. (2000). Grounded theory: Objectivist and constructivist methods. In N. K. Denzin & Y. Lincoln (Eds.), *Handbook in qualitative research* (2nd ed., pp. 509-535). Thousand Oaks, CA: Sage.

Chick, N., & Meleis, A. I. (1986). Transitions: A nursing concern. In P. Chinn (Ed.), *Nursing research methodology: Issues and implementation* (pp. 237-257). Rockville, MD: Aspen.

Clausen, J. A. (1995). Gender, contexts, and turning points in adults' lives. In P. Moen, G. H. Elder, & K. Luscher (Eds.), *Examining lives in context: Perspectives on the ecology of human development* (pp. 365-389). Washington, DC: American Psychological Association.

Commonwealth of Australia. (1999). *National diabetes strategy 2000-2004* (Australian Health Ministers' Conference). Canberra, Australia: Commonwealth Department of Health and Aged Care.

Dewar, A., & Lee, E. A. (2000). Bearing illness and injury. *Western Journal of Nursing Research, 22*(8), 912-926.

Dunstan, D., Zimmet, P., Welborn, T., Sieree, R., Armstrong, T., Atkins. R., et al. (2001). *Diabesity and associated disorders in Australia—2000: The accelerating epidemic*. Melbourne, Australia: International Diabetes Institute.

Lincoln, Y., & Guba, E. G. (1985). *Naturalistic inquiry*. Beverly Hills, CA: Sage.

Ellison, G., & Rayman, K. M. (1998). Exemplars' experiences of self-managing type 2 diabetes. *Diabetes Educator, 24*, 325-330.

Erikson, E. (1968). *Identity: Youth and crisis*. New York: W. W. Norton.

Glaser, B. G. (1992). *Basics of grounded theory analysis*. Mill Valley, CA: Sociology Press.

Glaser, B. G., & Strauss, A. (1967). *The discovery of grounded theory*. Chicago: Aldine.

Glasgow, R. E., Fisher, E. B., Anderson, B. J., & La Greca, A. M. (1999). Behavioral science in diabetes: Contributions and opportunities. *Diabetes Care, 22*(5), 832-843.

Glasgow, R. E., Hiss, R. G., Anderson, R., & Friedman, N. M. (2001). Report of the health care delivery work group: Behavioral research related to the establishment of a chronic disease model for diabetes care. *Diabetes Care, 24*(1), 124-129.

Gotlib, I. H., & Wheaton, B. (1997). *Stress and adversity over the life course: Trajectories and turning points*. Cambridge, UK: Cambridge University Press.

Hernandez, C. A. (1996). Integration: The experience of living with insulin-dependent diabetes. *Canadian Journal of Nursing Research, 28*, 37-56.

Joachim, G., & Acorn, S. (2000). Living with chronic illness: The interface of stigma and normalization. *Canadian Journal of Nursing Research, 32*(3), 37-48.

Kralik, D. (2002). The quest for ordinariness: Transition experienced by midlife women living with chronic illness. *Journal of Advanced Nursing, 39*, 146-154.

Liddle, J., Carlson, G., & McKenna, K. (2004). Using a matrix in life transition research. *Qualitative Health Research, 14*, 1396-1417.

Meleis, A. I., Sawyer, L. M., Im, E., Messias, D. K., & Schumacher, K. (2000). Experiencing transitions: An emerging middle-range theory. *Advanced Nursing Science, 23*(1), 12-28.

Moen, P. (1997). Women's role and resilience: Trajectories of advantage and turning points? In I. H. Gotlib & B. Wheaton (Eds.), *Stress and adversity over the life course: Trajectories and turning points* (pp. 133-158). Cambridge, UK: Cambridge University Press.

O'Connell, B. O., & Irurita, V. (2000). Facilitating the process of theory development by creating visual data analysis trail. *Graduate Research in Nursing On-line Journals, 2*(1). Retrieved 23 October, 2003, from http://www.graduatereserach.com

Paterson, B. L. (2001). The shifting perspectives model of chronic illness. *Journal of Nursing Scholarship, 3*(1), 21-26.

Paterson, B. (2003). The koala has claws: Applications of the shifting perspectives model in research of chronic illness. *Qualitative Health Research, 13*, 987-994.

Paterson, B. L., & Thorne, S. E. (2000a). Developmental evolution of expertise in diabetes self-management. *Clinical Nursing Research, 4*, 402-419.

Paterson, B. L., & Thorne, S. E. (2000b) Expert decision making in relation to unanticipated blood glucose levels. *Research in Nursing & Health, 23*(2), 47-57.

Paterson, B. L., Thorne, S. E., Crawford, J., & Tarko, M. (1999). Living with diabetes as a transformational experience. *Qualitative Health Research, 9*, 786-803.

Poirier-Solomon, L. (2002). A balancing act: Managing motherhood and diabetes (women's health exchange). *Diabetes Forecast, 55*(11), 46-49.

Rasmussen, B., Wellard, S., & Nankervis, A. (2001). Consumer issues in navigating health care services for type 1 diabetes. *Journal of Clinical Nursing, 10*, 628-634.

Rayman, K. M., & Ellison, G. C. (2000). The patient perspective as an integral part of diabetes disease management. *Disease Management Health Outcomes, 1*, 5-12.

Rayman, K. M., & Ellison, G. C. (2004). Home alone: The experience of women with type 2 diabetes who are new to intensive control. *Health Care for Women International, 25*, 900-915.

Sanden-Erikson, B. (2000). Coping with type-2 diabetes: The role of sense of coherence compared with active management. *Journal of Advanced Nursing, 31*(6), 1393-1397.

Schlossberg, N. K., Waters, E. B., & Goodman, J. (1995). *Counseling adults in transition: Linking practice with theory* (2nd ed.). New York: Springer.

Seiffge-Krenke, I. (2001). *Diabetic adolescents and their families: Stress, coping, and adaptation*. Cambridge, UK: Cambridge University Press.

Silverman, D. (2001). *Interpreting qualitative data: Methods for analysing talk, text and interaction* (2nd ed.). London: Sage.

Thorne, S. E., Nyhlin, K. T., & Paterson, B. L. (2000). Attitudes towards patient expertise in chronic illness. *International Journal of Nursing Studies, 37*(4), 303-311.

Thorne, S. E., Paterson, B., & Russell, C. (2003). The structure of everyday self-care decision making in chronic illness. *Qualitative Health Research, 13*(10), 1337-1352.

Weiss, J., & Hutchinson, S. A. (2000). Warnings about vulnerability in clients with diabetes and hypertension. *Qualitative Health Research, 10*, 521-537.

Wheaton, B. (1990). Life transitions, role histories, and mental health. *American Sociological Review, 55*, 209-223.

Bodil Rasmussen, PhD., is a lecturer at Deakin University, School of Nursing, Melbourne Campus, Burwood, Victoria, Australia.

Beverly O'Connell, PhD, is a professor at Southern Health and Deakin University, Melbourne, Victoria, Australia.

Patricia Dunning, PhD, is a professor at Deakin University, Melbourne, Victoria, Australia.

Helen Cox, PhD, is an emeritus professor at Deakin University, Melbourne, Victoria, Australia.

APPENDIX C

Coping and Depressive Symptoms in Adults Living With Heart Failure

Michael W. Vollman, PhD, RN; Lynda L. LaMontagne, DNSc, RN; Joseph T. Hepworth, PhD

Background and Research Objective: This study used process coping theory as the basis for investigating how coping strategies are associated with depressive symptoms in individuals living with heart failure (HF). Demographic factors also were examined as correlates of depressive symptoms. **Subjects and Methods:** The convenience sample of adults living with HF (n = 75) who participated in this study ranged in age from 27 to 82 years (*M* = 55). Sixty-nine percent of the participants were men, 59% were married or partnered, with the majority being Caucasian and from the middle class. Subjects were recruited from a comprehensive HF program located within an academic health science center in the southeastern United States. A single wave of data collection occurred. All study questionnaires were verbally administered in a clinic room selected for privacy during a routine HF clinic visit. **Results and Conclusion:** Individuals who used more planful problem-solving and social support seeking coping strategies had fewer depressive symptoms, whereas individuals who used more escape-avoidance coping (eg, wishful thinking) had more depressive symptoms. When demographic factors also were included in a regression analysis assessing depressive symptoms, marital status, functional impairment, and the coping strategies of planful problem-solving and escape-avoidance were all statistically significant predictors of depression. Single individuals, those who used more escape-avoidance, less planful problem-solving coping, and more functional impairment had more depressive symptoms. These results suggest that psychosocial factors, in addition to physical parameters, and the ways individuals cope with the stressors of living with heart failure may be important predictors of depressive symptoms.

KEY WORDS: coping, depression, heart failure

D epression is an independent risk factor of poor clinical outcomes in individuals living with heart failure (HF).[1-5] Prior research has demonstrated that perceptions of functional capacity, social interaction, and personal well-being influence the incidence and/or severity of depressive symptoms in individuals living with HF.[6-9] Depression negatively impacts general cardiac outcomes such as rehospitalization, nonadherence to therapeutic regimens, morbidity, and mortality.[10-14] In an attempt to increase our understanding of the role of depression in this population, HF researchers are beginning to expand their investigations beyond evaluating physical indi-

cators of HF alone to include factors such as the ways individuals psychologically cope with the demands of their illness.

Lazarus and Folkman's Process Theory of Coping[15] provided the theoretical underpinning for this study. The coping process perspective has 3 main features. First, the process approach is concerned with the way an individual appraises, or evaluates a specific stressor in terms of its impact on his or her well-being and the resources available to cope with the event. Second, an individual's evaluation of a specific stressor requires actions in response to the unique demands of the situation. Third, coping is presumed to be an unfolding process in which an individual's entire repertoire of emotion-focused coping and problem-focused coping strategies may be used to cope with the unique stressful demands of the situation. When viewed in this manner, the unfolding process of specific coping strategies are likely to vary, not only from one stressful situation to another but also as a function of an individual's changing appraisals (evaluations) of a specific stressful encounter.

Emotion-focused functions of coping consist of behaviors that are directed toward lessening emotional

Michael W. Vollman, PhD, RN
Assistant Professor, Vanderbilt University School of Nursing, Nashville, Tenn.

Lynda L. LaMontagne, DNSc, RN
Professor, Vanderbilt University School of Nursing, Nashville, Tenn.

Joseph T. Hepworth, PhD
Research Specialist, Principal, University of Arizona College of Nursing, Tucson, Ariz.

Corresponding author
Michael W. Vollman, PhD, RN, Vanderbilt University School of Nursing, 418 Godchaux Hall, Nashville, TN 37240 (e-mail: michael.vollman@vanderbilt.edu).

176

distress and include strategies such as escape-avoidance (eg, wishful thinking), distancing (eg, minimizing the significance of the event), positive reappraisals, and trying to keep negative feelings to self.[15] Emotion-focused functions of coping often rely on positive reappraisals (eg, reframing a situation in a more positive way) to reduce stress. For example, an individual living with HF may focus on the positive aspects of the situation such as being able to manage activities of daily living while minimizing the negative physical symptoms associated with the disease. According to Billings and Moos,[16] emotion-focused functions of coping also may help an individual maintain hope and optimism because minimizing the implications of reality (eg, functional impairment, insult to well-being) may effectively reduce distress in the short term.

However, the continued use of emotion-focused coping strategies may actually impede an individual's ability to use more active coping strategies,[15] such as solving problems of daily living and openly expressing negative feelings. Thus, minimizing the implications of the reality of living with HF may not effectively reduce distress over time. In contrast, problem-focused coping strategies consist of behaviors that focus on changing the self (eg, dietary change, adherence to therapeutic regimens), something in the environment (eg, simplifying home environment to minimize fatigue and shortness of breath), or both.[15,16] Strategies such as seeking social support, planful problem-solving, and actively confronting the event are behaviors that may have a beneficial impact on clinical outcomes over time. Individuals who used more emotion-focused coping strategies such as minimizing the significance of the stressor, denial, and wishful thinking (eg, hoping a miracle will happen) to mitigate their emotional distress were found in previous research to have more depressive symptoms.[17] According to Cohen and Lazarus,[18] both emotion-focused and problem-focused coping functions can occur simultaneously to either facilitate or impede the coping process.

Thus, the type of coping strategies individuals use to cope with daily stressors associated with their disease, such as depression, impaired physical function, and fatigue common in individuals living with HF, may be critically important to their clinical outcomes. Very little is known about how the coping processes described by Coyne, Aldwin, and Lazarus reflect the experience and response of patients living with HF. This study will address this deficiency.

Purpose

The purpose of this study was to investigate coping strategies and depressive symptoms in individuals living with HF. The research question addressed in this study was: What are the relationships between coping and depressive symptoms in individuals living with HF? Demographic factors, such as functional impairment and marital status, were also examined as potential correlates of depressive symptoms.

Methods

Research Design

A descriptive-correlational, cross-sectional design was used to examine the relationships among coping, depressive symptoms, and demographic factors in a convenience sample of adults living with HF. The sample size (n = 75) required for the planned analyses was determined based on a power analysis specifying a moderate effect size ($r = 0.30$) for the proposed relationships among study variables, a power of 0.75, and a two-tailed alpha level of .05.

Subjects

To be eligible for this study, participants met the following criteria: (*a*) ability to speak and understand English, (*b*) 21 years or older, (*c*) diagnosed with HF, (*d*) no recent evidence of acute cardiac decompensation, (*e*) no evidence of clinically significant psychopathology other than depression, (*f*) ability to complete study instruments, and (*g*) have access to a telephone.

Instruments

Beck Depression Inventory

Depression was measured using the Beck Depression Inventory II (BDI-II).[19] The BDI-II is a widely validated and reliable instrument used to measure the presence and intensity of depressive symptoms in study participants.

The BDI-II contains 21 items that are concerned with a particular aspect of the experience and symptoms of depression around 3 factors: negative attitude toward self, performance impairment, and somatic disturbance. Each item is rated on a 4-point intensity scale. A rating of 3 indicates the most severe symptoms, and zero indicates an absence of a problem in that area. Because the BDI-II requires a severity rating for each symptom, a more complete profile of the individual's depressive mood is obtained with this instrument than with other measures of depression.[19]

The psychometric properties of the BDI-II are widely reported. In nonpsychiatric samples, internal consistency scores (alpha) ranged from 0.73 to 0.95, and test-retest correlations range from 0.60 to 0.90.[19] In this study, instrument reliability of the

BDI-II was excellent with a Cronbach alpha coefficient of .86.

Ways of Coping Questionnaire

Individual coping was measured using the Ways of Coping Questionnaire—Research Edition (WCQ).[20] After self-identifying a predominant, stressful encounter during the preceding 7 days, each study participant completed the WCQ with the investigator.

The WCQ consists of 66 items with 8 subscales that represent generalized coping functions, namely, the use of problem-focused coping or emotion-focused coping. The problem-focused subscales include seeking social support, planful problem-solving, and confrontive coping. The emotion-focused subscales include positive reappraisal, self-controlling, distancing, escape-avoidance, and accepting responsibility. Examples of behaviors of each of these coping strategies are identified in Table 1. The psychometric properties of the instrument suggested a satisfactory degree of internal consistency for the 8 subscales of the WCQ, with alphas ranging from .61 to .79.[20] In this study, internal consistency was good with Cronbach alphas ranging from .55 to .93 across the 8 subscales.

Scoring the WCQ can produce both raw and relative scores for each of the 8 subscales.[20] Relative scores described the contribution of each coping scale relative to all of the subscales combined. Raw scores represent the sum of each individual's responses to the items that comprise a given subscale. The raw score provides a summary of the extent to which each type of coping is used in a particular encounter and, as such, describes coping effort for each of the 8 subscales. Because the type of coping strategies used by the participants in this study was of interest, the raw scoring method was used.

TABLE 1	**Ways of Coping Questionnaire**
Scales	**Examples**
Problem-focused	
Seeking social support	Efforts to seek tangible and emotional support
Planful problem-solving	Analytic approach to solving or managing problems
Confrontive	Expressing emotions such a hostility and anger
Emotion-focused	
Positive reappraisal	Focusing on the positive, personal growth, or religious faith
Self-controlling	Trying to keep feelings to self
Escape-avoidance	Wishful thinking (eg, hoping a miracle would happen)
Accepting responsibility	Acknowledging one's own role in the situation
Distancing	Minimizing significance of event

Adapted and reproduced by special permission of Lynda L. LaMontagne, DNSc, RN.

Demographic Information

Demographic information included level of functional impairment (New York Heart Association [NYHA] classification), age, gender, illness duration (months since original HF diagnosis), marital status, ethnicity, diagnosis of depression, antidepressant medication use, and socioeconomic status (Hollingshead Four-Factor Index of Social Status; A. S. Hollingshead, unpublished manuscript, 1975).

Procedure

Approval for conducting the study was obtained from the Institutional Review Board. Individuals referred to the heart institute with a diagnosis of HF who met study criteria were asked about study participation by a physician or nurse practitioner during a routine clinic visit. Seventy-seven individuals who met inclusion criteria were then approached by the PI about study participation, of whom 75 agreed to participate. Two individuals declined to participate because of other illnesses unrelated to their cardiac disease. Once an individual agreed to participate in the study, informed consent was obtained by the PI. A single wave of data collection occurred. All study questionnaires were verbally administered by the PI in a clinic room selected for privacy. Breaks also were offered to study participants every 10 minutes to avoid potential consequences of HF, such as fatigue and shortness of breath. Administration of the WCQ took approximately 30 minutes, whereas the administration of the BDI and demographic questionnaires took approximately 10 minutes each. Data from participant questionnaires and demographic information were identified using an anonymous descriptor, and maintained in the PI's office in a locked file cabinet. All study participant questionnaires and demographic information were destroyed after completion of the study.

Data Analysis

Study data were analyzed using the Statistical Package for Social Sciences (SPSS, Version 13.0). Pearson product-moment correlational analysis and multiple linear regression analyses were used to examine the relationships among coping strategies, depressive symptoms, and demographic factors.

Results

Sample Characteristics

Adults living with HF (n = 75) who participated in this study ranged in age from 27 to 82 years ($M = 54.6$, SD = 13.1). Sixty-nine percent were men (n = 52). Approximately 59% (n = 44) of participants were married or partnered, whereas the remaining participants were single (n = 12, 16.0%), widowed (n = 7, 9.3%), separated (n = 3, 4.0%), or divorced (n = 9, 12.0%). Most of the participants were Caucasian (n = 61, 81.3%), with the remaining participants being African American (n = 13, 17.3%) or Hispanic (n = 1, 1.3%). The Hollingshead Four-Factor Index of socioeconomic status indicated that 60% of the study participants were from the middle class (ie, skilled and semiskilled workers).

In terms of level of functional impairment (NYHA classification), 7% (n = 5) of the participants were classified as NYHA Class I, 36% (n = 27) as Class II, 48% (n = 36) as Class III, and 9.3% (n = 7) as Class IV. Further, ejection fractions derived from echocardiographic or ventriculographic studies ranged from 10% to 60% (M = 28.9, SD = 14.4). These data indicate that the majority of participants in this study experienced moderate to severe functional impairment. The length of time since the original diagnosis of HF was also recorded, and ranged from recently diagnosed (≤1 month) to 292 months (M = 49.2, SD = 50.4). Approximately 53% (n = 40) of participants had a clinically significant history of depression. Antidepressant medications were used by approximately 43% (n = 32) of participants, and depression scores ranged from 0 to 33 (M = 11.22, SD = 6.32). Based on these data, adults in this study experienced mild to moderate levels of depressive symptoms.

Correlational Analyses

The problem-focused coping strategies of seeking social support (r = −0.23, P = .04) and planful problem-solving (r = −0.27, P = .02) had direct, negative relationships with depressive symptoms. Thus, individuals who used more seeking social support coping, and who used more planful problem-solving coping had less depressive symptoms. The relationship between confrontive coping and depressive symptoms was not statistically significant.

The emotion-focused coping strategy of escape-avoidance (eg, wishful thinking) had a direct, positive relationship (r = 0.45, P < .001) with depressive symptoms. Individuals who used more escape-avoidance coping experienced more depressive symptoms. The relationships among distancing (minimizing the significance of the stressor), self-controlling, accepting responsibilities, positive reappraisal, and depressive symptoms were not statistically significant.

Multiple Regression Analyses

Multiple regression was used to examine the multivariate relationships among coping strategies, depressive symptoms, and demographic factors in individuals living with HF. Categorical variables were

dichotomized where necessary in order to meet the critical assumptions of regression analysis.

When regressing depressive symptoms on coping strategies and all demographic factors, 2 coping strategies and 2 demographic variables emerged as significant predictors of depressive symptoms: escape-avoidance (emotion-focused), planful problem-solving (problem-focused) coping, functional impairment (NYHA classification), and marital status (see Table 2). Single individuals with HF who used more escape-avoidance (emotion-focused) coping, less planful problem-solving (problem-focused) coping, and who experienced increased functional impairment were predicted to experience more depressive symptoms.

Discussion

The results of this study support the theoretical perspective of process coping,[15,16] in that individuals living with HF who used more problem-solving and seeking social support coping (problem-focused coping) had less depressive symptoms, whereas those who used more escape-avoidance (eg, hoped that a miracle would happen) (emotion-focused coping) had more depressive symptoms. This finding is consistent with other research studies of chronically ill individuals, including HF patients.[21,22] Perhaps the patients in this study who used more escape-avoidance (eg, wishful thinking) to cope with their situation had more depressive symptoms because they were too overwhelmed by the stressors of living with HF. In contrast, patients who use more problem-focused coping had less depressive symptoms because they were able to focus on changing the self or something in the environment for the better, such as dietary change, adherence to therapeutic regimens, or simplifying the home environment to minimize fatigue.

Individuals in this study who also sought social support had less depressive symptoms. This finding is consistent with earlier work by Coyne, Aldwin, and Lazarus, who indicated that individuals who used more problem-focused coping strategies to change the situation for the better, such as actively seeking social support to cope with problems, had fewer depressive symptoms.[18] Thus, patients who use more

TABLE 2	Summary of Regression Analysis		
Variable	**B**	**SE B**	**β**
Escape-avoidance coping	0.64	0.16	.38**
Planful problem-solving coping	−0.53	0.18	−.28*
Functional impairment (NYHA)	2.94	0.78	.36**
Marital status	−1.00	0.48	−.19**

NYHA indicates New York Heart Association.
$R^2 = 0.40$
*$P < .01$.
**$P < .001$.

emotion-focused coping may need additional support from healthcare providers to bolster their use of problem-focused strategies to actively cope with the situation.

The finding that individuals with more functional impairment had more depressive symptoms also is consistent with previous HF research.[6,21,23] The ability of functional impairment to predict depressive symptoms in this study likely stems from patients' limitations in physical functioning, decreased feelings of self-worth, changes in body image, loss of situational control, and strained social relationships.[24–27] There is some concern, however, that reliance on physical signs and symptoms of HF may preclude an accurate examination of the level of depressive symptoms in individuals living with HF, due largely to overlapping physical indicators such as fatigue, reduced energy, sleep disturbance, and weight changes. Therefore, the results of this study indicate that psychosocial factors, in addition to physical parameters, and the ways individuals living with HF cope with their disease may be important predictors of clinical outcomes, such as depressive symptoms, morbidity, and mortality.

Single individuals, individuals who used more escape-avoidance coping strategies (eg, hoped that a miracle would happen), and individuals who had increased functional impairment had more depressive symptoms. Perhaps those who were single may have felt more isolated and alone. This interpretation is supported by research that showed that the perception or belief that others are available to provide emotional, informational, and/or material resources when needed was beneficial for buffering negative emotions in individuals living with other chronic illnesses.[15,16,18] These findings also may be applicable to individuals with HF. This suggests that single individuals living with HF may be at higher risk for depressive symptoms, especially if they are more functionally impaired. Healthcare providers may need to be mindful that single individuals with HF would benefit from more information about what support resources are available to them in times of need.[15,16] More research is needed to provide a comprehensive view of the influence of expanded support networks in individuals living with HF.

Limitations

Limitations of this study include the research design and sample. The cross-sectional design used in this study provided limited insight into the complex relationships between coping strategies and depressive symptoms in HF patients because it restricts the ability to make causal inferences regarding the nature of these relationships. The specific relationships between

coping strategies and an individual's depressive symptoms have been found in previous research to be difficult to assess with any degree of clarity or precision. For example, the findings of these studies are not conclusive regarding whether avoidance coping is a symptom of psychological distress, a cause of psychological distress, or that it shares a bidirectional relationship with psychological distress.[17,18] Because of the time-sensitive nature of the coping process, coping should be assessed at multiple time points to determine whether specific coping strategies may be more efficacious for decreasing depressive symptoms at different times during the illness trajectory of individuals living with HF.

The use of a convenience sample in this study is a source of potential bias because study participants were recruited from a single comprehensive heart institute within an academic health science center. Further, including HF patients who live with minimal functional impairment (NYHA Class I) in this study could have been a potential sampling bias. This could have been avoided by only including individuals with moderate to severe functional impairment and who likely experience similar stressors and coping challenges. Thus, limiting the sample of patients in a narrower range of NHYA functional classifications should be considered in future research.

Summary

The findings of this study extend our understanding of the ways individuals with HF cope, and how coping is related to depressive symptoms. Further, the results of this study suggest that knowing how patients cope with their disease can help healthcare providers plan specific therapeutic approaches that could minimize the impact of functional impairment and psychological stressors over time. Because of the chronic and intractable nature of HF, however, alternative interventions should be directed at enhancing *both* emotion-focused and problem-focused coping strategies at different times during the illness trajectory. Helping patients self-identify activities they can realistically perform, encouraging patients to seek social support in times of need, and helping patients to become an active partner in their therapeutic care could be beneficial to achieving positive clinical outcomes over time.

REFERENCES

1. Freedland KE, Rich MW, Skala JA, Carney RM, Davila-Roma VG, Jaffe AS. Prevalence of depression in hospitalized patients with congestive heart failure. *Psychosom Med.* 2003;65:119–128.
2. Friedman MM, Griffin JA. Relationship of physical symptoms and physical functioning to depression in patients with heart failure. *Heart Lung.* 2001;30:98–104.

3. Jiang W, Kuchibhatla M, Cuffe M, et al. Prognostic value of anxiety and depression in patients with chronic heart failure. *Circulation.* 2004;110:3452–3456.

4. Murberg TA, Bru E, Aarsland T, Svebak S. Functional status and depression among men and women with congestive heart failure. *Int J Psychiatry Med.* 1998;28:273–291.

5. Vaccarino V, Kasl SV, Abramson J, Krumholz HM. Depressive symptoms and risk of functional decline and death in patients with heart failure. *J Am Coll Cardiol.* 2001;38:199–205.

6. Carels RA. The association between disease severity, functional status, depression, and daily quality of life in congestive heart failure patients. *Qual Life Res.* 2004;13:63–72.

7. Jiang W, Kuchibhatla M, Cuffe MS, et al. Prognostic value of anxiety and depression in patients with chronic heart failure. *Circulation.* 2004;110:3452–3456.

8. Koenig HG. Depression in hospitalized older patients with congestive heart failure. *Gen Hosp Psychiatry.* 1998;20: 29–43.

9. Westlake C, Dracup K, Creaser J, et al. Correlates of health-related quality of life in patients with heart failure. *Heart Lung.* 2003;31:85–93.

10. Clarke SP, Frasure-Smith N, Lesperance F, Bourassa MG. Psychosocial factors as predictors of functional status at 1 year in patients with left ventricular dysfunction. *Res Nurs Health.* 2000;23:290–300.

11. Medich C, Stuart E, Deckro J, Friedman R. Psycho-physiological control mechanisms in ischemic heart disease: the mind-heart connection. *J Cardiovasc Nurs.* 1991; 5:10–26.

12. Moser DK, Dracup K. Psychosocial recovery from a cardiac event: the influence of perceived control. *Heart Lung.* 1995;24:273–280.

13. Moser DK, Worster PL. Effect of psychosocial factors on physiologic outcomes in patients with heart failure. *J Cardiovasc Nurs.* 2000;14:106–115.

14. Thomas SA, Friedmann E, Khatta M, Cook LK, Lann AL. Depression in heart failure: physiologic effects, incidence, and relation to mortality. *AACN Clin Issues.* 2003;14: 3–12.

15. Lazarus RS, Folkman S. *Stress, Appraisal, and Coping.* New York: Springer; 1984.

16. Billings AG, Moos RH. Coping, stress, and social resources among adults with unipolar depression. *J Pers Soc Psychol.* 1984;46:877–891.

17. Coyne J, Aldwin C, Lazarus RS. Depression and coping in stressful episodes. *J Abnorm Psychol.* 1981;90:439–447.

18. Cohen F, Lazarus RS. Coping with the stresses of illness. In: Stone GC, Cohen F, Adler NE eds. *Health Psychology: A Handbook: Theories, Applications, and Challenges of a Psychological Approach to the Health Care System.* San Francisco: Jossey-Bass; 1979.

19. Beck AT, Steer RA, Brown GK. Beck Depression Inventory—II. *Behav Meas Lett.* 1996;3:3–5.

20. Folkman S, Lazarus RS. *Manual for the Ways of Coping Questionnaire.* Palo Alto, Calif: Consulting Psychologist Press; 1987.

21. Friedman MM, Griffin JA. Relationship of physical symptoms and physical functioning to depression in patients with heart failure. *Heart Lung.* 2001;30:98–104.

22. Monat A, Lazarus RS. *Stress and Coping: An Anthology.* 3rd ed. New York: Columbia University Press; 1991.

23. Riedinger MS, Dracup KA, Brecht M, Padilla G, Sarna L, Ganz P. Quality of life in patients with heart failure: do gender differences exist? *Heart Lung.* 2001;30: 105–116.

24. Stull DE, Starling R, Haas G, Young JB. Becoming a patient with heart failure. *Heart Lung.* 1999;28: 284–292.

25. Luttik ML, Jaarsma T, Moser D, Sanderman R, van Veldhuisen DJ. The importance of social support on outcomes in patients with heart failure. *J Cardiovasc Nurs.* 2005;20(3):162–169.

26. Chinn MH, Goldman L. Correlates of early hospitalization readmission or death in patients with congestive heart failure. *Am J Cardiol.* 1997;79:1640–1644.

27. Murberg TA, Bru E, Aarsland T, Svebak S. Social support, social disability and their roles as predictors of depression among patients with congestive heart failure. *Scand J Soc Med.* 1998;26:87–95.

PERSPECTIVES OF WOMEN WITH DEMENTIA RECEIVING CARE FROM THEIR ADULT DAUGHTERS

Catherine Ward-Griffin • Nancy Bol • Abram Oudshoorn

The caregiving experience within Alzheimer disease is fairly well documented. However, little research has been conducted from the perspective of the person living with dementia. The purpose of this study, part of a larger qualitative investigation of mother-daughter relationships within the care process of dementia, was to elicit the perceptions and experiences of mothers receiving care from their adult daughters. Guided by feminist and life-course perspectives, the researchers conducted in-depth, semi-structured interviews with a diverse sample of 10 community-dwelling women with mild to moderate cognitive impairment. In general, the health perceptions and experiences of the women were shaped by gender and how its meaning is constructed. While mothers reported mostly positive relationships with their daughters, cultural ideologies of individualism and familism manifested in feelings of "grateful guilt." Participants managed their contradictory experiences of receiving care from their daughters by *doing care, undemanding care, determining care*, and *accepting care*. The authors recommend changes in practice, policy, and research, with the aim of addressing relevant social determinants of health such as gender and social support, thereby promoting the health and well-being of women with dementia.
Keywords: aging, dementia care, women, health promotion

■ Background

Alzheimer's disease (AD) is an insidious, pervasive, debilitating disorder that destroys the affected person's capacity for self-care (Wuest, Ericson, & Stern, 1994). It not only has a profound impact on individuals diagnosed with the disease, but also affects the lives of family members caring for them (Wuest, Ericson, Stern, & Irwin, 2001). As Canada's elderly population grows, an increasing number of individuals will require care for AD. The prevalence of dementia nearly doubles with every 5-year increase in age from the age of 60, rising to 32% in those aged 90 to 94 (Hofman, Rocca, & Brayne, 1991). Studies have found that the prevalence of AD is higher in women (Evans, Ganguli, Harris, Kawas, & Larson, 1999). Moreover, the prevalence of AD in Canada is expected to increase from approximately 364,000 persons in 2000 to over 750,000 persons by 2030, with roughly half of those individuals living in the community (Canadian Study of Health and Aging [CSHA] Working Group, 1994).

There has been significant emphasis on the development of services that enable people with AD to remain in their own homes whenever possible. Although there is a growing commitment to assist the individual with dementia and his or her family, there are many challenges to achieving optimal dementia care in the home. Restructuring of hospital and social services, closure of long-term-care facilities, and underfunding of home care (Aronson, 2004; Chappell, 1999) have led to an increasing reliance on family care. The current trend towards the favouring of home care over care in a hospital or other institution is motivated in part by concerns about spiralling health-care costs (Armstrong & Armstrong, 2004; Neysmith, 1991; Strang & Koop,

2003). Only one in four people caring for a relative with dementia receives formal care services (CSHA Working Group, 1994). Consequently, families rather than paid caregivers assume and/or coordinate the majority of home-based care (Armstrong et al., 2003). Since most care recipients and family caregivers are women, these shifts in the delivery of health care tend to affect women to a greater degree than men (Armstrong & Armstrong, 2004; Gregor, 1997; Morris, 2004).

Given these challenges to the achievement of optimal home-based dementia care, the needs of women involved in dementia care, particularly those afflicted with AD, demand careful attention. The inclusion of the perspectives and voices of women who receive care is essential to the analysis of how social determinants, such as gender and social support, affect women's health. Health Canada identifies gender as one of the 12 determinants of health, because gender is a factor in both participation in and the consequences of health care (Armstrong, 2004). The purpose of this qualitative study, guided by feminist and life-course perspectives, was to explore the perceptions and experiences of women with mild to moderate dementia and their adult daughters in the giving and receiving of care. The aim of this paper is to report on the mothers' accounts of receiving care from their daughters, thereby bringing elderly women from the margin to the centre of the debate on dementia care. The daughters' perspectives on providing care to their mothers with dementia are reported elsewhere (Ward-Griffin & Bol, in press). The paper will conclude with recommendations for change in practice, policy, and research, with the aim of promoting the health and well-being of women with dementia.

■ Literature Review

RELATIONSHIPS BETWEEN PERSONS WITH AD AND FAMILY CAREGIVERS

The literature is replete with studies of the problems of caregiving, many of which view the individual with AD as a significant source of caregiver burden (Beeson, Horton-Deutsch, Farran, & Neundorfer, 2000; McCarty, 1996, Stevenson, 1990). Recently, however, researchers have focused on the relational aspects of dementia care (Globerman, 1994; Ward-Griffin & Bol, in press; Wuest, Ericson, & Stern, 1994). In a grounded theory study with 15 family caregivers, Wuest, Ericson, and Stern found that the interactions of persons with AD and family caregivers fell on a continuum from intimacy to alienation through dimensions of dawning, holding on, and letting go. Similarly, Ward-Griffin and Bol found that daughters caring for women with dementia reported difficulties in maintaining a reciprocal relationship with their mothers, using negotiating strategies such as "finding a balance," "leading the way," and "carrying the load." In another qualitative study with relatives of persons with dementia, Globerman suggests that families in crisis may find their usual roles and relationships inflexible and need help negotiating their relationships, particularly around their expectations of one another. Other investigations have found that the quality of interactions between persons with dementia and their family members prior to the onset of dementia is an important factor for predicting emotional strain, quality of life, and caregiving satisfaction (Mui, 1995; Spaid & Barusch, 1994). While the effects of the quality of this dyadic relationship on the well-being of the caregiver have been documented, a gap remains in the literature regarding the effect of such relationships on the health and well-being of the person with dementia.

Another limitation of the published research on individuals with dementia and their caregiving relatives is a tendency to distort the reciprocity in their relationships. Neufeld and Harrison (1995) report that 20 women caring for older family members with cognitive impairment described reciprocity as "give and take"; however, caregivers were unable to establish the same kind of reciprocal relationship with the person with dementia as they did with others. Keefe and Fancey (2002) also explored the importance, for caregiving daughters and their older mothers without dementia, of giving and receiving. They found that mothers and daughters had different perspectives on reciprocity, with mothers minimizing their past contributions. In contrast, Talbot (1990), in a study with 55 elderly widowed mothers without dementia, found that mothers gave much and received little, which may contribute to the negative effects of these relationships on the mothers. Finally, Carruth (1996) explored reciprocity among adult children of persons with and without dementia and found that the diagnosis of dementia did not contribute to the explained variance of caregiver reciprocity. These findings suggest that incongruent perspectives of reciprocity between mothers and their adult children may shape the experiences of giving and receiving dementia care. Clearly, further research in this area is warranted.

RESEARCH ON THE PERSPECTIVES OF PEOPLE WITH DEMENTIA

Although the aforementioned studies increase our knowledge about the process and outcomes of caregiving within dementia, we have limited knowledge about the relationships between individuals with dementia and their family caregivers, particularly from the perspective of the individual with AD. Most research in dementia has relied solely on the perspectives of the caregiver, whose stresses and coping strategies have been of much interest. Although there is a tendency to "bind together" the interests of individuals with dementia and their caregivers, especially within community care (Reid, Ryan, & Enderby, 2001), the interests of people with dementia and their caregivers do not always coincide (Askham, 1991). Rarely have the perceptions of the persons with AD been examined, because of their dementia (Cotrell & Schultz, 1993) and the difficulty in recruiting individuals with AD (Long, Sudha, & Mutran, 1998). However, the belief that it is impossible for people with dementia to express their views or describe their experiences has been increasingly rejected in recent

years (Clarke & Keady, 2002; Gilmour & Huntington, 2005; Whitlatch & Feinberg, 2001). Research has demonstrated that individuals with mild to moderate cognitive impairment are able to answer questions about their own care with a high degree of accuracy and reliability (Whitlatch & Feinberg) and are willing and able to share their personal narratives (Moore & Hollett, 2003; Svanstrom & Dahlberg, 2004; Usita, Hyman, & Herman, 1998). The exclusion of persons with dementia indicates a failure to acknowledge their ability to report accurately on their current situation (Cotrell & Shultz), rendering them as passive participants in the care process—as if they were the objects rather than the subjects of their circumstances (Aronson, 1991).

Although persons with dementia and their families are uniquely qualified to define priorities for improving dementia care, they have rarely been asked to do so. In recent years, however, there has been increasing interest in the experiences of people who have been diagnosed with dementia (Aggarwal et al., 2003; Gilmour & Huntington, 2005; Moore & Hollett, 2003; Morhardt, Sherrell, & Gross, 2003; Reid et al., 2001; Sabat, 1998; Svanstrom & Dahlberg, 2004; Werczak & Stewart, 2002). Gilmour and Huntington, in their qualitative study with five men and four women with dementia, found a need to maintain control and independence with the increasing need for support in everyday tasks. Similarly, Cox, Anderson, Dick, and Elgar (1998) found that individuals with dementia expressed a desire for reliable health-care workers who support their independence and treat them as individuals. Reid et al. interviewed 19 people with dementia as part of a larger study on unmet respite-care needs among caregivers and day-care attendees in England; they found that those who attended groups valued them for the support offered and provided, the potential for developing friendships, and the company offered. Similarly, Aggarwal et al, using a flexible, individualized approach, interviewed 27 people at all stages of dementia in residential and day-care settings, as well as their relatives, on the subject of care services and their experiences; the persons with dementia reported lack of choice and the need for independence and more social aspects of care, while their relatives were more positive about the services. This discrepancy in response between persons with dementia and their relatives suggests a need to approach people with dementia to elicit their views.

Based on two semi-structured interviews with each of three women and three men with dementia who lived at home with their spouses, Werczak and Stewart (2002) developed a theoretical framework outlining the continuous process of adjusting to early-stage dementia, which comprised five stages (antecedents, anticipation, appearance, assimilation, and acceptance). Similarly, Pearce, Clare, and Pistrang (2002) conducted separate interviews with 10 community-dwelling older men with dementia and their wives to elicit the men's appraisals of their illness and coping strategies. The participants' accounts suggested that the men were engaged in a process of attempting to manage their sense of self. The ways in which the men attempted to manage sense of self were thus affected by their appraisals of and reactions to their difficulties, which in turn had an influence on and were influenced by their relationships and social identities. As previous studies suggest (Evans et al, 1999), women and men may cope with dementia differently, which warrants a more detailed gender analysis of dementia care.

Proctor (2001), in a qualitative study with elderly women with dementia, focused on relationships, gender, and issues of power. Using Brown and Gilligan's (1993) Voice Relational Method, Proctor interviewed four women twice about their experiences with health services. The findings illuminated the situation of power in the women's relationships, particularly their relationships with health professionals. The women felt that they could not challenge doctors and nurses about decisions regarding their welfare, thereby illustrating how gender and (dis)ability shape interactions between caregivers and care recipients.

Although dementia is usually seen as an older person's disease, a grounded theory study (Harris & Keady, 2004) with younger people with dementia in the United States ($n = 23$) and families of younger people with dementia in the United Kingdom ($n = 15$) resulted in the emergence of eight inductively generated themes: (1) difficulty obtaining a diagnosis, (2) issues of self-hood and self-esteem, (3) changing relationships within the family structure, (4) awareness of changes in self, (5) workforce and retirement/financial issues, (6) feelings of extreme social isolation and exclusion, (7) "off-time" dependency, and (8) lack of meaningful occupation. While the findings suggest that people with dementia and their families are confronted with unique social issues, there is a need to explore common experiences among people of any age diagnosed with dementia, such as the feelings of isolation associated with the loss of social roles. It is also important that the life course not be segmented, as this can lead to divisive conceptualizations of care and service provision between and among those receiving care and those giving it. Moreover, the tendency in the literature to focus on static life stages indicates a failure to capture the continuity of gender identity and experience over the life course, particularly for women (Aronson, 1991).

In summary, despite increasing interest in the experiences of people who have been diagnosed with dementia, there is still a dearth of research into the ways in which persons with dementia negotiate relationships in their social world. In particular, little is known about the specific relationship between women with AD and their adult daughters, and how the care process influences their health and well-being, particularly from the mother's perspective. If we are to broaden our understanding of the complexities of the care process in AD, research will have to consider the perspectives of both the caregiver and the care recipient (Cox & Dooley, 1996). Finally, we need to increase our knowledge about gender and how it shapes intergenerational care within the mother-daughter relationship. This information will help us to identify those societal conditions that require change, with the aim of promoting the health of women with dementia.

■ Method

As part of a larger qualitative investigation of mother-daughter dyads within the care process of dementia, we were interested in developing a better understanding of the experiences of community-dwelling women with AD receiving care from their daughters. Evidence suggests that the care experience differs by gender, family relation, and health status of the care recipient (Dupuis & Norris, 2001). Therefore, this study focused exclusively on women with mild to moderate cognitive impairment receiving care from their adult daughters. Specifically, we were interested in addressing the following research questions: (1) *How do women with AD and their adult daughters describe their experiences of receiving/providing care?* (2) *How do women with AD and their adult daughters describe their relationship?* (3) *What contextual factors influence the care provided/received?*

THEORETICAL FRAMEWORK

This qualitative study was guided by socialist-feminist theory and a life-course perspective. This type of inquiry gives primacy to individual subjective perceptions of care experiences, while at the same time seeking to understand the fluctuating nature of the mother-daughter relationship over time. Feminist scholars have identified the importance of the tie between mother and daughter. Given their skills and expectations in maintaining social ties, it is not surprising that, in adulthood, mothers and daughters share stronger relationships than fathers and sons (Fingerman, 2001). Feminist theorists have also questioned the premise that autonomy is the final virtue to be equated with maturity. Thus the emphasis in feminist writing has been on the bond between mothers and daughters (Fingerman).

Social-feminist scholars, most notably Stoller (1993) and Ungerson (1990), have provided explanations for the ways in which caring is defined and how it is organized. Since a feminist perspective views women's everyday caring experiences as inextricably connected to the larger political, social, and economic environment (Hall & Steyens, 1991), elicitation of women's narratives about the intergenerational care process identifies larger cultural values and ideologies. As discussed earlier, the caregiving literature tends to portray elderly mothers as burdensome to their overworked daughters. Feminist inquiry offers an alternative view—that caring is an intergenerational process between two women. Finally, the goal of feminist research is to develop knowledge, thereby creating positive changes with the aim of improving the lives of women in this intergenerational relationship.

This study also took a life-course perspective in order to understand the interactions and exchanges between mothers and adult daughters throughout their lives. This perspective is appropriate since it assumes that the meaning of care (giving and receiving) is based on a lifetime of experiences rather than on the current event or situation (i.e., dementia) (Fingerman, 2001). A life-course perspective also captures the care relationship between two generations of women and its shaping of women's health and well-being.

RECRUITING AND SAMPLING METHODS

After approval had been secured from the Ethics Review Board of the affiliated university, multiple recruitment strategies (e.g., key community agencies, doctors' offices, community centres) were used to obtain a diverse sample of community-dwelling women with mild to moderate cognitive impairment and their adult daughters. In an attempt to reach participants who may not have had access to these services, colourful flyers and notices about the study were sent out and posted in the offices of family physicians and at community sites such as libraries and seniors' centres. Also, health professionals providing services to women with dementia and/or their families, such as clinical nurse specialists, community nurses, and social workers, were contacted by telephone or in person to enlist their help in identifying potential participants. Follow-up letters and telephone calls to community agencies were made 2 to 3 weeks later. Finally, through use of the snowball technique, some daughter participants indicated that their sister(s) would be interested in taking part in the study. Consequently, three mothers had two or more adult daughters participating in the study.

Inclusion criteria for mothers and daughters were consent to participate, ability to speak English, and receiving/providing at least 2 hours of care per week. In addition, mothers had to score 17 or higher on the Standardized Mini-Mental Status Examination (SMMSE) and to demonstrate good verbal and comprehension skills (e.g., ability to state date of birth). According to Molloy and Clarnette (1999), a SMMSE score of 21 to 24 is indicative of early dementia and a score of between 10 and 20 is indicative of moderate dementia. Based on the clinical experience of one of the investigators, the cutoff score was set at 17, to ensure accurate, reliable interview data. In the end, of the 20 mothers with dementia in the larger study, 10 were unable to participate in the interview due to low SMMSE scores.

All potential participants were given written information about the purpose and nature of the study and were asked to take part in two interviews 6 to 9 months apart. Multiple interviews are often necessary with persons with dementia, to ensure sufficiently rich data and to compensate for the day-to-day fluctuations in their abilities (Moore & Hollett, 2003). Moreover, since we were interested in understanding how the progress of dementia may shape the mother-daughter relationship, we selected an intermediate time frame, one that would potentially capture this aspect of the relationship without risking participant attrition. However, two mothers who were interviewed at time 1 could not be interviewed at time 2 due to a low SSME score.

Written consent was obtained immediately prior to the first interview and all participants were assured of confidentiality (e.g., use of pseudonyms). The assent of each participant was reaffirmed at the beginning of the second interview.

SAMPLE

The participants ranged in age from 75 to 98 years (mean age = 88) and obtained SMMSE scores of 18 to 28 out of a possible 30 (mean = 22). Six of the women identified as Canadian, seven were widowed, and most had two or more adult children involved in their care. Four of the women had not completed secondary school. Incomes ranged from less than \$20,000/year ($n = 4$) to \$60,000/year ($n = 1$). All but one of the mothers lived in the same city as at least one of her daughters. At the time of the first set of interviews, four of the mothers lived in their own home, four lived in their daughter's home, and two lived in a retirement home in the community.

On average, the mothers and daughters saw one another 3 days per week. The daughters reported that they had been providing daily to weekly assistance to their mothers for an average of 49 months, with a range of less than 1 year to more than 6 years. All mothers received some degree of help, such as personal care, transportation, housekeeping, or meal preparation, from their daughters.

DATA COLLECTION

If both mother and daughter in a dyad consented to participate in the study, separate indepth interviews were arranged at a mutually convenient time and place. The decision to not conduct conjoint mother/daughter interviews was largely based upon the belief that the participants would be more forthcoming in their reports if interviewed alone. Furthermore, there is considerably less research documentation on the perspectives of persons who receive care (Allen & Walker,

1992), and the research team believed it was important to capture voices previously unheard. On three occasions, however, mothers required or requested the presence of a relative, usually the daughter or a granddaughter. During these interviews, one of the two parties occasionally drew the other into the conversation to confirm or verify some information. Therefore, it is possible that the mother's responses in these situations were influenced by the presence of her relative. One advantage of the conjoint interviews was the opportunity to collect observational data with respect to mother-daughter interactions. Thus, interviewing the mother and daughter together did not necessarily yield a less complete picture of the relationship, although it did yield a different one.

Audiotaped interviews, lasting approximately 45 minutes, were conducted initially, followed by a second set of interviews with a total of eight mothers (the SMMSE scores of two of the original 10 participants were below 17). One mother was interviewed twice because she needed extra time to fully discuss her relationships with her four daughters. All of these interviews were held at the mother's residence. At the end of the first interview, all participants completed a brief demographic questionnaire. Finally, full field notes were written after each interview.

Using an in-depth, focused interviewing approach (Merton, Fiske, & Kendall, 1990), the interviewer asked the participant non-directive questions designed to trigger dialogue about her experiences in providing/receiving care, the mother-daughter relationship, and the factors influencing the process of care. Through this approach, the participants were encouraged to discuss what they considered to be the most important aspects of the care process and of their relationships. The research team's use of this approach to interviewing was informed by the work of feminist scholars (Oakley, 1982; Reinharz, 1992) and other researchers who interview persons with dementia (McKillop & Wilkinson, 2004; Moore & Hollett, 2003; Reid et al., 2001). All three investigators strove to build rapport with the participant and to provide support

and information during the interview. Guided by clinical evidence in dementia care, the research team employed additional interview strategies for use with individuals with AD (e.g., using visual aids, providing questions on yellow paper, ensuring a quiet environment). Thus, the study sought to include people with dementia in research about their experiences, creating the potential for personal empowerment consistent with feminist goals.

DATA ANALYSIS

The major procedures for qualitative data analysis followed the guidelines of Lofland and Lofland (1995). After each interview, full field notes were written to record perceptions, insights, and observations (Morse & Field, 1995). The field notes, a method commonly used in qualitative research, added richness and depth to the data and also guided the planning of interviews. As data analysis proceeded, memos or notes were used to keep track of the researchers' insights and included justifications for making analytic decisions.

Gathering and analyzing data were simultaneous processes (Lofland & Lofland, 1995). Transcription and analysis of the interviews began immediately after the first interview and proceeded as data were collected. Shortly after each interview, individual researchers read the transcription and independently made a preliminary data analysis. Team analysis was used to clarify concepts (e.g., guilt, gratitude) and themes (e.g., undemanding care). Ultimately, the principal investigator explored the connections among the themes and prepared an overarching conceptual interpretation of participants' experiences, which was finalized through team analysis.

Throughout data analysis, Guba and Lincoln's (1989) criteria for establishing credibility, transferability, dependability, and confirmability were used. Credibility was established through prolonged engagement with the data, persistent observation, and audiotaping and verbatim transcription of all interviews. Transferability of the findings to other settings was promoted by providing a rich description of the context and methods entailed in generating the data. Dependability and confirmability of the data were promoted by maintaining an extensive audit trail.

■ Findings

Building on the theoretical perspectives outlined above, the accounts of mothers and daughters were treated as both individual perceptions of caregiving and care receiving and "points of entry" into social processes far beyond the realities of the participants (Smith, 1987). In adopting a method that addresses both sides of the care relationship, the research team sought to uncover a number of features that are not addressed in policy, such as the relationship itself, emotional labour, and the complex exchanges of care (Henderson & Forbat, 2002). The goal of the study was to explore the perceptions and experiences of community-dwelling women with dementia and their daughters. In this paper we report only on the perspectives of the mothers. A full account of the different types of mother-daughter relationship, using the dyad as the unit of analysis, will be published elsewhere.

Based on our interview and field-note data, the mothers' perceptions and experiences of receiving care from their daughters are conceptualized in the form of a flower (see Figure 1). The familiar AD logo, the forget-me-not, was purposely selected to depict how mothers managed their contradictory experience of needing care. Each petal of the flower represents one of four responses: *doing care, undemanding care, determining care*, and *accepting care*. The appraisal of the situation, the conceptualization of need, and the acceptability of the care received were all subject to negotiation between the mother and daughter. Implicit in the process of negotiation is the recognition that people are active participants, capable of constructing their actions to deal with social situations (Gerson & Peiss,

1985). All mothers spoke of feeling grateful for the care received, but at the same time they felt guilty for being a burden to their daughters. While the mothers reported mostly positive relationships with their daughters, the findings revealed that cultural ideologies and constraints manifested in feelings of "grateful guilt." The two major underlying ideologies, individualism and familism, appeared to be at the root of these responses. The mothers' experiences of receiving care from their daughters and the contextual factors shaping those experiences will now be described and illustrated through the use of comments by the participants.

MOTHERS' EXPERIENCES OF RECEIVING CARE

Analysis of the mothers' experiences of receiving care from their daughters illuminated four interrelated responses.

Doing care The first response was *doing care*. Simply stated, this was the mothers' perceived ability to perform self-care. Although the focus of the study was care *received* by the mothers, this finding highlighted how mothers' *provided* care, primarily to themselves. Most of the mothers asserted that they continued to live independently, apart from their daughters. They claimed that they would not "do that" to their daughters, implying that they did not wish to be "a burden" to their children. When the mothers were asked if they felt it was better to live with or apart from their daughters, many were explicit in their views about being independent:

I think it [living apart] is better. We each have our own sense of independence. . . . I think people need their independence as much as possible. . . . I think it's better to be apart if it's at all possible. (Margaret)

I wouldn't want to live with my kids, not one of them. I'd go into a home first. I've been independent. I wouldn't want to interfere with their lives. . . . I was brought up to be independent. (Georgina)

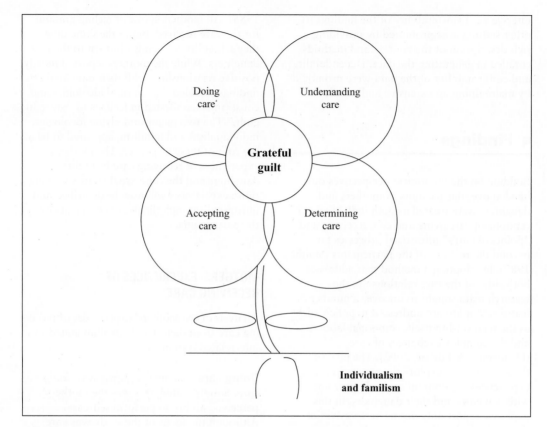

FIGURE 1 Receiving Care within Dementia: Mothers' Perspectives.

Adherence to cultural values of independence was driven mostly by the need to be productive and self-reliant:

> I clean my own windows, do my own house-work... When I have to stop doing that, then it's time to go. (Anne)

> I try not to give up the things that I'm interested in, and things that I do, to keep myself busy. (Helen)

> I don't ask her [daughter] to do anything for me. I'm an independent person and I do things for myself. (Bess)

> Never ask anybody for anything and you have nobody to thank. (Georgina)

Undemanding care   Closely aligned with doing care, *undemanding care* emerged from the women's accounts as a second thematic response. Withholding requests for assistance

was the predominant response reported by the participants. Consistent with Aronson's (1990a) finding of mothers appreciating their daughters' "busy family and work lives" and not wanting to add to their burden, many of the mothers in this study attempted to prevent their daughters from doing too much by suppressing their own wishes and needs. This was particularly noticeable with respect to their need for social interaction:

> It's very, very difficult for me to stay here all the time by myself... there's always this empty feel-ing of sitting by yourself... But I don't complain. I never tell her I'm lonely. (Helen)

> I don't want to take her life away from her. I've had mine. But I hate when she goes, when she says, "I'll just lock up the door, you know, for security." Oh yeah, now I'm all by myself again. (Anne)

For fear of asking too much of their children, the mothers sometimes found it easier to ask for nothing. The following comments also shed light on the Western cultural belief that the family of procreation takes primacy over the family of origin:

I don't bother them. I never call them. [If] they come, they come, if they don't, they don't. They're busy and they have families. . . I can't expect them to. . . they all have responsibilities and families. . . I don't demand nothing from them. (Georgina)

I don't see her as often as I'd like, but she's busy, like all young people are. Her time is taken up with important things now and you have to respect that. . . She's grown up and has a lot of responsibility. . . She needs to take care of her own home. I don't ask her to do anything for me. (Bess)

Determining care Torn between wanting to be independent and needing assistance, the participants actively responded to the dilemma by *determining* the extent and type of care they would receive from their daughter. They tended to ask for or were prepared to accept care only under certain conditions, thereby maintaining some degree of control over the care received, as well as addressing the tensions they experienced in needing help. Moreover, all of the participants accepted assistance from their daughter only if it did not restrict or jeopardize the daughter's independence. As illustrated in the following comments, the mothers were mindful of the demands on their daughters' lives and made an effort to restrict care to the absolute minimum:

I know that if I called and said, "Hey I'd like to see you—I'm lonely," she would be here. But I don't do that. She has her own life to lead. (Helen)

You want your daughter to have a full life. You want her to have time to do what she wants to do. . . so I feel better when I know she has her things to do too. (Margaret)

I mustn't bother her too much. She's a busy lady. (Bess)

Determining care also entailed decisions about what types of assistance were acceptable. Shopping, laundry, and banking were considered "normal" daily chores for adult daughters to perform for their mothers:

It's part of her day to come and take me shopping, like it would be if my mother was around. (Margaret)

She's been kind enough to do some of my laundry, because I hate to send my good clothes to the laundry here. So if I have two or three pieces of laundry, she does it for me and brings it back. (Helen)

She helps me with the banking. It's not because I can't do it myself. She has a car and it's handier for her to get my stuff than for me to do it. (Bea)

However, some participants realized that, due to deteriorating memory, they needed their daughter's assistance with other activities, such as dispensing medication and keeping doctors' appointments:

She sometimes gets my pills out. . . but I quite often do them myself. . . I think last week I goofed. I don't know I think I missed a couple of pills. I think it mixed me up. I was trying to think, how can I do this to get the right ones in? So sometimes she helps me with that. (Elizabeth)

When I was in the hospital she was able to talk to the doctors and the nurses in a way that I couldn't. . . Sometimes when I wasn't getting the drift she would get that across. . . She also goes to the doctor's [office] with me. She listens. She keeps it all straightened in my mind. (Margaret)

She took me to the eye doctor's today, but I don't like to put too much on her shoulders because she's got enough to do already. . . I try not to bother her because God only knows. . . how she does what she does. I hate to be a pest or a nuisance. . . so I make that [requests] a minimum. (Helen)

Finally, the participants not only exercised their right to restrict the care being provided currently, but also spoke about the future. Moreover, such responses seemed to serve the purpose of lessening their sense of dependency and preserving their sense of pride:

I'll ask for help when I need it. . . If I was at that stage [of needing more help], I'd put myself in a nursing home. (Ethel)

Accepting care The final response, *accepting care*, occurred when mothers passively accepted assistance from their daughter regardless of whether, in their opinion, they needed it or not. This response was particularly common among mothers who were receiving regular, almost daily, care from their daughter. In fact, some daughters occasionally reminded their mothers of the care that they received:

My kids tell me, "You never had it so good, Ma." (Helen)

I know that I'm not really with it. . . so I know that she helps me out, which is fine. Sometimes we joke about it. I think that was what she was saying when she came home last night. She said, "You know what, Mom? You got it made, really." (Elizabeth)

Clearly, many participants were well aware of the time and energy their daughters spent providing care and did not want to appear ungrateful. In response, they gradually relinquished control of their care to their daughters:

I really do rely more on her. When she makes a plan or something like that, I try to make sure I go along with it because that's something she's spent some thought on. . . Now she just goes ahead and does things for me. (Margaret)

I'm lucky. I'm lucky to have the help when I need it. [Daughter] was right here when I needed her. She took care of me like a little sister, which was wonderful. (Helen)

I see her quite frequently and she is very, very good. . . She brings me my meals. . . She does all she possibly can and I look forward to her coming over. I can depend on her. (Georgina)

Other participants were aware of their reliance on others and did not want to risk losing their assistance. This placed the mothers in a precarious position, which often led to their relinquishing the right to control their lives:

My daughter is my mainstay and I accept what she tells me. (Sarah)

If she thinks it's better for me [living with daughter], then it's alright. . . I take her word for it. She should know more than I do. . . and I'm exceedingly grateful to her for doing what she does, because a lot of young people that I know of nowadays wouldn't be so willing. . . She takes care of everything here and everything I need is
covered. *She takes the money out of the bank if she thinks I need it. And I don't have any responsibilities like that. Sometimes I wish I had, but if that's what she wants to do, then I don't care. All my life I took care of myself and all of a sudden I don't have to, but now I realize how wonderful it is, that I don't have to do anything.* (Helen)

CONTEXT OF RECEIVING/PROVIDING CARE

Two factors tended to account for and shape the mothers' responses to the care they received from their daughters: individualism and familism. The personal values and belief systems that we develop and follow throughout our lives are rooted in the societal ideologies of individualism and familism (Hooyman & Gonyea, 1995). An ideology is a set of beliefs and attitudes about our social reality, as well as the practices and motives they manifest. Ideologies are powerful in that they are often invisible and therefore difficult to contest (Anderson, 1990). In othet words, since care provided and received between mothers and daughters is viewed as "natural," ideologies often hinder our ability to imagine otherwise.

The values of individualism include self-reliance, self-determinism, privacy, living one's life independently, freedom from intrusion, and freedom from dependence on the will of others (Dalley, 1996). Many of the accounts described above reflect these values. Self-reliance and resisting dependency on others were the attributes of individualism most commonly described by the participants:

I think I'm independent, very independent. We were brought up to be like that. One thing that Daddy used to say, "Don't ask for favours, then you don't have to return them." (Georgina)

I do the dishes. . . she didn't like how I did them but I still went ahead and did them anyway. I don't care if she gets mad or not, I'm gonna do it!. . . She doesn't need to have all this to do. (Elizabeth)

The following comment illustrates the women's attempts to resolve the tension between being independent and being dependent, while also being grateful for any assistance offered:

> She would do anything I ask her, and I don't ask her because I'm an independent person and I can do it myself. But if they want to do some little thing for me, I'm always very happy and genuinely grateful. . . I wouldn't ask them to. . . They're ready to help me in any way, shape, or form if I said the word, but I try to be independent. (Bess)

The ideology of individualism depends on familism (Dalley, 1996), the second contextual factor that shaped the women's responses. When the emphasis is on family commitment and obligation, family members are expected to "care for" one another because they "care about" one another. With the notion of privacy of the family unit and minimal state interference, women's caring role within the family is perceived as "natural" and freely given. The participants respected these prevailing assumptions and values with regard to women's role as primary caregiver within the family. Iris, who had both daughters and sons, quoted a common saying to explain her son's limited ability to assist her, thus illustrating the intertwining of gender-role expectations and "family" caregiving:

> A daughter is a daughter for life. A son is a son 'til he takes a wife.

Indeed, another participant noted her good fortune in having a daughter who cared about her and sympathized with those who did not:

> It's a wonderful feeling to know that your daughter cares enough about you to do these things, because I've met some people who don't have anybody to do anything for them and it's pitiful, but whatever she does for me seems to be of her own free will, and if I need anything. . . she's there for me, and you really can't ask for much more. (Helen)

This comment also illustrates the participants' internalizing of ideologies—judging others and oneself against normative rules of conduct. Nourished by the strong roots of individualism and familism, "grateful guilt" was at the centre of the mothers' experiences in receiving care from their daughters. Conflicting emotions, such as guilt and gratitude, illustrate the invisible process of social

control described by Hochschild (1979). Covert forms of power, particularly at the ideological level, reflect and reinforce dominant cultural assumptions about women and care. The following comments illustrate the mothers' questioning of whether they deserved or were entitled to the care they received from their daughters:

> I don't want my daughter to feel that I'm going to be an anchor underneath. . . It makes me feel so guilty. . . I'm happy when she helps me, but at the same time I feel guilty. (Anne)

> She's very thoughtful. She brings me little dinners and stuff like that. I have no complaints...but I hope I deserve it. (Georgina)

Most of the participants refrained from asking for their daughters' help for fear of "being a burden." The provision of assistance frequently led to feelings of guilt, mixed with gratitude. Some mothers reported that others reinforced these feelings of gratitude:

> I'm very lucky, and many people have told me that too. (Margaret)

■ Discussion

Despite the limitations of a small, homogeneous sample of women with mild to moderate dementia, the findings from this study extend our knowledge of the perceptions and experiences of older women living with dementia, with a particular focus on mothers' relationships with their caregiving daughters. The findings highlight a number of areas that need to be addressed by practitioners, policymakers, and researchers as they work together to promote the health of older women with dementia. Specifically, we need to better understand how social determinants of health, such as gender, income, and social support, influence the health of women living with dementia.

First and foremost, we need to listen closely to what women with dementia have to say. Similar to the findings of other investigators (Aronson, 1991; Proctor, 2001), the accounts of women in this study revealed that their needs for care and social support were stifled by the internalization of dominant societal ideologies of individualism and familism. The findings affirm the wish of most people with disabilities not to be a burden to their families. Since there are few publicly funded supports to assist with the care of older women with dementia and other chronic conditions (Dalley, 1996; Guberman, 2004; Krogh, 2004), the mothers in this study had little choice but to depend on their daughters to meet their needs, which led to feelings of "grateful guilt." Nurses and other health professionals need to be aware of the extent to which they may perpetuate these feelings. For instance, praising the efforts of care-giving daughters may inadvertently reinforce the mothers' feelings of guilt and unworthiness. Changes in health-care practice have the potential to address older women's sense of disentitlement and marginal social status.

Second, the findings affirm the need to radically alter the home-care system to better meet the needs of community-dwelling women and their families. We must challenge the pervasive gendered ideologies of familism that undergird the implicit and explicit policies of family care (Hooyman & Gonyea, 1995) and develop alternative types of care. Policies that view families as the cornerstone of home care and women's proper role as caregiver within the family are harmful to women's health, both as caregivers and as care recipients (Guberman, 2004). References to "the family" in home-care policies that hide the gendered nature of family caregiving must be openly criticized, while alternative models of care based on the belief that the care of disabled members of society is a social responsibility, such as those models proposed by Neysmith (1991) and Guberman, must be developed. Empowerment, genuine choice, and partnerships between all concerned stakeholders are central to this approach to community care. Since public services are available to people who need them within this innovative approach to community care, mothers with dementia would have their needs met without having to rely solely on their daughters.

Third, genuine partnerships among care recipients, family caregivers, professionals, and policy-makers will be possible only when all voices are heard. Although the perspectives of women—as either providers or receivers of care—are seldom considered central to the policy debates on health and social care in an aging society (Aronson, 1990b), women with dementia are beginning to speak up about their personal experiences in living with AD (Sterin, 2002; Truscott, 2003). Morris (2002) urges the disability movement to adopt the feminist perspective of "the personal is political" by giving voice to the subjective experiences of individuals with a disability. A feminist perspective runs counter to the individualist ethic inherent in the focus on personal health behaviour by situating women's health within current social, economic, and political conditions. It fosters a collective rather than an individual response and challenges governments and other social institutions to assume responsibility for the health of women and the population as a whole (MacDonald, 2002).

Pringle (2003) makes a strong case for not only deepening our understanding of the lives of severely cognitively impaired people but also finding ways of "making moments matter" in the activities of daily living of those with dementia. Pringle asks, "How do we get nurses to sew a tapestry using multiple colours and strands?" with the aim of improving the quality of life of persons with dementia. One response would be for nurses to sit down with persons with dementia and their families and sew this tapestry together. In other words, women with AD not only need to be heard, but need to actively contribute to the construction of equitable policies that promote their health and well-being. Policy rarely reflects the voices of both sides of the care relationship, and indeed often fails to acknowledge the role of the relationship itself in how people construct meanings of their situation (Henderson & Forbat, 2002). Only when we acknowledge the overriding importance of this relationship in the provision of care, allowing for relationship-based social policy, will we be able to create a representative, colourful tapestry that promotes the health and well-being of women.

The fourth and final area that needs to be addressed in light of the present findings relates to future research directions. We need to explore how other social determinants of health, such as income and social inclusion, shape women's health experiences. Previous research shows that elderly people of financial means generally buy services and hire people to meet their needs, instead of choosing to be cared for by family and friends (Guberman, 2004). Most of the women in the present study lacked the financial resources to purchase caregiving assistance. This may have contributed to their sense of lack of control and their ambiguous relations with their daughters. It is essential that nurses and other health professionals understand the complex dynamics inherent in the relationship between the social determinants of health and inequities and address those inequities by speaking out against poverty, social exclusion, and gender-based discrimination.

It is also important that a variety of research methods be used to increase our understanding of the health experiences of women with dementia. According to Perry (2005), the biomedical model that guides the assessment and diagnosis of dementia is based on assumptions and approaches that, while critical to medicine, may be less consequential for nursing. Although screening tools are often employed in dementia research, Perry recommends that we consider extending our views of assessment and evaluation to include the individual's narrative. The present study collected narratives from individuals with dementia and their daughters, making it possible for us to hear the voices of both care recipients and caregivers. Regrettably, however, it included only those women with an SMME score of 17 or higher. Since those individuals in the later stage of dementia still possess an intact sense of personal identity (Sabat, 1998), future research in dementia care should include stories by individuals at all stages of dementia, thereby recognizing and supporting their personhood.

In conclusion, this study explored the perceptions and experiences of older women with mild to moderate dementia receiving care from their daughters. A feminist perspective helped us to uncover the ideological roots of dementia care and further our understanding of how these gendered ideologies shape the lives and health of older women with dementia. As well, we have suggested changes in practice, policy, and research, with the aim of transforming older women's feelings of "grateful guilt" into feelings of self-worth and dignity. These health-promoting practices and policies represent optimal growing conditions, which will ultimately support and nourish older women with dementia and their families.

REFERENCES

Aggarwal, N., Vass, A. A., Minaardi, H. A., Ward, R., Garfield, C., & Cybyk, B. (2003). People with dementia and their relatives: Personal experiences of Alzheimer's disease and of the provision of care. *Journal of Psychiatric and Mental Health Nursing, 10*(2), 187–201.

Allen, K., & Walker, A. (1992). A feminist analysis of interviews with elderly mothers and their daughters. In J. Gilgun, K. Daly, & G. Handel (Eds.), *Qualitative methods in family research* (pp. 198–214). Newbury Park, CA: Sage.

Anderson, J. (1990) Home care management in chronic illness and the self-care movement: An analysis of ideologies and economic processes of influencing policy decisions. *Advances in Nursing Science, 12*(2), 71–83.

Armstrong, P. (2004). Health, social policy, social economies and the voluntary sector. In D. Raphael (Ed.), *Social determinants of health: Canadian perspectives* (pp. 331–343). Toronto: Canadian Scholars' Press.

Armstrong, P., & Armstrong, H. (2004). Thinking it through: Women, work and caring in the new millennium. In K. R. Grant, C. Amaratunga, P. Armstrong, M. Boscoe, A. Pederson, & K. Willson (Eds.), *Caring for/caring about: Women, home care and unpaid caregiving* (pp. 5–43). Aurora, ON: Garamond.

Armstrong, P., Boscoe, M., Clow, B., Grant, K., Pederson, A., & Willson, K. (2003). *Reading Romanow: The implications of the final report of the Commission on the Future of Health Care in Canada for women.* Winnipeg: Canadian Women's Health Network.

Aronson, J. (1990a). Women's perspectives on informal care of the elderly: Public ideology and personal experience of giving and receiving care. *Aging and Society, 10,* 610–84.

Aronson, J. (1990b). Old women and care: Choice or compulsion? In P. Leonard & B. Nichols (Eds.), *Gender, aging and the state* (pp. 17–43). Montreal: Black Rose.

Aronson, J. (1991). Dutiful daughters and undemanding mothers: Constraining images of giving and receiving care in midlife and later life. In C. Baines, P. Evans, & S. Neysmith (Eds.), *Women's caring: Feminist perspectives on social welfare* (pp. 138–168). Toronto: McClelland & Stewart.

Aronson, J. (2004). "Just fed and watered": Women's experiences of the gutting of home care in Ontario. In K. R. Grant, C. Amaratunga, P. Armstrong, M. Boscoe, A. Pederson, & K. Willson (Eds.), *Caring for/caring about: Women, home care and unpaid caregiving* (pp. 167–183). Aurora, ON: Garamond.

Askham, J. (1991). The problem of generalizing about community care of dementia sufferers. *Journal of Aging Studies, 5,* 137–146.

Beeson, R., Horton-Deutsch, S., Farran, C., & Neundorfer, M. (2000). Loneliness and depression in caregivers of persons with Alzheimer's disease or related disorders. *Issues of Mental Health Nurse, 21*(8), 779–806.

Brown, L. M., & Gilligan, C. (1993). Meeting at the crossroads: Women's psychology and girls' development. *Feminism and Psychology, 3*(1), 11–35.

Canadian Study of Health and Aging Working Group. (1994). CSHA: Study methods and prevalence of dementia. *Canadian Medical Association Journal, 150,* 899–913.

Carruth, A. (1996). Motivating factors, exchange patterns and reciprocity among caregivers of parents with and without dementia. *Research in Nursing and Health, 19,* 409–419.

Chappell, N. (1999). Editorial: Canadian Association on Gerontology policy statement on home care in Canada. *Canadian Journal on Aging, 18*(3), i–iii.

Clarke, C. L., & Keady, J. (2002). Getting down to brass tacks: A discussion of data collection with people with dementia. In H. Wilkinson (Ed.), *The perspectives of people with dementia—Research methods and motivation* (pp. 25–46). London: Jessica Kingsley.

Cotrell, V., & Schultz, R. (1993). The perspective of the patient with Alzheimer's disease: A neglected dimension of dementia research. *Gerontologist, 33*(2), 205–211.

Cox, E. O., & Dooley, A. C. (1996). Care-receivers' perception of their role in the care process. *Journal of Gerontological Social Work, 26*(1/2), 133–152.

Cox S., Anderson, I., Dick, S., & Elgar, J. (1998). *The person, the community and dementia: Developing a value framework.* Stirling, UK: Dementia Services Development Centre.

Dalley, G. (1996). *Ideologies of caring: Rethinking community and collectivism* (2nd ed.). London: Macmillan.

Dupuis, S., & Norris, J. (2001). Roles of adult daughters in long-term care facilities: Alternative role manifestations. *Journal of Aging Studies, 15*(1), 27–50.

Evans, D., Ganguli, M., Harris, T., Kawas, C., & Larson, E. (1999). Commentary: Women and Alzheimer disease. *Alzheimer Disease and Associated Disorders, 13*(4), 187–189.

Fingerman, K. (2001). *Aging mothers and their adult daughters: A study in mixed emotions.* New York: Springer.

Gerson, J. M., & Peiss, K. (1985). Boundaries, negotiation, consciousness: Reconceptualizing gender relations. *Social Problems, 32*(4), 317–331.

Gilmour, J. A., & Huntington, A. D. (2005). Finding the balance: Living with memory loss. *International Journal of Nursing Practice, 11,* 118–124.

Globerman, J. (1994). Balancing tensions in families with Alzheimer's disease: The self and the family. *Journal of Aging Studies, 8*(2), 211–232.

Gregor, F. (1997). From women to women: Nurses, informal caregivers and the gender dimension of health care reform in Canada. *Health and Social Care in the Community, 5*(1), 30–36.

Guba, E., & Lincoln, Y. (1989). Judging the quality of fourth generation evaluation. In E. Guba & Y. Lincoln (Eds.), *Fourth generation evaluation* (pp. 228–251). Newbury Park, CA: Sage.

Guberman, N. (2004). Designing home care for women with disabilities: A call for citizenship. In K. R. Grant, C. Amaratunga, P. Armstrong, M. Boscoe, A. Pederson, & K. Willson (Eds.), *Caring about/caring for: Women, home care, and unpaid caregiving* (pp. 75–90). Aurora, ON: Garamond.

Hall, J. M., & Steyens, P. E. (1991). Rigor in feminist research. *Advances in Nursing Science, 13*(3), 16–29.

Harris, P. B., & Keady, J. (2004). Living with early onset dementia: Exploring the experience and developing evidence-based guidelines for practice. *Alzheimer's Care Quarterly, 5*(2), 111–122.

Henderson, J., & Forbat, L. (2002). Relationship-based social policy: Personal and policy constructions of care. *Critical Social Policy, 22*(4), 669–687.

Hochschild, A. (1979). Emotion work, feeling rules, and social structure. *American Journal of Sociology, 85,* 551–575.

Hofman, A., Rocca, W. A., & Brayne, C. (1991). The prevalence of dementia in Europe: A collaborative study of 1980–1990 findings. *International Journal of Epidemiology, 20*(3), 736–748.

Hooyman, N., & Gonyea, J. (1995). *Feminist perspectives on family care: Policies for gender justice.* Thousand Oaks, CA: Sage.

Keefe, J. M., & Fancey, P. J. (2002). Work and eldercare: Reciprocity between older mothers and their employed daughters. *Canadian Journal on Aging; 21*(2), 229–241.

Krogh, K. (2004). Redefining home care for women with disabilities: A call for citizenship. In K. R. Grant, C. Amaratunga, P. Armstrong, M. Boscoe,

A. Pederson, & K. Willson (Eds.), *Caring about/caring for: Women, home care, and unpaid caregiving* (pp. 115–146). Aurora, ON: Garamond.

Lofland, J., & Lofland, L. (1995). *Analyzing social settings: A guide to qualitative observation and analysis* (3rd ed.). Belmont, CA: Wadsworth.

Long, K., Sudha, S., & Mutran, E. (1998). Elder-proxy agreement concerning the function status and medical history of the older person: The impact of caregiver burden and depressive symptomatology. *Journal of the American Geriatrics Society, 46*, 1103–1111.

MacDonald, M. (2002). Health promotion: Historical, philosophical, and theoretical perspectives. In L. E. Young & V. Hayes (Eds.), *Transforming health promotion practice: Concepts, issues and application* (pp. 22–45). Philadelphia: F.A. Davis.

McCarty, E. F. (1996). Caring for a parent with Alzheimer's disease: Process of daughter caregiver stress. *Journal of Advanced Nursing, 23*(4), 792–803.

McKillop, J., & Wilkinson, H. (2004). Make it easy on yourself! Advice to researchers from someone with dementia on being interviewed. *Dementia: International Journal of Social Research and Practice, 3*(2), 117–126.

Merton, R. K., Fiske, M., & Kendall, P.L. (1990). *The focus interview: A manual of problems and procedures* (2nd ed.). New York: Free Press.

Molloy, D. W., & Clarnette, R. (1999). Standardized Mini-Mental State Examination: A user's guide. Troy, ON: New Grange Press.

Moore, T. F., & Hollett, J. (2003). Giving voice to persons living with dementia: The researcher's opportunities and challenges. *Nursing Science Quarterly, 16*(2), 163–167.

Morhardt, D., Sherrell, K., & Gross, B. (2003). Reflections of an early stage memory loss support group for persons with Alzheimer's disease and their family members. *Alzheimer's Care Quarterly, 4*(3), 185–188.

Morris, J. (2002). Personal and political: A feminist perspective on researching physical disability. *Disability, Handicap and Society, 7*(2), 157–166.

Morris, M. (2004). What research reveals about gender, home care and care-giving: Overview and the case for gender analysis. In K. R. Grant, C. Amaratunga, P. Armstrong, M. Boscoe, A. Pederson, & K. Willson (Eds.), *Caring for/caring about: Women, home care and unpaid caregiving* (pp. 89–113). Aurora, ON: Garamond.

Morse, J. M., & Field, P.A. (1995). *Qualitative research methods for health professionals* (2nd, ed.). London: Sage.

Mui, A. (1995). Caring for frail elderly parents: A comparison of adult sons and daughters. *Gerontologist, 35*, 86–93.

Neufeld, A., & Harrison, M. (1995). Reciprocity and social support in caregivers' relationships: Variations and consequences. *Qualitative Health Research, 5*(3), 348–365.

Neysmith, S. (1991). From community care to a social model of care. In C. Baines, P. Evans, & S. Neysmith (Eds.), *Women's caring: Feminist perspectives on social welfare* (pp. 272–299). Toronto: McClelland & Stewart.

Oakley, A. (1981). Interviewing women: A contradiction in terms. In H. Roberts (Ed.), *Doing feminist research* (pp. 30–61). Boston: Routledge.

Pearce, A., Clare, L., & Pistrang, N. (2002). Managing sense of self: Coping in the early stages of Alzheimer's disease. *Dementia, 1*(2), 173–192.

Perry, J. (2005). Expanding the dialogue on dementia: (Re)positioning diagnosis and narrative. *CJNR, 37*(2), 3–6.

Pringle, D. (2003). Discourse: Making moments matter. *CJNR, 35*(4), 7–13.

Proctor, G. (2001). Listening to older women with dementia: Relationships, voices and power. *Disability and Society, 16*(3), 361–376.

Reid, D., Ryan, T., & Enderby, P. (2001). What does it mean to listen to people with dementia? *Disability and Society, 16*(3), 377–392.

Reinharz, S. (1992). *Feminist methods in social research*. Toronto: Oxford University Press.

Sabat, S.R. (1998). Voices of Alzheimer's disease sufferers: A call for treatment based on personhood. *Journal of Clinical Ethics, 9*, 35–48.

Smith, D. E., (1987). *The everyday world as problematic: A feminist sociology*. Boston: Northeastern University Press.

Spaid, V., & Barusch, A. (1994). Emotional closeness and caregiver burden in the marital relationship. *Journal of Gerontological Social Work, 21*(3/4), 197–211.

Sterin, G.J. (2002). Essay on a word: A lived experience of Alheimer's disease. *Dementia, 1*(1), 7–10.

Stevenson, J. P. (1990). Family stress related to home care of Alzheimer's disease patients and implications for support. *Journal of Neuroscience Nursing, 22*(3), 179–188.

Stoller, E. P. (1993). Parental caregiving by adult children. *Journal of Marriage and the Family, 45*(4), 851–858.

Strang, V., & Koop, P. (2003). *Family caregivers waiting placement of cognitively impaired persons.* Unpublished paper.

Svanstrom, R., & Dahlberg, K. (2004). Living with dementia yields a heteronomous and lost existence. *Western Journal of Nursing Research, 26*(6), 671–687.

Talbot, M. (1990). The negative side of the relationship between older widows and their adult children: The mothers' perspective. *Gerontologist, 30*(5), 595–603.

Truscott, M. (2003). Life in the slow lane. *Alzheimer's Care Quarterly, 4*(1), 11–17.

Ungerson, C. (1990). The language of care. In C. Ungerson (Ed.), *Gender and caring* (pp. 8–32). Harlow, UK: Pearson Higher Education.

Usita, P. M., Hyman, I. E., & Herman, K. C. (1998). Narrative intentions: Listening to life stories in

Alzheimer's disease. *Journal of Aging Studies, 12*(2), 185–197.

Ward-Griffin, C., & Bol, N. (in press). Mother-daughter relationships within Alzheimer disease: Daughters' perspectives. In I. Paoletti (Ed.), *Family care-giving to older disabled people: Relational and institutional issues*. New York: Nova Science Publishing.

Werczak, L., & Stewart, N. (2002). Learning to live with early dementia. *Canadian Journal of Nursing Research, 34*(1), 67–85.

Whitlatch, C., & Feinberg, L. (2001). Are persons with cognitive impairment able to make consistent choices? *Gerontologist, 41*(3), 374–382.

Wuest, J., Ericson, P., & Stern, P. (1994). Becoming strangers: The changing family caregiving relationship in Alzheimer's disease. *Journal of Advanced Nursing, 20*, 437–443.

Wuest, J., Ericson, P., Stern, P., & Irwin, G. (2001). Connected and disconnected support: The impact on the caregiving process in Alzheimer's disease.

Health Care for Women International, 22, 115–130.

AUTHORS' NOTE

Comments or queries may be directed to Catherine Ward-Griffin, School of Nursing, University of Western Ontario, London, Ontario N6A 5C1 Canada. Telephone: 519-661-2111, ext. 86584. Fax: 519-661-3928. E-mail: cwg@uwo.ca

---

Catherine Ward-Griffin, RN, PhD, is Associate Professor, School of Nursing, University of Western Ontario, London, Ontario, Canada. Nancy Bol, RN, MScN, is Clinical Nurse Specialist, St. Joseph's Health Care, London, Ontario. Abram Oudshoorn, RN, BScN, is a doctoral student in the School of Nursing, University of Western Ontario.

Translating Best Practices in Nondrug Postoperative Pain Management

Susanne Tracy ▼ Marlene Dufault ▼ Stephen Kogut ▼ Valerie Martin
Susan Rossi ▼ Cynthia Willey-Temkin

► **Background:** The research-to-practice gap is at the heart of the problem in the underuse of nondrug complementary methods to manage postoperative pain.

► **Purpose:** To show how the six steps of the Collaborative Research Utilization (CRU) model can be used to translate research into practice, using an example of nondrug pain management protocols.

► **Methods:** The CRU model was used to translate empirically tested nondrug interventions for surgical pain management enhancement into cost-effective, easy-to-use, best-practice nursing interventions, using tailored patient teaching.

► **Results:** The preliminary findings of the substudy in the context of the CRU model are reported.

► **Discussion:** The CRU model was successful in changing patients' knowledge, attitudes, and use of nondrug interventions for pain management. Further research is needed in heterogeneous populations. Organization receptivity to research and a well-integrated computerized documentation system for cueing clinicians' pain management practices are key for effectiveness of change.

► **Key Words:** collaborative research utilization model · complementary pain management · tailored teaching

Older adults frequently minimize pain and endure it with stoicism. Their pain is often not communicated or well documented (Brown, 2004; McDonald, Thomas, Livingston, & Severson, 2005; Nikolaus & Zeyfang, 2004; Vallerand, Fouladbakhsh, & Templin, 2005). Even reported pain has been found to be undertreated with drugs in older adults (Ardery, Herr, Titler, Sorofman, & Schmitt, 2003; Bell & Reeves, 1999; Brockopp et al., 2004; Sauaia et al., 2005), and the use of complementary, nondrug strategies is not integrated fully into standard postoperative pain management practices in most hospitals (United States Department of Health and Human Services, Agency for Healthcare Research and Quality [AHRQ], 2001). Indeed, nondrug methods are underused in the postoperative older adult (Bell, 1997; Bell & Reeves, 1999; Ferrell, Whedon, & Rollins, 1995; Zalon, 1997). In one study, only 4 of 177 nurses reported using nondrug methods for pain relief with their patients (Wessman & McDonand, 1999). Further, nursing knowledge about pain and pain relief has not improved over time, a factor that continues to impede the relief of pain in older adults (Kelly, 2003; MacLellan, 2004; McMillan, Tittle, Hagan, & Small, 2005; Watt-Watson, Chung, Chan, & McGillion, 2004). Nurses have reported they do not know enough about pain and pain relief methods (Holley, McMillan, Hagan, Palacios, & Rosenberg, 2005; McCaffery & Robinson, 2002).

Nondrug methods of relieving pain for which there is a strong body of empirically validated knowledge are massage, music, and the cognitive behavioral interventions of self-guided imagery and patient education (AHRQ, 2001). The American Geriatrics Society (AGS) and other organizations support the use of nondrug methods of pain relief for older adults and have published pain management guidelines for using these methods (AGS Panel on Persistent Pain in Older Persons, 2002; Horgas & McLennon, 2003). The advantages are many: Nondrug strategies promote self-care and enhance personal control for one's own health. Although use of some nondrug methods is not reimbursable, many are readily available, inexpensive, and associated with few adverse side effects. They can be used alone or in combination with drug treatment and frequently minimize drug side effects. They are within the scope of independent nursing practice and older adults are usually receptive to their use (Ebener, 1999). Despite the empirical evidence, integrating these guidelines into standards of pain

Susanne Tracy, PhD, RN, is Assistant Professor, University of New Hampshire, Durham.

Marlene Dufault, PhD, RN, is Professor, College of Nursing, University of Rhode Island, Kingston; and is Research Consultant, Newport Hospital, Rhode Island.

Stephen Kogut, PhD, MBA, is Assistant Professor; Cynthia Willey-Temkin, PhD, is Professor, College of Pharmacy; and Susan Rossi, PhD, RN, is Adjunct Research Professor of Nursing, College of Nursing, University of Rhode Island, Kingston.

Valerie Martin, MS, RN, is Director of Surgical Nursing, Newport Hospital, Rhode Island.

Reprinted with permission from *Nursing Research* 2006; 55(2):S57–S67.

199

management care and translating them into everyday nursing interventions has posed a significant challenge.

Patient Teaching and Pain Management

Patient teaching is an important medium for communicating self-care information about nondrug enhancements for managing postoperative pain. Effective patient teaching may improve patient satisfaction with nursing care (Innis, Bikaunieks, Petryshen, Zellermeyer, & Ciccarelli, 2004; Sherwood, McNeill, Starck, & Disnard, 2003). Teaching goes beyond imparting knowledge; the primary aim is to effect behavioral change in patients (Saarman, Daugherty, & Riegel, 2000). There are problems with patient teaching, including poor adherence; lack of understanding of materials presented, associated with poor readability of materials; and general difficulties in getting patient education materials to *stick*. Nurses have identified that staffing, time constraints, and lack of patients' receptiveness inhibit patient teaching (Marcum, Ridenour, Shaff, Hammons, & Taylor, 2002). Teaching sessions are recalled inconsistently by patients, interfering with their ability to use valuable health information (Momtahan, Berkman, Sellick, Kearns, & Lauzon, 2004; Ni et al., 1999).

Customizing information enhances client attentiveness and recall (Kreuter, Strecher, & Glassman, 1999). Customization may improve patient recall of teaching materials, enhance the usability of the information, and improve patient outcomes. Tailoring teaching information to individual characteristics makes a difference in the ways in which people cope with information in situations of uncertainty and may influence patient responses to health directives (Fang, Miller, Daly, & Hurley, 2001; Miller, 1987; Miller, Fang, Diefenbach, & Bales, 2001; Miller, Sherman, Buzaglo, & Rodoletz, 2001). However, little is known about the relationship between information-coping style and tailoring patient teaching (Kwekkeboom, 2003; Suls & Wan, 1989; Watkins, Weaver, & Odegaard, 1986).

Barriers to Translating Research

Major barriers to using research to attain best-practice pain management are organizational climate, clinician and patient attitudes, and clinician lack of knowledge (Clarke et al., 1996; Dufault, Bielecki, Collins, & Wiley, 1995; McMillan, Tittle, Hagan, Laughlin, & Tabler, 2000; White, 1999). As noted earlier, nurses' pain management knowledge is lacking in depth and nursing school curricula in pain management are only fairly adequate (Clarke et al., McCaffery & Robinson, 2002). There remain organizational barriers to research utilization (Fink, Thompson, & Bonnes, 2005; Rappolt, Pearce, McEwen, & Polatajko, 2005; Reed, 2005; Scott-Findlay & Golden-Biddle, 2005) and a lack of standards, policies, and protocols used to integrate research innovations into practice (Brown, 2000; Dufault & Willey-Lessne, 1999; Dufault & Sullivan, 2000; Dufault, Willey-Temkin, Schwager, & Hockhausen, 2002). Based on this evidence, it was believed that an innovative, cost-effective approach was needed to translate research effectively on nondrug interventions into practice and to change clinician practice.

Such change is intended to improve patient outcomes while also integrating the use of innovative nondrug interventions into the practices of future clinicians (i.e., students).

Use of the Collaborative Research Utilization Model

The use of the Collaborative Research Utilization (CRU; Table 1) model to translate pain management innovations into practice is well documented (Dufault, 2004; Dufault et al., 2002; Dufault & Sullivan, 2000; Dufault & Willey-Lessne, 1999). The model served as the backdrop for this parent project and the substudy, and is adapted from the Conduct and Utilization of Research in Nursing Project that was used to generate best-practice standards, policies, and protocols (Horsley, Crane, & Bingle, 1978). Underpinned by Roger's Diffusion of Innovations Theory, Janken and Dufault (2002) describe how Dufault's six-step CRU model for translation of research within organizations is operationalized. In the model's early development, research roundtables were first used as a technique to improve staff nurse and student's awareness of the relevancy of research to their practice (Janken, Dufault, & Yeaw, 1988). By 1992, the model was expanded to involve student and staff nurses in each step.

The use of nursing students to evaluate the strength of the empirical evidence in the context of their coursework and assist clinicians and scientists in generating best-practice protocols is unique to the model. Clinicians are linked with students and scientists in a system that results in changes in each member of the partnership, subsequent changes in practice, and, ultimately, changes in patient outcomes. A major advantage of using the CRU model was that it can be used to target improvements in the clinical environment by facilitating research-driven changes in practice, as well as to develop present and future clinicians competent in these skills.

Approach

The preliminary work and the first three steps of the approach to be taken were completed in December of 2003. Funding was received for Steps 4, 5, and 6 of the model that began in January 2004 and ended in June 2005.

Preliminary Work

The principal investigator conducted interviews at hospitals throughout the state interested in participating in a *translating best practice in pain management* study. Of five hospitals indicating interest, the study site was selected based on a strong commitment to improving pain management, a well-integrated information system, and established documentation forms for cueing clinician's pain management practices. These organizational features have been essential to success in other translational studies (Dufault, 2004).

Step 1. Identify a Clinical Problem and Assess the Research Bases for Evidence of a Solution

Focus groups with unit-level staff nurse council members were led by the hospital's nurse researcher to identify common problematic areas of pain management care for which

TABLE 1. Steps in the CRU Model

CRU Step	Explanation	Estimated Timeline
1. Identify a clinical problem and assess the research bases for evidence of a solution	Connect with nursing administration, nursing staff, organizational nursing research committee, and other interested parties to identify common problematic areas for which there is a strong body of empirical evidence. Determine the extent of the problem and search for new research evidence in the literature.	2–3 months
2. Evaluate the relevance of the research as it relates to the selected problem, agency values, standards, and potential cost and benefits	Critically analyze new research evidence; judge strength of evidence; and critique evidence for applicability, usefulness, and potential for translation into the agency's best-practice standards, policies, and care protocols. Discuss findings with nurses involved in translation project. Jointly develop recommendations for development of best-practice protocols.	5–9 months
3. Design evidence-based best-practice standards, policies, or protocols	Transform recommendations into best-practice protocols and standards that meet the organization's specific needs. Design research study to pilot recommended best practices.	2–4 months (depending on IRB schedules)
4. Implement and evaluate innovative standards, policies, or protocols related to nondrug interventions for feasibility, usefulness, and effectiveness	Implement pilot study, analyze evidence, and prepare written reports of project implementation.	8–12 months
5. Decide to sustain, alter, or discontinue the standards, policies, or protocols	Presentation of pilot results to nursing administration, nursing staff, and other interested parties for decisional consideration regarding continuation of practice innovations.	1–2 months
6. Develop a way to disseminate and extend the innovation to other appropriate settings	Seek publication of results, prepare presentations, and seek inclusion at conferences and scholarly events. Begin work to discover other settings where innovations may be applied to practice.	As soon as project is complete

Note. CRU = Collaborative Research Utilization Model.

there is a strong body of validated empirical evidence. The underuse of nondrug interventions for pain management was a common theme cited in 80% of the focus groups.

Next, a 3-month chart audit was conducted on the use of nondrug interventions; none of the 91 charts audited contained documentation that nondrug interventions were used to complement drug therapy for surgical patients. Throughout the organization, the need and desire for translating research into better pain management practices using nondrug complementary interventions was recognized and supported.

The three interventions (massage, music, and the cognitive behavioral interventions of self-guided imagery and patient education) were selected based on the determination in the AHRQ's (2001) Evidence Summary that they have a strong evidence base, and are low in cost and complexity, but were underused in practice. The chosen interventions are effective in improving the outcomes of interest (AHRQ, 2001).

A reference librarian assisted the principal investigator in guiding 48 undergraduate nursing students to conduct literature searches from 1992 (the publication year of the pain management guidelines; AHRQ, 1992) to 2004 on massage, music, and guided imagery. Under the guidance of the course faculty and project director, 48 studies were critiqued in depth by 48 students for strength of evidence (AHRQ, 2001), including methodological strengths and

weaknesses. Patient education literature was examined also in the context of these interventions by the co-investigator, at the time a doctoral student in the College of Nursing.

Step 2. Evaluate the Relevance of the Research as it Relates to the Selected Problem, Agency Values, Standards, and Potential Cost and Benefits

Critiques of the research evidence on massage, music, guided imagery, and patient education were used by clinicians and senior baccalaureate students in four research roundtable discussions held on the surgical and rehabilitative care units. Tools for utilization of focused reviews (Stetler et al., 1998) were used to guide the roundtable discussions. The studies critiqued in Step 1 were evaluated for their clinical applicability, usefulness, and potential for translation into the experimental hospital's best-practice standards, policies, and protocols to be used by the nurse-led pain service. Twenty-two recommendations specific to the protocols for massage, music, and guided imagery were generated from 27 of the 48 studies critiqued in Step 1.

Step 3. Design Evidence-Based Best-Practice Standards, Policies, or Protocols

In Step 3, recommendations generated in the research roundtables were translated to conform to the organization's specific needs. The principal investigator led a team of clinicians, research associates, and others in developing three best-practice protocols for the use of massage, music, and guided imagery. A 12-member, unit-based nursing Comfort Therapy Service was formed and trained in the use of the best-practice protocols. The pool of caregivers trained in the use of the protocols was later expanded to include all registered nurses on the two units involved in the substudy and the student nurses affiliating on the units. Patient teaching materials tailored to patients' information-coping styles were developed for the three nondrug protocols, and a videotape was developed to complement the printed teaching materials. Nursing Care Plans were revised to include a segment on the use of the comfort therapies to integrate and individualize the plan for each patient.

Step 4. Implement and Evaluate Innovative Standards, Policies, or Protocols Related to Nondrug Interventions for Feasibility, Usefulness, and Effectiveness

In Step 4, the best-practice protocols for massage, music, and self-guided imagery, and the related tailored patient teaching intervention were implemented and evaluated. When this publication was submitted, the parent study was in progress; only the preliminary report of substudy data is described here.

Design

The parent project was composed of: (a) a primary efficacy study ($n = 137$) using a two-group, quasi-experimental design to determine the impact of nondrug interventions on pain intensity, functional ability, and patient satisfaction; and (b) a (pilot) substudy, using a single-group ($n = 46$) pretest–posttest descriptive design to evaluate the tailored teaching intervention (the independent variable) and to describe the changes in the patients' knowledge, attitudes, ability to use, as well as patient's actual use of the three nondrug best-practice protocols (the dependent variables).

Sample

The parent study sample included 137 surgical patients, age 50 years or older, who were undergoing elective joint replacement surgery, able to speak English, cognitively intact, with no history of mental illness involving reality disturbances, and able to respond to questions concerning their pain. Forty-six of these patients were selected by convenience sample to be used in the substudy. Baseline data were provided for 45 (98%) patients, Postoperative Day 3 data for 37 (80.4%) patients, and day-of-discharge data for 35 (76.0%) patients; composition of the initial sample of 46 patients changed only slightly at each assessment point.

Setting

The setting was a 148-bed urban community Magnet hospital serving tourists, military personnel, and adults from an island community, similar in percentage of minorities, gender, and socioeconomic status to other community hospitals in the state. At the hospital, nursing care hours per patient day were 6.1 hours, the average length of stay for surgical patients was 4 days, and the Press Ganey (2002) Patient Satisfaction with Pain Management Index score was 87.2 at the start of the study. Standards of pharmaco-

logical pain management care included the use of intravenous patient-controlled analgesia as the method of choice for pain control during the immediate postoperative period (first 3 days). There was a striking lack of nondrug pain interventions used to enhance pharmacological interventions in postoperative patients. At the hospital, older joint replacement patients typically are admitted to a surgical unit for the first 3 days of their stay, followed by transfer to a subacute unit where unit-based rehabilitation services are provided.

Instruments

Knowledge, attitudes, and ability to use music and guided imagery were assessed using the Non-Drug Complementary Pain Interventions Survey (NDCPI), a 38-item instrument developed for and piloted in this study to assess patient knowledge, attitudes, and behaviors associated with each of the three best-practice protocols (Tracy, 2005). Before study use, a group of 15 well adults (60 years of age or older) were asked to review the original 45-item survey for readability, user-friendliness, and length. Reading level was modified and the survey shortened to 38 items. A panel of four nursing experts in complementary methods and patient education was asked then to review the survey for content validity. The panel established content validity, finding that survey items were sampled adequately from the empirical evidence on best practices for the three methods chosen and were consistent with both conceptual and operational definitions of knowledge, attitudes, and behaviors.

The Audit Instrument, an adapted version of Ferrell's standard of care audit instrument used in previous studies (Dufault & Willey-Lessne, 1999; Ferrell et al., 1995), was used to assure that each patient's complementary pain service nurse followed the best-practice protocols. An audit was conducted on each study patient's chart and determined to provide sufficient detail to facilitate judgment about whether the individualized pain treatment plans and protocols were followed.

The short form of the Miller Behavioral Style Scale (MBSS; Miller, 1987) was used to determine patients' preferred method for receiving information, also known as the patient's information-coping style. In the short form of the MBSS, two hypothetically stressful vignettes are presented, each with eight corresponding behavioral statements for dealing with the stressful situation. The patient is asked to read the vignettes and then each of the eight statements under the vignettes, marking *yes* if they would respond using a proposed behavior or *no* if they would not respond using a proposed behavior. Using a key furnished with the instrument, the researcher sums the number of *yes* and *no* responses across both vignettes. A total instrument score of 0 to 8 represents a *monitoring* information-coping style; a score of -1 to -8 represents a *blunting* information-coping style. The psychometric properties of the MBSS, to include construct, discriminant, and convergent validity, as well as reliability, have been documented in naturalistic, laboratory, and hypothetical settings (Cheng, Hui, & Lam, 2000; Miller, 1996; Rees & Bath, 2000; Ross & Maguire, 1995). In previous studies, Cronbach's alpha coefficients for MBSS subscales in medical settings ranged from .69 to .80 (monitoring) and .61 to .64 (blunting; Rees & Bath, 2000). Test–retest reliability has been reported as favorable ($r = .71$, $p < .05$); the monitoring subscale displayed the most utility in terms of its predictive value (Rees & Bath, 2000).

Databases for data collection and analysis were constructed using the Statistical Package for the Social Sciences (SPSS, version 12, Chicago, IL) and instruments for demographic data collection were developed for this substudy.

Procedures

Following approval of the institutional review board, data collection began. During preadmission testing, the research assistant explained the project to each patient and obtained informed consent. Demographic data, including prior use of several nondrug methods, were collected, and patients were assessed for information-coping style using the short form of the MBSS (Miller, 1987).

Patients then completed the 38-item NDCPI (Tracy, 2005). They were shown a videotape describing the use of music, imagery, and massage, and were given a teaching pamphlet that matched their scored information coping style. Content of the teaching pamphlet on music, imagery, and massage was based on best practice protocols developed in Step 3 of the CRU. Patients were reassured that best practice comfort measures would not replace any pharmacological pain interventions, but would be used as enhancements to the standard plan of postoperative care ordered by their physician.

Before departing, patients were asked to read the pamphlet at home and to practice preparatory techniques described in the pamphlet before returning for surgery. The night before surgery, each patient was contacted by telephone to assess his or her experiences with reading the pamphlet and practicing preparatory techniques, and to give the patient another chance to ask questions about involvement in the study.

On the day of surgery, patients were followed by a Comfort Therapy Service nurse when they returned to the unit following surgery. Each patient received use of a CD player and selected music, CDs for guided imagery, and requested massages. Patients were reassessed and evaluated by a Comfort Therapy Service nurse throughout the hospital stay.

Each evening during the hospital stay, specific data on the use of music, imagery, and massage were collected from patients using the Use of Non-Drug Complimentary Interventions (UNDCPI) Form (Tracy, 2005). The UNDCPI was a 9-item instrument developed and piloted in this study and used to track actual patient use of comfort enhancements during the 3-day hospital stay. To ensure that best-practice protocols were followed, the site coordinator, also the unit's clinical manager, monitored all patients, and a study-specific audit instrument was used to measure nurses' compliance to study protocols. On Postoperative Day 3, patients' knowledge, attitudes, and behaviors were reassessed using the NDCPI (Tracy, 2005).

Analysis of Substudy Data

Using SPSS, descriptive statistics (including frequencies, measures of central tendency, and standard deviations) were calculated for each of the demographic and dependent

TABLE 2. Characteristics of Sample Patients Undergoing Knee or Hip Total Joint Replacement Surgery ($N = 46$)

	n	%	M	SD
Information-coping style				
Monitors	40	87.0		
Blunters	6	13.0		
Age (years)			70.39	10.77
50–59	9	19.6		
60–69	10	21.8		
70–79	15	32.6		
80–89	12	26.0		
Gender				
Male	15	32.6		
Female	31	67.4		
Race				
White, non-Hispanic	45	97.8		
Black, non-Hispanic	1	2.2		
Marital status				
Married	21	45.7		
Single	4	8.7		
Divorced	7	15.2		
Widowed	14	30.4		
Education*			3.17	1.23
<High school diploma	4	8.7		
High school diploma	11	23.9		
Some college	12	26.1		
College graduate	11	23.9		
Graduate school	8	17.4		

Note. *Scale score for education: 1 = <HS diploma; 2 = HS diploma; 3 = some college; 4 = college graduate; 5 = graduate school.

variables of interest. Pearson r and Spearman rho correlations were calculated to determine relationships between each of the demographic and dependent variables of interest. Paired-sample t tests were used to evaluate changes in patients' knowledge, attitudes, and behaviors before (at preadmission testing time) and after the tailored teaching intervention (on the Postoperative Day 3). Statistical significance was set at $p < .05$.

Substudy Results

Demographic data (Table 2) and experience in using 12 of the most commonly used complementary pain management methods (Table 3) were collected. The three most commonly used nondrug interventions were prayer and meditation (58.8%), music (54.4%), and heat or cold (50%). Only 21.6% of the sample reported previously using massage and 13% reported previously using self-guided imagery.

There were significant relationships between age and information-coping style (Table 4). Also, education and

TABLE 3. Frequencies on Prior Use* of Nondrug Measures During Month Preceding Surgery (N = 46)

	n	%	M	SD
Prayer or meditation			1.89	1.65
No use	17	37.0		
Seldom	1	2.2		
Occasionally	9	19.6		
Frequently	9	19.5		
Very frequently	10	21.7		
Music			1.78	1.62
No use	17	37.0		
Seldom	4	8.7		
Occasionally	7	15.2		
Frequently	8	17.4		
Very frequently	10	21.7		
Heat or cold			1.41	1.31
No use	17	37.0		
Seldom	6	13.0		
Occasionally	13	28.3		
Frequently	7	15.2		
Very frequently	3	6.5		
Massage			0.63	1.14
No use	33	71.7		
Seldom	3	6.5		
Occasionally	6	13.0		
Frequently	2	4.4		
Very frequently	2	4.4		
Self-help education			0.57	1.13
No use	36	78.3		
Seldom	0	0.0		
Occasionally	5	10.8		
Frequently	4	8.7		
Very frequently	1	2.2		
Herbs			0.46	1.13
No use	38	82.6		
Seldom	2	4.3		
Occasionally	2	4.4		
Frequently	1	2.2		
Very frequently	3	6.5		
Acupressure			0.26	0.80
No use	41	89.1		
Seldom	0	0.0		
Occasionally	4	8.7		
Frequently	0	0.0		
Very frequently	1	2.2		
Aromatherapy			0.26	0.71
No use	40	86.9		
Seldom	1	2.2		

TABLE 3. (continued).

	n	%	M	SD
Occasionally	4	8.7		
Frequently	1	2.2		
Very frequently	0	0		
Acupuncture			0.22	0.66
No use	41	89.1		
Seldom	1	2.2		
Occasionally	3	6.5		
Frequently	1	2.2		
Very frequently	0	0		
Yoga			0.22	0.66
No use	41	89.1		
Seldom	1	2.2		
Occasionally	3	6.5		
Frequently	1	2.2		
Very frequently	0	0		
Reiki or therapeutic touch			0.13	0.54
No use	43	93.4		
Seldom	1	2.2		
Occasionally	1	2.2		
Frequently	1	2.2		
Very frequently	0	0		

Note. *Scale score for prior use: 0 = no use; 1 = seldom; 2 = occasional; 3 = frequently; 4 = very frequently.

prior use of music, imagery, and massage were found to be significantly correlated (Table 4).

Changes in Knowledge After using the teaching intervention, patients' knowledge scores on the Non-Drug Complementary Pain Intervention Survey increased on items related to the purposes and benefits of non-drug interventions (Table 5). A comparison of the means of specific knowledge related to each protocol showed that, following the tailored teaching intervention, there were statistically significant positive changes in patients' postintervention knowledge about each of the methods. For 12 of the 17 pairs of knowledge items on the NDCPI, the mean knowledge score changed from 57.82 (SD = 7.24) to 61.05 (SD = 4.39). A paired-samples *t* test was performed to compare the mean scores for total knowledge before and after the teaching intervention. A statistically significant positive difference in preintervention and postintervention means [total *t* score: $t(34) = 2.95$, $p < .05$] was obtained.

Changes in Attitudes Likewise, a paired samples *t* test was also performed to compare differences in the pre-intervention and post-intervention means for patient attitudes about using non-drug methods to complement pharmacological pain relief interventions (Table 5). Results showed that for 12 of the 13 items, patients had a statistically significant positive

TABLE 4. Bivariate Analysis of Prior Use of Music, Imagery, and Massage Against Age, Educational Level, Information-Coping Style (N = 46)

	Age (years)	Education	Prior Use of Nondrug Methods	Information-Coping Style
Age (years)	1.00			
Education	−.159	1.00		
Prior use of nondrug methods	−.143	.344*	1.00	
Information-coping style	−.420**	.156	.022	1.00

Note. r = Pearson r.
*Correlation is significant at the .05 level (two-tailed).
**Correlation is significant at the .01 level (two-tailed).

change ($p < .05$) in attitudes about using nondrug methods for pain management after the tailored teaching intervention. The mean score on the attitude survey changed from 48.36 (SD = 4.19) prior to the teaching intervention to 52.41 (SD = 6.23) after the teaching intervention. A statistically significant difference in attitude mean scores [$t(32) = 3.81$, $p < .01$] was obtained.

Changes in Use Data suggest that patients perceived they had the psychomotor ability to use the best-practice protocols, although they were unable to control lighting and environmental noise in the hospital setting. Patients used massage, music, and self-guided imagery with increasing frequency over the 4-day hospital stay, and became increasingly satisfied with the choices of nondrug enhancements (Table 6).

On the day of surgery and Postoperative Days 1, 2, and 3, correlations between patients' prior use of nondrug methods and use of the three nondrug methods during hospitalization showed there was a significant relationship ($\rho = .533$, $p < .01$) between prior use and current use only on the day of surgery (Table 7). Significant relationships were also found between Days 1 and 2 of postoperative recuperation, and Days 2 and 3 of recovery.

Finally, on a scale of 1 (*very dissatisfied*) to 5 (*very satisfied*), the overall satisfaction mean increased from 3.68 on the day of surgery to 4.16 on the third postoperative day [$t(30) = −3.03$, $p < .01$].

Discussion of Substudy

The CRU model was an essential component of the translation project and formed the critical framework of the project within which substudy results were obtained. The substudy sample was drawn from a population of older adults, mostly White, well educated with a predominantly monitoring information-coping style; generalizations are limited to patients with similar characteristics. The inverse correlation between age and information-coping style suggests that age may not be a good indicator of coping style. Perhaps as people get older, they seek more information regarding health matters. The positive correlation between education and prior use of nondrug methods suggests that individuals who have experienced more formal learning may be more inclined to seek out and use information about nondrug measures for pain relief.

Changes in Knowledge Patients increased in overall and specific knowledge scores about the purposes, benefits, and use of massage, music, and self-guided imagery to enhance pain management after using the tailored teaching intervention. This finding suggests that the tailored teaching intervention may play a distinct role in changing patients' knowledge related to the use of nondrug methods for pain management. Information-coping style may have played some role in the knowledge patients gained from the multimodal teaching approach used to inform and support patients' use of the best-practice nondrug protocols. This finding is useful as nurses seek to develop consistent approaches to overcoming the ongoing problems of poor retention and inattentiveness in teaching patients.

Changes in Attitudes The finding of significant improvement in patients' attitudes toward the best-practice protocols suggests that the teaching intervention may have positively influenced their attitudes about using the nondrug methods. Changes in attitudes are often underpinned by changes in knowledge and manifested by changes in behavior (Epstein, 1998). As a result, the findings about

TABLE 5. Changes in Knowledge and Attitudes Towards Music, Self-Guided Imagery, and Massage After Tailored Teaching Intervention

	N	Pretest Mean Score	N	Posttest Mean Score	Change Score	Paired Samples t test	p Value
Knowledge	45	57.82	35	61.05	3.23	2.95	<.01
Attitudes	44	48.36	34	52.41	4.05	3.81	<.01

TABLE 6. Frequencies and Descriptive Statistics for Patients' Use of Music, Self-Guided Imagery, and Massage for Day of Surgery and Days 1, 2, and 3 of Postoperative Recuperation

	n	M	SD
How many times during the past 24 hours have you used music to help relieve your pain?*			
Day of surgery	38	1.63	1.22
Post op Day 1	40	2.55	1.63
Post op Day 2	40	3.08	1.53
Post op Day 3	37	3.08	1.67
How many times during the past 24 hours have you used imagery to help relieve your pain?			
Day of surgery	38	1.34	0.994
Post op Day 1	40	1.78	1.42
Post op Day 2	39	1.92	1.46
Post op Day 3	36	2.14	1.78
How many times did you use music and imagery together over the past 24 hours?			
Day of surgery	37	1.35	1.01
Post op Day 1	39	1.77	1.42
Post op Day 2	36	1.94	1.53
Post op Day 3	32	2.03	1.67
How many times did you request a massage over the past 24 hours?			
Day of surgery	37	1.38	0.545
Post op Day 1	38	1.63	0.714
Post op Day 2	40	1.73	0.751
Post op Day 3	36	1.61	0.803

Note. *Use rubric: 1 = none; 2 = one; 3 = two; 4 = three; 5 = four; 6 = five or more (times); Post op day = day of postoperative recuperation.

changes in attitudes are believed to amplify the findings on knowledge.

Changes in Use The inclusion of specific information in the teaching pamphlet on how to use the nondrug methods appeared to be sufficient for patients to use each method successfully. The significant correlations between patients' prior use of nondrug methods and use of massage, music, and imagery on the day of surgery was an unexpected finding because it was believed that they would be too sleepy from anesthesia to want to use the complementary interventions on the day of surgery. The finding suggests that patients relied on their positive past experiences with nondrug methods to aid them on the day of surgery, or they were motivated to use the protocols on the day of surgery when they anticipated having a great deal of pain, or both.

The strong correlations between use and day of hospitalization suggests that patients found the use of the best practices to be beneficial in managing their pain and were motivated to use them progressively more each day of their stay. This finding supports the notion that beneficial outcomes tend to create a self-satisfying cycle of continuous use, thereby enhancing patient comfort and reinforcing patient attitudes about using complementary measures for pain management in the future. Confirmation of use findings was also demonstrated by patients' increasingly positive satisfaction scores with their pain management plans over the first 3 days of the hospital stay.

Temporal Issues During the substudy, questions were raised about whether such best-practice protocols could be integrated into the everyday caregiving activities of nurses on a busy acute care unit. Nurse managers and researchers were concerned about the time it would take for nurses to carry out the protocols. As the study proceeded, it became clear that there were not enough nurses from all shifts trained in the use of the best-practice protocols. As a result, all staff members were oriented to the project and trained in the protocols. Nurses reported that implementation of study protocols did not interfere with their other nursing responsibilities, and the interventions took, on average, only 12 to 15 minutes.

Step 5. Decide to Sustain, Alter, or Discontinue the Standards, Policies, or Protocols
Following completion and analysis of primary efficacy study findings, Step 5 consists of staff and nursing administration deciding to adopt the best-practice protocols and integrate them into practice, or to reject them. Results of the primary efficacy study will be published later, although the decision whether or not to adopt the best-practice protocols may be made tentatively by nursing staff and administration using the results of the substudy. Within the organizational structure of the hospital, through the Policy and Procedure Committee and Joint Practice Committee, staff members will collaborate to make a decision about the ongoing use of the tailored teaching intervention for future patients.

Recently, the principal investigator met with the Director of Volunteers at the hospital who inquired about the project and volunteered to assist in ensuring that patients and nurses have the supplies they need to carry out the comfort protocols. The volunteers have chosen to do this as one of their major projects in the coming year. In January 2005, 13 volunteers were trained and supplies were purchased so that all of the patients at the study site can receive the services of the Comfort Therapy Service. Beginning in February, the volunteers began to make regular rounds with a Comfort Therapy Cart to offer changes in the selection of music and guided imagery tapes and lotions for use during massage. In addition to the patients in the study, over 300 patients have used the comfort therapy services as of June 2005.

Step 6. Develop a Way to Disseminate and Extend the Innovation to Other Appropriate Settings
The comfort service protocols have been integrated into continuing education and in-service programs at the hospital. Findings will be shared also with clinicians at the hospital through presentations at an upcoming major

TABLE 7. Bivariate Correlations Between Patients' Prior Use of Music, Self-Guided Imagery, and Massage, and Actual Use by Day of Postoperative Hospital Stay

	Day of Surgery	Postoperative Day 1	Postoperative Day 2	Postoperative Day 3	Prior Use
Day of surgery	1.00				
Spearman ρ	–				
n	36				
Postoperative Day 1	.443**	1.00			
Spearman ρ	.009	–			
n	34	37			
Postoperative Day 2	.432**	.831**	1.00		
Spearman rho	.015	.000	–		
n	31	32	35		
Postoperative Day 3	.436*	.571**	.694**	1.00	
Spearman rho	.023	.002	.000	–	
n	27	26	27	31	
Prior use	.533**	.159	.120	.043	1.00
Spearman rho	.001	.346	.493	.818	–
n	36	37	35	31	31

Note. *Correlation is significant at the .05 level (two-tailed). **Correlation is significant at the .01 level (two-tailed).

conference sponsored by the hospital. The study was presented in 2005 at the Eastern Nursing Research Conference held in New York City, the Sigma Theta Tau International Research Conference held in Hawaii, and a local chapter of Sigma Theta Tau in Rhode Island. Additional manuscripts on the project are in progress and will be submitted to leading journals.

Conclusions and Recommendations

Future studies with the tailored teaching intervention should be conducted where populations are more heterogeneous in terms of race, educational experience, and information-coping style. Tailoring patient teaching interventions about the use of nondrug pain interventions to their information-coping style may have the power to transform the patient's role from one of passive recipient of care to one of active participant and regulator of his or her own care.

Additional testing and refinement of survey instruments is needed to demonstrate reliability and further demonstrate construct and content validity, and to obtain more information about the survey's internal consistency. Future survey work might also include a Delphi study of experts in perioperative teaching and complementary pain interventions to determine the verifiability of the best-practice protocols in a larger nursing practice arena.

The validity of the process of tailoring the teaching pamphlets to patients' information-coping styles requires additional attention. Results of the substudy suggest that the use of tailored teaching interventions may improve patients' knowledge, attitudes, and use of nondrug methods to enhance pain management. The increased use of music, self-guided imagery, and massage throughout the hospital stay demonstrates the ease of use and the desire patients have to play a part in managing their own pain.

The climate of receptivity to research that characterizes the organization in which the study was conducted cannot be overstated. A critical element in the conduct and translation of research using the CRU model is administrative support for research and an attitude of scientific inquiry. Such attitudes transcend the routinization of care and empower nurses to advance practice through the discovery, validation, and integration of new practices that improve patient care. Characteristics of the study hospital, staff commitment to improving pain management care, and the proactive nursing department staff contributed substantially to the development and use of a complementary pain service.

Finally, a well-integrated computerized documentation system for cueing clinicians' pain management practices was in place and further strengthened the potential for changing practice at this hospital. Selection of sites for future translation research studies should include examining such organizational features to provide clearly defined environments for study and facilitate adoption and integration of novel approaches to care. Effectiveness of the CRU model provides for connections among research faculty, students, and members of the nursing community and facilitates the synergy for change essential to advancing practice. Student involvement facilitates future incorporation of complementary interventions into patient care and provides students and clinicians with an experiential opportunity to learn the process of translating research findings to solve day-to-day clinical problems. The use of this translation research model to change clinician practice and sustain organizational change incorporates directions established by the National Institute of Nursing Research, *Healthy People 2010*, and AHRQ to create meaningful change resulting in clinical interventions to reduce the toll of physical pain, especially on older people. ▼

Accepted for publication November 21, 2005.

The research was funded by The Mayday Fund, Delta Upsilon Chapter of Sigma Theta Tau, and the New Hampshire State Nurses Association.

The authors thank the Newport Hospital Comfort Therapy Service and nursing staff of Turner 2 and Vanderbilt Rehabilitation who had the courage to open their practice to the eyes of research. Without an organization that invites innovation, we would not have been able to explore and reveal the nature of practices related to complementary pain management interventions. Appreciation is extended to Mary Lavin, FNP, RN, and Patricia Stout, FNP, RN, Clinical Assistant Professors; to Sandra McPherson, MS, RN, and Lisa Sullivan, MS, RN, former graduate assistants; and to the Class of 2004 undergraduate nursing students in the College of Nursing at the University of Rhode Island.

Corresponding author: Marlene Dufault, PhD, RN, College of Nursing, University of Rhode Island, 133 White Hall, Kingston, RI 02881 (e-mail: marlened@uri.edu).

References

American Geriatrics Society Panel on Persistent Pain in Older Persons. (2002). The management of persistent pain in older persons. *Journal of the American Geriatrics Society, 50*(6 Suppl.), S205–S224.

Ardery, G., Herr, K. A., Titler, M. G., Sorofman, B. A., & Schmitt, M. B. (2003). Assessing and managing acute pain in older adults: A research base to guide practice. *Medsurg Nursing, 12*(1), 7–19.

Bell, M. L. (1997). Postoperative pain management for the cognitively impaired older adult. *Seminars in Perioperative Nursing, 6*(1), 37–41.

Bell, M. L., & Reeves, K. A. (1999). Postoperative pain management in the non-Hispanic white and Mexican-American older adult. *Seminars in Perioperative Nursing, 8*(1), 7–11.

Brockopp, D. Y., Downey, E., Powers, P., Vanderveer, B., Warden, S., Ryan, P., et al. (2004). Nurses' clinical decision-making regarding the management of pain. *International Journal of Nursing Studies, 41*(6), 631–636.

Brown, D. (2004). A literature review exploring how healthcare professionals contribute to the assessment and control of postoperative pain in older people. *Journal of Clinical Nursing, 13*(6B), 74–90.

Brown, S. T. (2000). Outcomes analysis of a pain management project for two rural hospitals. *Journal of Nursing Care Quality, 14*(4), 28–34.

Cheng, C., Hui, W.-M., & Lam, S.-K. (2000). Perceptual style and behavioral pattern of individuals with functional gastro-intestinal disorders. *Health Psychology, 19*(2), 146–154.

Clarke, E. B., French, B., Bilodeau, M. L., Capasso, V. C., Edwards, A., & Empoliti, J. (1996). Pain management knowledge, attitudes and clinical practice: The impact of nurses' characteristics and education. *Journal of Pain and Symptom Management, 11*(1), 18–31.

Dufault, M. (2004). Using a collaborative research utilization model to translate best practices in pain management. *Worldviews on Evidence-Based Nursing, 1*(Supplement), S26–32.

Dufault, M. A., Bielecki, C., Collins, E., & Willey, C. (1995). Changing nurses' pain assessment practice: A collaborative

research utilization approach. *Journal of Advanced Nursing, 21*(4), 634–645.

Dufault, M. A., & Sullivan, M. (2000). Using a research utilization model to develop and test research-based pain management standards. *Journal of Professional Nursing, 16*(4), 240–250.

Dufault, M. A., & Willey-Lessne, C. (1999). Using a collaborative research utilization model to develop and test the effects of clinical pathways on pain management. *Journal of Nursing Care Quality, 13*(4), 19–33.

Dufault, M., Willey-Tempkin, C., Schwager, J., & Hockhausen, K. (2002, March). Improving outcomes in home care pain management. Presentation at the Eastern Nursing Research Society, State College, PA.

Ebener, M. K. (1999). Older adults living with chronic pain: An opportunity for improvement. *Journal of Nursing Care Quality, 13*(4), 1–7.

Epstein, S. (1998). Personal control from the perspective of cognitive-experiential self-theory. In M. Kofta, G. Weary, & G. Sedek (Eds.), *Personal control in action: Cognitive and motivational mechanisms* (pp. 5–26). New York: Plenum.

Fang, C. F., Miller, S. M., Daly, M. B., & Hurley, K. (2001). The influence of attentional style and risk perceptions on intentions to undergo prophylactic oophorectomy among FDRs. *Psychology and Health, 17*, 365–376.

Ferrell, B., Whedon, M., & Rollins, B. (1995). Pain and quality assessment/improvement. *Journal of Nursing Care Quality, 9*(3), 69–85.

Fink, R., Thompson, C. J., & Bonnes, D. (2005). Overcoming barriers and promoting the use of research in practice. *Journal of Nursing Administration, 35*(3), 121–129.

Holley, S., McMillan, S. C., Hagan, S. J., Palacios, P., & Rosenberg, D. (2005). Pain resource nurses: Believing the patients, and believing in themselves. *Oncology Nursing Forum, 32*(4), 843–848.

Horgas, A. L., & McLennon, S. M. (2003). Pain management. In M. Mezey, T. Fulmer, I. Abraham, & D. A. Zwicker (Eds.), *Geriatric nursing protocols for best practice* (2nd ed., pp. 229–250). New York: Springer.

Horsley, J. A., Crane, J., & Bingle, J. (1978). Research utilization as an organizational process. *Journal of Nursing Administration, 8*(7), 4–6.

Innis, J., Bikaunieks, N., Petryshen, P., Zellermeyer, V., & Ciccarelli, L. (2004). Patient satisfaction and pain management: An educational approach. *Journal of Nursing Care Quality, 19*(4), 322–327.

Janken, J. K., & Dufault, M. A. (2002). Improving the quality of pain assessment through research utilization. *Online Journal of Knowledge Synthesis for Nursing, 9*, 2C.

Janken, J. K., Dufault, M. A., & Yeaw, E. M. (1998). Research roundtables: Increasing student/staff nurse awareness of the relevancy of research to practice. *Journal of Professional Nursing, 4*(3), 186–191.

Kelly, A. (2003). Integrating Joint Commission on Accreditation of Healthcare Organizations Standards into pain management practices. *Home Health Care Management & Practice, 15*(3), 231–236.

Kreuter, M. W., Strecher, V. J., & Glassman, B. (1999). One size does not fit all: The case for tailoring print materials. *Annals of Behavioral Medicine, 21*(4), 276–283.

Kwekkeboom, K. L. (2003). Music versus distraction for procedural pain and anxiety in patients with cancer. *Oncology Nursing Forum, 30*(3), 433–440.

Marcum, J., Ridenour, M., Shaff, G., Hammons, M., & Taylor, M. (2002). A study of professional nurses' perceptions of patient education. *Journal of Continuing Education in Nursing, 33*(3), 112–118.

McCaffery, M., & Robinson, E. S. (2002). Your patient is in pain: Here's how you respond. *Nursing, 23,* 327–333.

MacLellan, K. (2004). Postoperative pain: Strategy for improving patient experiences. *Journal of Advanced Nursing, 46*(2), 179–185.

McDonald, D. D., Thomas, G. J., Livingston, K. E., & Severson, J. S. (2005). Assisting older adults to communicate their postoperative pain. *Clinical Nursing Research, 14*(2), 109–126.

McMillan, S. C., Tittle, M., Hagan, S., Laughlin, J., & Tabler, R. E., Jr. (2000). Knowledge and attitudes of nurses in veterans hospitals about pain management in patients with cancer. *Oncology Nursing Forum, 27*(9), 1415–1423.

McMillan, S., Tittle, M., Hagan, S., & Small, B. (2005). Training pain resource nurses: Changes in their knowledge and attitudes. *Oncology Nursing Forum, 32*(4), 835–842.

Miller, S. M. (1987). Monitoring and blunting: Validation of a questionnaire to assess styles of information seeking under threat. *Journal of Personality and Social Psychology, 52*(2), 345–353.

Miller, S. (1996). Monitoring and blunting of threatening information: Cognitive interference and facilitation in the coping process. In I. G. Sarason, G. R. Pierce, & B. R. Sarason (Eds.), *Cognitive interference: Theories, methods, and findings* (pp. 175–190). Mahwah, NJ: Lawrence Erlbaum.

Miller, S. M., Fang, C. Y., Diefenbach, M. A., & Bales, C. (2001). Tailoring psychosocial interventions to the individual's health information processing style: The influence of monitoring versus blunting in cancer risk and disease. In A. Baum, & B. Anderson (Eds.), *Psychosocial interventions in cancer* (pp. 343–362). Washington, DC: American Psychological Association.

Miller, S. M., Sherman, K., Buzaglo, J., & Rodoletz, M. (2001). Monitoring–blunting behavioral signatures in coping with health threats: The example of cancer. *Psicologia della Salute, 3,* 37–48.

Momtahan, K., Berkman, J., Sellick, J., Kearns, S. A., & Lauzon, N. (2004). Patients' understanding of cardiac risk factors: A point-prevalence study. *Journal of Cardiovascular Nursing, 19*(1), 13–20.

Ni, H., Nauman, D., Burgess, D., Wise, K., Crispell, K., & Hershberger, R. E. (1999). Factors influencing knowledge of and adherence to self-care among patients with heart failure. *Archives of Internal Medicine, 159*(14), 1613–1619.

Nikolaus, T., & Zeyfang, A. (2004). Pharmacological treatments for persistent non-malignant pain in older persons. *Drugs & Aging, 21*(1), 19–41.

Press Ganey. (2002). *Health care satisfaction report.* Indianapolis, IN: Author.

Rappolt, S., Pearce, K., McEwen, S., & Polatajko, H. J. (2005). Exploring organizational characteristics associated with practice changes following a mentored online educational module. *Journal of Continuing Education in the Health Professions, 25*(2), 116–124.

Reed, J. (2005). Using action research in nursing practice with older people: Democratizing knowledge. *Journal of Clinical Nursing, 14*(5), 594–600.

Rees, C. E., & Bath, P. A. (2000). The psychometric properties of the Miller Behavioural Style Scale with adult daughters of women with early breast cancer: A literature review and empirical study. *Journal of Advanced Nursing, 32*(2), 366–374.

Ross, C. J. M., & Maguire, T. O. (1995). Informational coping styles: A validity study. *Journal of Nursing Measurement, 3,* 145–158.

Saarman, L., Daugherty, J., & Riegel, B. (2000). Patient teaching to promote behavioral change. *Nursing Outlook, 48*(6), 281–287.

Sauaia, A., Min, S.-J., Leber, C., Erbacher, K., Abrams, F., & Fink, R. (2005). Postoperative pain management in elderly patients: Correlation between adherence to treatment guidelines and patient satisfaction. *Journal of the American Geriatrics Society, 53*(2), 274–282.

Scott-Findlay, S., & Golden-Biddle, K. (2005). Understanding how organizational culture shapes research use. *Journal of Nursing Administration, 35*(7–8), 359–365.

Sherwood, G. D., McNeill, J. A., Starck, P. L., & Disnard, G. (2003). Changing acute pain management outcomes in surgical patients. *AORN Journal, 77*(2), 374, 377–380, 384–390.

Stetler, C. B., Brunell, M., Guiliano, K. K., Morsi, D., Prince, L., & Newell-Stokes, G. (1998). Evidence-based practice and the role of nursing leadership. *Journal of Nursing Administration, 28*(7–8), 45–53.

Suls, J., & Wan, C. K. (1989). Effects of sensory and procedural information on coping with stressful medical procedures and pain: A meta-analysis. *Journal of Consulting and Clinical Psychology, 57*(3), 372–379.

Tracy, S. (2005). A pilot study of tailored teaching on nondrug enhancements for managing post-operative pain. Unpublished doctoral dissertation, University of Rhode Island, Kingston.

United States Department of Health and Human Services, Agency for Healthcare Research and Quality. (1992). Clinicians' quick reference guide to postoperative pain management in adults. *Journal of Pain and Symptom Management, 7,* 214–228.

United States Department of Health and Human Services, Agency for Healthcare Research and Quality. (2001, July). Making health care safer: Critical analysis of patient safety practices. *Evidence Report/Technology Assessment No. 43,* AHRQ Publication No. 01-E058, Rockville, MD: U.S. Department of Health and Human Services.

Vallerand, A. H., Fouladbakhsh, J., & Templin, T. (2005). Patients' choices for the self-treatment of pain. *Applied Nursing Research, 18*(2), 90–96.

Watkins, L. O., Weaver, L., & Odegaard, V. (1986). Preparation for cardiac catheterization: Tailoring the content of instruction to coping style. *Heart & Lung, 15*(4), 382–389.

Watt-Watson, J., Chung, F., Chan, V. W. S., & McGillion, M. (2004). Pain management following discharge after ambulatory same-day surgery. *Journal of Nursing Management, 12*(3), 153–161.

Wessman, A. C., & McDonald, D. D. (1999). Nurses' personal pain experiences and their pain management knowledge. *Journal of Continuing Education in Nursing, 30*(4), 152–157.

White, L. (1999). Competence: The basis of pain management. *Journal of Nursing Care Quality, 13*(4), 86–89.

Zalon, M. L. (1997). Pain in frail, elderly women after surgery. *Image: The Journal of Nursing Scholarship, 29,* 21–26.

**Western Journal of
Nursing Research**
Volume 29 Number 3
April 2007 344-356
© 2007 Sage Publications
10.1177/0193945906296564
http://wjn.sagepub.com
hosted at
http://online.sagepub.com

A Meta-Analysis of
Interventions for Informal
Stroke Caregivers

JuHee Lee
Karen Soeken
Sandra J. Picot
University of Maryland School of Nursing, Baltimore

The purpose of this study is to examine the effectiveness of the interventions for improving mental health of caregivers of people with stroke by synthesizing individual studies. A meta-analysis was performed to summarize findings of intervention studies of caregivers of elderly stroke patients. Additionally, a sensitivity analysis and a publication bias were tested. The overall mean weighted effect size (MWES) for the four studies is 0.277 ($Z = 3.432$, $p = .001$) with a 95% CI .118 to .435 ($N = 718$) indicating that the intervention was effective in improving the mental health of informal stroke caregivers. The MWES for the education program was 0.354 ($Z = 2.613$, $p < .01$) and for the support program was .234 ($Z = 2.335$, $p = .02$). The MWES for the Europe study was .219 ($Z = 2.613$, $p < .01$) and for the United States was .922 ($Z = 3.287$, $p = .001$). The results show that overall interventions improved mental health of informal stroke caregivers. The small number of studies included in the meta-analysis limits the generalizability of results while supporting the need for more research in this area.

Keywords: *stroke; informal caregiver; intervention; mental health; meta-analysis*

Since the late 1970s, there have been studies of interventions for caregivers designed to reduce the negative impact of caregiving (Acton & Kang, 2001). Despite the high prevalence of stroke and the high potential burden of family caregiving for caregivers of stroke patients (Wright et al., 1999), most of the study populations have been caregivers of dementia patients.

Authors' Note: Please address correspondence to JuHee Lee, University of Maryland, School of Nursing, Room 311R, 655 West Lombard Street, Baltimore, MD, 21201; e-mail: jlee@son.umaryland.edu.

At least 50 to 75% of stroke patients are left with chronic neurological or cognitive impairments (American Heart Association, 2005) and almost half need the assistance of unpaid informal caregivers, such as family members (Horner, 1998). Many studies have focused on the determinants of psychological outcomes of caregivers such as burden, stress, strain, costs, hassles, or depression from the caregiving experience. Based on these findings, researchers have tested interventions designed to improve the mental health of caregivers. The authors, however, were unable to locate any study reporting a comprehensive evaluation of the effects of these interventions on the mental health of stroke caregivers.

Purpose, Research Question, and Variable Definitions

The purpose of this meta-analysis was to examine the effectiveness of interventions for improving the mental health of caregivers of stroke patients by synthesizing across studies. The research question was: What are the effects of interventions on the mental health of informal stroke caregivers?

In this meta-analysis, mental health was defined as a psychological state as measured by the Short Form Health Survey (SF-36). The SF-36 is one of the most widely used measures of health status that has been used with stroke patients and caregivers (Anderson, Laubscher, & Burns, 1996; Bakas & Champion, 1999; Hoabart, Williams, Moran, & Thompson, 2002; Hobson, Bhowmick, & Meara, 1997). Hoabart and colleagues (2002) stated, "The Medical Outcomes Study 36-item Short-Form Health Survey (SF-36) is a widely used, generic, patient-report, health status measure. In neurology, the SF-36 has been used in stroke—a MEDLINE search indicates more than 30 articles."

The specific outcome was the difference in the SF-36 mental health score between the experimental group and the control group. The independent variable included any type of intervention that was implemented for informal stroke caregivers to improve their mental health.

Methods

Literature Search

Searches were performed using MEDLINE (1966-2005) and Cumulative Index for Nursing and Allied Health Literature (CINAHL, 1982-2005) computerized databases. The searches were limited to articles published in the English language using combinations of the keywords caregiving, stroke caregiver, stroke caregiving, control group, and interventions. For the keyword search, the author wanted to identify experimental studies with stroke caregivers. The database searches of MEDLINE and CINAHL revealed a total of 30 articles. A citation search of the Social Sciences Citation Index and Science Citation Index yielded one additional article for inclusion. In addition, the Cochrane library search to find additional studies resulted in the same finding as that found in the computerized database searches. Unpublished studies were not included in this meta-analysis because they have not undergone peer review.

Study Selection

Abstracts of the 31 studies identified through the search were independently reviewed by the first author for inclusion in this meta-analysis. The inclusion criteria were (a) sample included informal caregivers of stroke patients; (b) intervention for stroke caregivers to improve their mental health; (c) outcome variables include the SF-36; (d) quantitative study; and (e) use of a comparison group on the outcome measure. From the 31 abstracts, only 11 articles met the inclusion criteria.

Based on a review of the 11 studies, 7 articles were excluded due for various reasons including: (a) using the SF-36 outcome, but not reporting the data (Dennis, O'Rourke, Slattery, Staniforth, & Warlow, 1997; Printz-Feddersen, 1990); (b) inadequate descriptive statistics (Grant, 1999); (c) not presenting caregivers' data in results section (Forster & Young, 1996; Lincoln, Francis, Lilley, Sharma, & Summerfield, 2003; Mayo et al., 2000); and (d) only reporting qualitative data (Stewart, Doble, Hart, Langille, & MacPherson, 1998). Finally, 4 studies were retained for this meta-analysis.

Data Collection Methods

After initially reviewing the four studies to be included in this meta-analysis, variables were selected for inclusion in the codebook. Coded were: first author, year, design, number of subjects in each group (experimental and control), intervention characteristics, theoretical background for the intervention, intervention period, setting, data collection period, attrition rate, and statistical results. The first author and a second coder independently extracted data from all four studies. Coder agreement was initially 95.8%. Coders then reviewed items for which there was lack of agreement. After discussion, consensus was reached on all items. The data extracted were entered into an EXCEL file.

For the quality rating, several items were selected from a quality measure previously used by Soeken and colleagues (2002). These items assessed study aim, randomization, blinding, attrition, statistical testing, and the discussion section. Using this quality rating scale, the range of total quality points is 0 to 16. Because all the studies used a randomized design, and treatment personnel conducted the interventions, the quality assessment scale specifically addressed blinding of caregivers, treatment personnel, or data collector. Studies with scores of 0 to 9 were considered *low quality* and those with scores 10 to 16 were considered *high quality*.

All studies were assessed for quality by two independent raters. The agreement rate between the two raters was 90%. Following discussion, the raters reached consensus for all items. Quality scores for four studies ranged from 9 to 13. One study was rated *low quality* because no one was blinded (Van den Heuvel et al., 2002). The remaining three were rated *high quality* (Grant, Elliot, Warver, Bartolucci, & Giger, 2002; Mant, Carter, Wade, & Winner, 2000; Rodgers et al., 1999).

Statistical Methods

An effect size (d) was calculated for each of the individual studies converting the reported statistics into the standardized effect size. The raw effect sizes were weighted for study sample size because raw effect sizes from studies with small samples are prone to overestimate the population effect size (Shadish & Haddock, 1994). An overall mean weighted effect size for the four studies was calculated. Additionally, 95% confidence intervals were calculated for each effect size.

To assess sensitivity of the results, mean weighted effect sizes were computed by study quality rating. Subgroup analyses examined differences regarding types of intervention (*education/support*), presence of a theoretical background for creating the intervention (*yes/no*), and study setting (*Europe/United States*). Finally, potential publication bias was assessed using the fail-safe N.

Results

General Descriptions

The four study samples included 718 individuals with a large proportion of women (71.7%). The mean age of the subjects was 61.1 years. All of the studies used randomized controlled designs.

Three studies (Mant et al., 2000; Rodgers et al., 1999; Van den Heuvel et al., 2002) were conducted in Europe (U.K. and the Netherlands) and only one study (Grant et al., 2002) was done in the United States. The interventions were held in community settings and were either an education program (Grant et al., 2002; Rodgers et al., 1999) or a support program (Mant et al., 2000; Van den Heuvel et al., 2002) for caregivers. One study (Van den Heuvel et al., 2002) used the stress, appraisal, and coping theory by Lazarus & Folkman (1984) for creating the intervention, and another (Grant et al., 2002) used D'Zurilla and Nezu's (1999) work on problem-solving therapy. The remaining two studies did not specify the theoretical framework used.

The intervention period varied between studies (Table 1). Two studies were conducted over 6 to 12 weeks (Grant et al. 2002; Van den Heuvel et al., 2002). One study did not report the intervention period but counted the frequency for caregivers' participating in the program as greater than three times (Rodgers et al., 1999).

For the education program, interventions consisted of identifying and defining problems, determining what needs to be done, possible solutions, selecting the best solution, and assessing outcomes of problem solving. Regarding knowledge of stroke, topics included nature of stroke, role of physical and occupational therapy, psychological effects of stroke, and care for a stroke patient such as communication with the patient, management of swallowing problems of patient, and reduction of stroke recurrence. In the support program, expressing emotions, receiving information, and learning how to use active coping strategies, discussing emotions regarding stroke occurrence, dealing with social networks, and handling caregiver stress and health promotion were included.

The data collection period varied. Final data collection occurred 13 weeks postdischarge (Grant et al., 2002), 6 months after the stroke (Mant, Carter, Wade, & Winner, 2000; Rodgers et al., 1999), and 7 months after the completion of the program (Van den Heuvel et al., 2002).

Pooled Results

Effect sizes and 95% confidence intervals for each individual study and for the overall mean weighted effect size (MWES) were calculated (Figure 1). Effect sizes ranged from 0 to .92. The four studies had varied effect with an overall MWES of 0.277 ($p < .001$) with a 95% CI from .118 to .435 ($N = 718$). Thus, across the four studies the results indicate that the intervention was effective in improving the mental health of informal stroke caregivers (Table 2).

Table 1
Summary of Sample Studies

First Author	Mean Age	Intervention	Interview Period
Grant (2002)	Men 58 ± 12 Women 56 ± 12	3–4 weeks poststroke, initial 3 hour meeting in home; thereafter weekly telephone sessions 2–4 weeks postdischarge, and biweekly weeks 6, 8, 10, and 12 postdischarge.	1–2 days predischarge, 5–9 weeks postdischarge, and 13 weeks postdischarge.
Van den Heuvel (2002)	Group program 66.4 Home visits 63.2 Control 60.8	6 months to 3.5 (3.81) years poststroke. Group support consists of 8 weeks group program (8 meetings, 16 hrs of education), or an 8–10 weeks home visit program (4 visits, 8 hrs of education)	Started within 4 weeks following the baseline interview, second interview was approximately 14 weeks postbaseline and final interview 6 months after second interview.
Mant (2000)	Family support 65.1 Control 63.7	Intervention began within 6 weeks of stroke. Nature and frequency of interaction was based on the judgment of the family support organizer. Included an average of one hospital visit, one home visit, and three telephone calls, and referral to one other service.	6 months after stroke and intervention, subjects were interviewed.
Rodgers (1999)	Stroke Education Program 58 Control 60	One hour inpatient small group educational session, followed by 6-hourly sessions postdischarge. A minimum of three session attendances required for completion.	6 months poststroke participants were interviewed.

Study Guide for Essentials of Nursing Research: Appraising Evidence for Nursing Practice, 7e

Figure 1
Effect Sizes and 95% Confidence Intervals

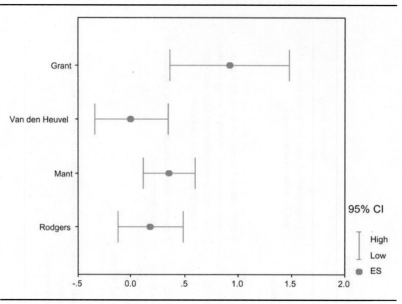

Table 2
Study Effect Sizes

First Author	Exp (n1)	Control (n2)	Total (N)	Effect Size (d)	95%CI Lower	95%CI Upper	p Value
Grant (2002)	42	21	63	0.922	0.361	1.482	0.001
Van den Heuvel (2002)	170	42	212	0	−0.34	0.34	1
Mant (2000)	130	137	267	0.355	0.112	0.597	0.004
Rodgers (1999)	107	69	176	0.181	−0.124	0.487	0.24
Combined	449	269	718	0.277	0.118	0.435	0.001

Subgroup Analyses

The variability of effect sizes was examined using the Q-statistic and found to be significant ($Q = 8.65$, $df = 3$, $p = .05$). Heterogeneity was partitioned according to the types of intervention characteristics. Between the education and support programs, there was no variability. However, the two studies with an education program differed significantly from one another because one study (Grant et al., 2002) had an effect size of .922. For the two studies with a support program, the effect sizes did not differ statistically. Interestingly, the two studies that used a theory-based intervention had the largest and smallest effect sizes (.92 and 0, respectively).

To describe the effectiveness of the different characteristics of intervention combined in this meta-analysis, a MWES was calculated for subgroups of studies for descriptive purposes (Figure 2). The MWES for the education programs was 0.354 ($p < .01$) with 95% CI of .087 to .621. The MWES for the support programs was .234 ($p = .02$) with 95% CI of .037 to .432. The MWES for studies having theory-based intervention studies was .253 ($p = .09$) with 95% CI of $-.036$ to .542. For atheoretical intervention studies, the MWES was .287 ($p < .01$) with 95% CI of .098 to .477. The MWES for studies conducted in Europe was .219 ($p < .01$) with 95% CI of .053 to .384 and for the one United States study was .922 ($p = .001$) with 95% CI of .360 to .1.482.

Sensitivity Analyses

A sensitivity analysis was performed based on the study quality rating to assess the judgment while doing research synthesis. Three of the four studies scored between 11 and 13 on the quality assessment and were considered a *high quality* study whereas the one remaining study was considered a *low quality* study. The MWES for the high quality studies was .354 ($p < .001$) with a 95% CI of .175 to .534 whereas the MWES for the low quality study that did not use the blinding method was 0 with a 95% CI of -.340 to .340 (Figure 2). Results indicate that interventions in high quality studies that used blinding were significant in improving mental health of stroke caregivers whereas the low quality study did not.

Publication Bias

A fail-safe N = 13 was calculated for the four studies using the Rosenthal's (1984) formula. This reflects the number of studies having an average effect of zero needed to decrease the overall effect to nonsignificance (Becker, 1994). Because $N_F S$ was less than the "reasonable" value, there is evidence of publication bias according to Rosenthal (1984). These biases might reflect editors' acceptance for publication, authors' decision not to submit an article, nonsignificant findings, or study design issues (Conn, Valentine,

Figure 2
Subgroup Analyses Results: Mean Effect Sizes and 95%
Confidence Intervals

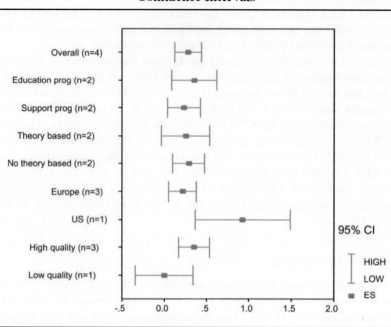

Cooper, & Rantz, 2003; Soeken & Sripusanapan, 2003). An additional source of bias in this meta-analysis might be the inclusion of only bias in favor of significant findings, which tend to be introduced in English language studies (Egger & Smith, 1998).

Discussion

The purpose of this meta-analysis was to examine the effectiveness of interventions for improving the mental health of caregivers of stroke patients. This meta-analysis indicated that, overall interventions improved mental health of informal stroke caregivers. The results are important because mental health decline, such as burden, depression, and strain, is one of the most commonly reported problems with informal caregivers (Pinquart & Sorensen, 2003; White, Lauzon, Yaffe, & Wood-Dauphinee, 2004).

There were several limitations in this study. First, as noted previously, this study included only published studies, which had undergone peer review. Restricting the meta-analysis to published literature may overestimate effect sizes. Second, only English language studies were included. Third, we used only one specific outcome measure, SF-36, as the measure of mental health. Whereas this approach may increase the precision of estimates, it limits generalizability to other outcome measures. With these decisions, the meta-analysis included only a small number of studies focused on stroke caregivers.

In this study, the effect and quality ratings of education program interventions were larger than support programs. The goal of support program might have been too broad, whereas education programs used more focused content. Moreover, most participants were recruited after discharge from the hospital. At that time, caregivers with stroke patients might primarily need information such as expectations related to recovery of function, assistance with physical activities of daily living (e.g., lifting techniques), communication strategies, and other useful information resources.

The effect size for the atheoretical intervention studies was larger than that for the theory-based intervention studies. Fidelity to the theoretical background is relevant to the quality of an intervention (Resnick et al., 2005) and interpretation of its effect (Lipsey, 1990). Theories specify the ingredients, required dose, timing, and correct implementation of the intervention (Lipsey, 1990; Sidani & Braden, 1998). Consequently, they help to explain the why and how interventions work. For example, both Grant et al. (2002; theoretically guided) and Mant et al. (2002; atheoretical) provided individually tailored interventions. Grant and colleagues (2002) used theory to structure the contents of the intervention. In contrast, Mant and colleagues (2000) permitted the full discretion of the family support organizer (liaison) to determine the frequency and content of the interactions. As a result, it was unclear exactly which ingredients worked and the correct "dosage" to obtain effective mental health outcomes.

The drawback of not having theory-guided effective doses, protocols, and timing is that it makes replication of the intervention on a larger scale cost prohibitive. Nevertheless, it must be remembered that the assessment in this study addressed whether the intervention reflected a theory and not these other details. Yet the use of theory is critical to interpreting intervention results. Finally, in this meta-analysis the studies with atheoretical interventions had larger sample sizes compared to theory-based intervention studies. Thus, the atheoretical intervention studies carried more weight in the analysis. Therefore, these meta-analysis results, including the publication bias, limit the generalizability of the findings and interpretation should be done cautiously.

The effect of the one study conducted in the United States was larger than those for Europe. The study in the United States, however, required a smaller sample size because of the repeated measures design. In the future, more studies are needed using different ethnicities or cultures, such as the Asian population.

When the studies were categorized by quality rating, the effect sizes were larger with higher quality studies (see Table 2). The rigorous design can make researchers more confident of the results. We recommend that future intervention studies use the double-blind method.

Based on the overall effect size and the limited number of studies, more studies are needed to analyze the long-term effects of interventions to improve mental health of caregivers. More definitive studies that clearly describe the intervention dosage, period, and content guided by theory are needed. Future studies should be conducted sooner, for example, immediately postdischarge. More controlled intervention designs are needed. Based on the consistent results from two high-quality randomized studies with an educational intervention, more education programs are needed for addressing the mental health of stroke caregivers.

Future meta-analyses may discover the effect of different types of intervention access to caregivers such as using the telephone, the Internet, or home visits. In addition, meta-analysis with different outcome variables, such as depression or burden, can indicate whether the intervention program is effective for this population. In conclusion, the small number of studies included in this meta-analysis limits the generalizability of results while supporting the need for more research in this area.

References

Acton, G. J., & Kang, J. (2001). Interventions to reduce the burden of caregiving for an adult with dementia: A meta-analysis. *Research in Nursing & Health, 24,* 349-360.

American Heart Association. (2005). *Heart disease and stroke statistics, 2005 update.* Dallas, TX: American Heart Association.

Anderson, C., Laubscher, S., & Burns, R. (1996). Validation of the Short Form 36 (SF-36) health survey questionnaire among stroke patients. *Stroke, 27,* 1812-1816.

Bakas, T., & Champion, V. (1999). Development and psychometric testing of the Bakas Caregiving Outcomes Scale. *Nursing Research, 48*(5), 250-259.

Becker, B. J. (1994). Combining significance levels. In, H. Cooper & L.V. Hedges (Eds.), *The handbook of research synthesis* (pp. 215-230). New York: Russell Sage Foundation.

Conn, V. S., Valentine, J. C., Cooper, H. M., & Rantz, M. J. (2003). Grey literature in meta-analyses. *Nursing Research, 52*(4), 256-261.

Dennis, M., O'Rourke, S., Slattery, J., Staniforth, T., & Warlow, C. (1997). Evaluation of a stroke family care worker: Results of a randomised controlled trial. *British Medical Journal, 314* (7087), 1071-1076.

D'Zurilla, T. J., & Nezu, A. (1999). *Problem-solving therapy* (2nd ed.). New York: Springer.

Egger, M., & Smith, G. D. (1998). Bias in location and selection of studies. *British Medical Journal, 316*, 61-66.

Forster, A., & Young, J. (1996). Specialist nurse support for patients with stroke in the community: A randomised controlled trial. *British Medical Journal, 312*(7047), 1642-1646.

Grant, J. S. (1999). Social problem-solving partnerships with family caregivers. *Rehabilitation Nursing, 24*(6), 254-260.

*Grant, J. S., Elliott, T. R., Weaver, M., Bartolucci, A. A., & Giger, J. N. (2002). Telephone intervention with family caregivers of stroke survivors after rehabilitation. *Stroke, 33*, 2060-2065.

Hoabart, J. C., Williams, L. S., Moran, K., & Thompson, A. J. (2002). Quality of life measurement after stroke: Use s and abuses of the SF-36. *Stroke, 33*(5), 1348-1356.

Hobson, P., Bhowmick, B., & Meara, J. (1997). Use of the SF-36 questionnaire in cerebrovascular disease. *Stroke, 28*(2), 464-465.

Horner, R. D. (1998). The high cost of stroke to society, the family, and the patient. *Pharmacotherapy, 18*(3 Pt 2), 87S-93S; Discussion 85S-86S.

Lazarus, R. S., & Folkman, S. (1984). *Stress, appraisal, and coping*. New York: Springer.

Lincoln, N. B., Francis, V. M., Lilley, S. A., Sharma, J. C., & Summerfield, M. (2003). Evaluation of a stroke family support organiser: A randomized controlled trial. *Stroke, 34*, 116-121.

Lipsey, M. W. (1990). *Design sensitivity: Statistical power for experimental research*. Newbury Park, CA: Sage.

*Mant, J., Carter, J., Wade, D. T., & Winner, S. (2000). Family support for stroke: A randomised controlled trial. *Lancet, 356* (9232), 808-813.

Mayo, N. E., Wood-Dauphinee, S., Cote, R., Gayton, D., Carlton, J., Buttery, J. et al. (2000). There's no place like home: An evaluation of early supported discharge for stroke. *Stroke, 31*(5), 1016-1023.

Pinquart, M., & Sorensen, S. (2003). Differences between caregivers and non-caregivers in psychological health and physical health: A meta-analysis. *Psychology & Aging. 18*(2), 250-267.

Printz-Feddersen, V. (1990). Group process effect on caregiver burden. *Journal of Neuroscience Nursing, 22*(3), 164-168.

Resnick, B., Inguito, P., Orwig, D., Yahiro, J. Y., Hawkes, W., Werner, M., et al. (2005). Treatment fidelity in behavior change research: A case example. *Nursing Research, 54*(2), 139-143.

*Rodgers, H., Atkinson, C., Bond, S., Suddes, M., Dobson, R., & Curless, R. (1999). Randomized controlled trial of a comprehensive stroke education program for patients and caregivers. *Stroke, 30*(12), 2585-2591.

Rosenthal, R. (1984). *Meta-analysis procedures for social research*. Beverly Hills, CA: Sage.

Shadish, W. R., & Haddock, C. K. (1994). Combining estimates of effect size. In H. M. Cooper & L. V. Hedges (Eds.), *The handbook of research synthesis* (pp. xvi, 573). New York: Russell Sage Foundation.

Sidani, S., & Braden, C. J. (1998). *Evaluating nursing interventions: A theory-driven approach*. Thousand Oaks, CA: Sage.

Soeken, K. L., Lee, W., Bausell, R. B., Agelli, M., & Berman, B. M. (2002). Safety and efficacy of S-adenosylmethionine (SAMe) for osteoarthritis. *Journal of Family Practice, 51*(5), 425-430.

Soeken, K. L., & Sripusanapan, A. (2003). Assessing publication bias in meta-analysis. *Nursing Research, 52*(1), 57-60.

Stewart, M. J., Doble, S., Hart, G., Langille, L., & MacPherson, K. (1998). Peer visitor support for family caregivers of seniors with stroke. *Canadian Journal of Nursing Research, 30*(2), 87-117.

*Van den Heuvel, E. T., Witte, L. P., Stewart, R. E., Schure, L. M., Sanderman, R., & Meyboom-de Jong, B. (2002). Long-term effects of a group support program and an individual support program for informal caregivers of stroke patients: Which caregivers benefit the most? *Patient Education & Counseling, 47*(4), 291-299.

White, C. L., Lauzon, S., Yaffe, M. J., & Wood-Dauphinee, S. (2004). Toward a model of quality of life for family caregivers of stroke survivors. *Quality of Life Research, 13*(3), 625-638.

Wright, L. K., Hickey, J. V., Buckwalter, K. C., Hendrix, S. A., & Kelechi, T. (1999). Emotional and physical health of spouse caregivers of persons with Alzheimer's disease and stroke. *Journal of Advanced Nursing, 30*, 552-563.

*Articles included in this meta-analysis

JuHee Lee, PhD, RN, is a postdoctoral fellow at the University of Maryland School of Nursing.

Karen Soeken, PhD, is a professor at the University of Maryland School of Nursing.

Sandra J. Picot, PhD, RN, FAAN, is an associate professor at the University of Maryland School of Nursing.

Strangers in Strange Lands
A Metasynthesis of Lived Experiences of Immigrant Asian Nurses Working in Western Countries

Yu Xu, PhD, RN, CTN

Nurses from Asian countries make up the majority of immigrant nurses globally. Although there are a limited number of studies on the lived experiences of Asian nurses working in Western countries, the development of nursing science will be impeded if the rich understanding gleaned from these studies is not synthesized. Using Noblit and Hare's (*Metaethnography: Synthesizing Qualitative Studies*. Newbury Park, Calif: Sage; 1988) procedures, a metasynthesis was conducted on 14 studies that met preset selection criteria. Four overarching themes emerged: (*a*) communication as a daunting challenge; (*b*) differences in nursing practice; (*c*) marginalization, discrimination, and exploitation; and (*d*) cultural differences. Based on the metasynthesis, a large narrative and expanded interpretation was constructed and implications for nursing knowledge development, clinical practice, and policy making are elaborated. **Key words:** *adaptation, Asian nurses, foreign nurses, lived experiences, metasynthesis*

NURSE SHORTAGE is a global issue.[1,2] Asian nurses from the Philippines and India have been the major targets of international recruitment.[3] For instance, internationally educated nurses made up 3.5% of the estimated 2.9 million US nurse workforce in 2004 and among them 50.2% were from the Philippines alone.[4] Buchan reported that India and the Philippines were the top 2 source countries for internationally recruited nurses (IRNs) in the United Kingdom during 2004–2005.[5]

Author Affiliation: University of Nevada, Las Vegas.

Funding for this research was provided by the Small Faculty Fund, University of Connecticut. The author thanks Drs Barbara Jacobs, Carolyn Yucha, Cheryl Bowles, Michele Clark, and Nancy Menzel for critiquing an earlier version of this manuscript. Thanks also go to Drs Ola Fox, Paulette Williams, Barbara Schneider, and Tish Smyer for sharing their insight and to the 3 anonymous reviewers for their valuable comments.

Corresponding Author: *Yu Xu, PhD, RN, CTN, University of Nevada at Las Vegas School of Nursing, 4505 Maryland Parkway, Las Vegas, NV 89154 (mailto:yu.xu@unlv.edu).*

Both published literature and anecdotal evidence suggest that Asian nurses working in Western countries encounter unique challenges that profoundly affect their relationships with their patients, coworkers, physicians, supervisors, employers, and the host country at large. In addition, these challenges impact their relationships with peers from their home countries, their own immediate and extended families, and most importantly, their inner most selves. Because these challenges and associated issues are intertwined with gender, race, and culture, the dynamics of the interactions among these factors significantly affect the work and life experiences of Asian nurses and deserve a serious and rigorous examination.

As early as the 1970s, researchers started documenting and examining the experiences of Asian nurses working in the United States.[6-9] Most of the early studies were concentrated on Filipino nurses in the United States, primarily because they were the predominant subgroup of international nurses. In the last decade and particularly in recent years, qualitative studies on Asian

Reprinted with permission from *Advances in Nursing Science* 2007; 30:246–265.

223

nurses working in Western countries have flourished.[6,10-20] These studies not only "renewed" the previously little-heard voices of Asian nurses but also expanded the geographical boundary beyond the United States.

However, systematic searches revealed no scholarly efforts to synthesize the available research except one systematic review that evaluated studies on black (African and Caribbean) and minority ethnic (Asian) nurses in the United Kingdom.[21] Essentially, this review concludes that the experiences of black and minority ethnic nurses is "generally poorly researched"[21(p50)] and there is a "lack of comprehensive literature concerning experiences of overseas black and minority ethnic nurses in the UK."[21(p54)] In addition, it identifies "a notable lack of empirical studies with gaps in knowledge, theory, and methodology"[21(p54)] and suggests a need for "rigorous, high-quality research."[21(p53)] However, the limitations of this review in context of the purpose of this metasynthesis are apparent: (*a*) its focus on how to conduct a rigorous systematic review rather than the substantive issues encountered by black and minority ethnic nurses; (*b*) its exclusion of studies conducted outside the United Kingdom; and (*c*) its inclusion of nonresearch literature.

The absence of a metasynthesis of the experiences of Asian nurses working in Western countries indicates a cross-disciplinary knowledge gap. The purpose of this metasynthesis is to provide cumulative insight into the collectively lived experiences of these Asian nurses in order to advance nursing knowledge and to inform practice, policy, and future research. For the purpose of this study, *Asian nurses* are defined as nurses whose home countries are in Asia.

METHODS

Metasynthesis is a method of synthesizing findings from qualitative studies. According to Sandelowski and colleagues, metasynthesis refers to "the theories, grand narratives, generalizations, or interpretative translations produced from the integration or comparison of findings from qualitative studies."[22(p366)] Specifically, metasynthesis refers to translating qualitative studies into each other so that a grand narrative or interpretation can emerge that is more than a sum of the parts.[22] Unlike meta-analysis where the purpose is to reduce findings (ie, data), the purpose of metasynthesis is to allow for an enlarged interpretation.[22]

Procedures

Systematic searches through the Cumulative Index to Nursing and Allied Health Literature (CINAHL), MEDLINE, PsychINFO, Sociological Abstracts, and ERIC were performed in consultation with an experienced health sciences librarian. To minimize bias against nonpublished research literature, a search through ProQuest Dissertations and Theses was also conducted. The following terms and their variations and combinations were used as search terms: "Asian nurses," "foreign nurses," "foreign-born nurses," "internationally educated nurses," "internationally recruited nurses," "international nurses," "immigrant nurses," and names of a half dozen Asian countries or regions such as Korea and Taiwan. These electronic searches did not set any specific cutoff dates; the last search was performed in July of 2006. In addition, ancestral searches (ie, tracing relevant studies through references in qualified studies) were conducted. Finally, targeted journals that had published studies on the topic were hand-searched. Two criteria were set for inclusion in this metasynthesis: (*a*) empirical studies published in English that had a qualitative research design or contained qualitative data and (*b*) studies that focused on the experiences of Asian nurses working as clinicians in Western countries.

Types of qualitative research designs had no effect on selection. For a qualified study using a mixed method design or an overall quantitative design with a qualitative component, only data from the qualitative portion of the study were included for synthesis. For studies that included both Asian nurses and nurses from other countries, only data specifically identified from Asian nurses were incorporated. When the nationalities of included nurses could not be determined, efforts were made to contact the primary author of the original study for clarification to make an inclusion or exclusion decision. As a result, a few qualitative studies had to be excluded because of the inability to separate the qualitative data among groups of international nurses, even though the author(s) had a blanket statement indicating nurses from Asian countries made up part of the samples. For one study, the primary author refused to disclose the national origins of participating nurses because of concern with confidentiality since the sample was very small.

Sample

Sampling in the real world is rarely simple and clear-cut. For this metasynthesis, studies based on the same sample but reporting different aspects of research findings were counted separately; however, they were grouped together in analyses to conserve space. This situation applied to several studies.[9-11,20] When it was impossible to differentiate data from Asian nurses and data from nurses coming from other countries in the original report of 2 studies,[10,11] an inquiry was made. Based on an e-mail reply from the primary author (O. Alexis, [oalexis@brookes.ac.uk] e-mail, July 28, 2006) indicating the applicability of all the identified themes to Asian nurses, both studies were included in this metasynthesis. Despite repeated efforts, one master of science thesis study from the University of Birmingham in the United Kingdom could not be obtained to evaluate for inclusion. The final sample for this metasynthesis included 14 studies.

Data analysis

The established 7-phase procedures proposed by Noblit and Hare[23(pp26-29)] were employed in this metasynthesis. In phase 1, this researcher determined the studies to include on the basis of the above 2 selection criteria. In phase 2, the researcher identified what was relevant to the purpose of this metasynthesis. In phase 3, the researcher read and re-read all the selected studies to become engaged with the results and contexts. In phase 4, how the selected studies were related to one another was examined. Several procedures were undertaken in this phase: (*a*) making a list of key metaphors (ie, "themes," "concepts," or "phrases") from each study; (*b*) identifying relations among these metaphors (ie, "reciprocal," "refutational," or presenting a "line of argument"); and (*c*) making initial assumptions of the relationships among the selected studies. After comparing all the metaphors from the selected studies, it was determined that the relationships among these metaphors were reciprocal because they were about similar things in similar "directions." In phase 5, the selected studies were translated into each other by juxtaposing the key metaphors. "Translations are especially unique syntheses, because they protect the particular, respect holism, and enable comparison. An adequate translation maintains the central metaphors and/or concepts of each account *in their relation to other key metaphors or concepts in that account*" (original emphasis).[23(p28)] In phase 6, the translations were synthesized. This involved "putting together" a whole that was more than what the each individual study implied. In phase 7, this researcher expressed the synthesis through written word. During the working process of the 7 steps, the advice from Sandelowski and colleagues was kept in mind:

Qualitative metasynthesis is not a trivial pursuit, but rather a complex exercise in interpretation: Carefully peeling away the surface layers of studies to find their hearts and souls in a way that does the least damage to them. Synthesists must analyze studies in sufficient detail to preserve the integrity of each study and yet not become so immersed in detail that no useable synthesis is produced.[22(p370)]

RESULTS

Demographic and methodological characteristics of all the studies included in this metasynthesis are provided in Tables 1 and 2.

Table 1. Demographic characteristics of the participants of individual studies in the metasynthesis[a]

study	Sample size	Age	Marital status	Gender	Time in host country	Religion	Type of program graduated from	Nationality of Asian nurses
Alexis & Vydelingum (2004, 2005a)	12[b]	...	...	F = 7 M = 5	...	...	...	Philippines
Allen & Larsen (2003)[c]	67 (11 Asians)	25–61	...	F = 58 M = 9	Mean = 3.8 y	...	...	Philippines India Pakistan
Daniel et al (2001)	24	...	...	F = 23 M = 1	Group 1 = 3 mo Group 2 = 2 wk	...	...	Philippines
Davison (1993)	10	42–59	...	F = 10	5–24 y	Mainly Catholic	BSN = 6 MSN = 2 PhD = 2	Philippines
Dicicco-Bloom (2004)	10	40–50	M = 10	F = 10	20–25 y	Christian	Diploma	India
Lopez (1990)	10	...	M = 7 S = 3	F = 9 M = 1	<2 y = 4 4–6 y = 3 >10 y = 3	Catholic	Mostly BSN	Philippines
Matti & Taylor (2005)	12[d]	...	...	7 M = 5	9 mo–2 y	...	...	India Philippines
McGonagle et al (2004)	10	...	...	F & M	>3 mo	...	...	Philippines
Miraflor (1976)[e]	405	21 to >60	M = 205 S = 190 Sp = 3 W = 6	F = 384 M = 21	A few mo	Mainly Catholic	5-yr BSN = 112 4-yr BSN = 53 4-yr diploma = 238	Philippines
Spangler (1991)	26	25–51	...	F & M	<5 y = 14 5–10 y = 7 >10 y = 5	Mainly Catholic	BSN = 23 Diploma = 3	Philippines
Withers & Snowball (2003)[f]	45	25–39	...	F = 31 M = 12	3–18 mo	...	...	Philippines
Yi (1993) Yi & Jezewski (2000)	12	25–57	M = 8 D = 1 S = 3	F = 12	1–23 y	Christian = 10	MSN = 3 BSN = 5 Diploma = 4	Korea

[a]Under "Marital Status": M = married; S = single; Sp = separated; D = divorced; W = widowed. Under "Gender": F = female; M = male.
[b]This figure included an unspecific number of nurses from South Africa, the Caribbean, and Sub-Saharan Africa.
[c]The demographical profile reported here is for the total sample (N = 67) due to the unavailability of specific demographical data on the 11 Asian nurses.
[d]This figure included an unspecified number of non-Asian nurses.
[e]Sum of subcategory figures under "Marital Status" is not equal to 405 due to missing data in the original study.
[f]Sum of subcategory figures under "Gender" is not equal to 45 due to missing data in the original study.

Table 2. Methodological characteristics of included studies in the metasynthesis

Study	Discipline published in	Country	Data analysis method	Research design and data-collection method
Alexis & Vydelingum (2004, 2005a)	Nursing	United Kingdom	Thematic analysis	Phenomenology (focus group)
Allen & Larsen (2003)	Nursing	United Kingdom	Thematic analysis	Phenomenology (focus group)
Daniel (2001)	Nursing	United Kingdom	Thematic analysis	Phenomenology (focus group)
Davison (1993)	Asian American studies	United States	Thematic analysis	Oral history (interview)
Dicicco-Bloom (2004)	Nursing	United States	Content analysis and critical case analysis	General descriptive design (interview)
Lopez (1990)	Education	United States	Thematic analysis	General descriptive design (interview)
Matti & Taylor (2005)	Nursing	United Kingdom	Thematic analysis	General descriptive design (semistructured interview)
McGonagle et al. (2004)	Allied health	Ireland	Thematic analysis	Phenomenology (focus group)
Miraflor (1976)[a]	Education	United States	Thematic analysis	Quantitative design with qualitative component (open-ended questions in questionnaire)
Spangler (1991)	Nursing	United States	Leininger's Ethnonursing Phases of Qualitative Data Analysis (Thematic analysis via induction)	Ethnonursing (ethnonursing interview, observation)
Withers & Snowball (2003)[b]	Nursing	United Kingdom	Thematic analysis	Mixed method design (semistructured interview)
Yi (1993) and Yi & Jezewski (2000)	Nursing	United States	Constant comparative method	Grounded theory

[a] Only qualitative data from this quantitative study were included for analysis.
[b] Only qualitative data from this mixed method study were included for analysis.

Study Guide for Essentials of Nursing Research: Appraising Evidence for Nursing Practice, 7e

Out of the 14 studies, 4 were doctoral dissertations, 1 was master's thesis, and the rest (9) were research reports. The disciplines or fields represented by the selected studies were nursing, education, Asian American studies, and allied health. These studies took place in 3 countries (United States, United Kingdom, and Ireland), involving nurses from 4 Asian countries (India, Korea, Pakistan, and the Philippines). The most frequently used research design was phenomenology ($n = 5$) and general descriptive design (ie, qualitative descriptive studies without identifying a specific research design) ($n = 3$), followed by grounded theory ($n = 2$), ethnonursing ($n = 1$), oral history ($n = 1$), mixed method design ($n = 1$), and quantitative design with a qualitative component ($n = 1$). In addition, a detailed table of metaphors, themes, and concepts from the 14 studies was constructed and translated into each other, using Noblit and Hare[23] as outlined above (Table 3). What follows is a descriptive and interpretive report of the lived experiences of Asian nurses under 4 overarching themes.

Theme 1: Communication as a daunting challenge

Communication is critical in healthcare settings, especially for nurses who work with patients around the clock to conduct assessment, plan, coordinate, and deliver care, and evaluate interventions. By definition, communication is the creation of *shared* meaning and understanding. However, because of a variety of factors, Asian nurses encounter an array of difficulties that hinder their ability to communicate.

Unfamiliarity with accents and informal language usage

All of the included studies except one[16] documented language difficulties of Asian nurses, including agonizing experiences, especially during the initial period following their arrival in a new country. No matter how well Asian nurses thought they were prepared

linguistically, they still found themselves not prepared enough to meet the communication needs in a foreign country. For many Asian nurses, language was a major obstacle for survival, both at work and in other aspects of their lives, particularly during the initial time after arrival.

The communication difficulties came from unfamiliar accents; usage of slang, idioms, jargon, abbreviations; recorded shift reports; and idiosyncratic physicians' handwriting.[6–12,15,17,19,20] Difficulties also rose from differences between the "book English" they learned formally in their home countries and the "street English" used in the new country.[7] For instance, to newly arrived Filipino nurses, the euphemistic use of "potty" (for "bedpan") was new; the British use of "theater" for "operating room" was unheard of; and the idiomatic use of the words such as "hell" as in "You are a hell of a good worker" was seemingly paradoxical and puzzling to their linear interpretation. Another example was the response "Uh-huh" because different tones had different and even opposite meanings.

Frequently, communication difficulty was compounded by frustration, stress, and psychological breakdown, and prevented Asian nurses from performing at their best, especially with regard to patient care, leaving them with a deeply saddened feeling of inadequacy, shame, and self-pity. From time to time, they questioned their ability to "handle" the new job and wondered "Why am I here?" Somatic symptoms were also reported from the associated distress.[9] At its worst, communication deficiency led to downward psychological spiral such as depression and resulted in job termination.[7]

Communication deficiency not only affected the effectiveness and efficiency of care delivery to patients but also impacted patients' families and the healthcare team in a variety of ways. In extreme cases, patients refused care by Asian nurses merely because of their inability to create mutual understanding.[7] Such incidents were painful, humiliating, and devastating because such

Table 3. Individual study metaphors as related to 4 overarching themes[a]

Study	Communication challenges	Differences in nursing practice	Marginalization, discrimination, and exploitation	Cultural differences
Alexis & Vydelingum (2004, 2005a)	Communication difficulties with patients and peers	Organization of care and its delivery; not prepared to provide ADLs for patients; focus on paperwork rather than delivery of care	Being seen as "other"; feeling unwelcome, not appreciated, and not belonging; no one would listen to complaints; lack of support from British peers & training opportunities; unfair treatment; lack of equal opportunity for promotion; had to prove self; being bullied & fear of being reported and reprisal	Lack of cultural preparation for United Kingdom and what to expect; feeling of being displaced and thrown into a different world
Allen & Larsen (2003)	Communication compromised by dialects, accents, colloquialism, intonation and style of talking; communication issue as stigma; being labeled "different" and "difficult" due to language deficiency	Nursing qualifications unrecognized; narrower scope of practice leading to feeling of being deskilled; humiliated to provide ADLs; different legal framework; focus on paperwork rather than care	Language barrier as vehicle for discrimination; felt exploited during induction and adaptation period; continuing exploitation after registration when negotiating employment status; being paid for one grade while being asked to take on responsibilities of a higher grade; undesirable working hours; backstabbing and policed by carers; not being accepted by patients—lack of appreciation, respect & trust; feeling of discrimination; manipulated & bullied by care assists	Negative UK attitude and treatment of the elderly; unaware of existence of care homes; tiers of bureaucracy to get registered; high living cost and tax
Dicicco-Bloom (2004)			Discrimination for being immigrant nonwhite female nurses in a gendered profession; alienation at work; marginalization, exploitation, and racism at workplace	Culturally uprooted; valuing family less by Americans; struggle to retain women's traditional role in Asian family

(continues)

Table 3. Individual study metaphors as related to 4 overarching themes[a] *(Continued)*

Study	Communication challenges	Differences in nursing practice	Marginalization, discrimination, and exploitation	Cultural differences
Davison (1993)	Communication barriers; language as an area of tension		Marginalization/discrimination as "foreigners": substandard wage, undesirable shifts, passed over for promotion; not allowed to speak Tagalog during work break, treated with hostility and retaliation, demotion for speaking Tagalog; nursing as a gendered profession: Asian women as exotic and sexual objects; constant fight against stereotyping	Hard-to-understand "American way of life" and culture: elderly abandonment, loose moral, lack of discipline, and "crumbling" of families; culture as another area of tension
Daniel (2001)	Difficulty understanding jargons, medications, abbreviations, and accents of staff and patients	Different role of family; nursing physically demanding; common use of verbal orders; different names of medications; different procedures for dispensing medications; specialization in nursing; legal issues in nursing practice.		Low social status of the elderly
Lopez (1990)	Communication deficiency: slang, "street English" vs "book English," fear of phone conversation; difficulty expressing self	Differences in nurses' role: bedside care vs paperwork; doing vs talking; respect and gratitude vs disrespect and lack of respect from patients; rejection from patients; risk of being sued	No one at airport to meet newly arrived Filipino nurses; lack of trust; frustration with "testy" US nursing aides; suffering quietly; had to earn right to be heard; differential treatment; hostility toward foreign nurses; jealousy; favoritism; rejection by patients and physicians	Lack of understanding of US culture, social skills, and assertiveness; hard to admit "Don't know;" speaking up as challenge

Study Guide for Essentials of Nursing Research: Appraising Evidence for Nursing Practice, 7e

Matti & Taylor (2005)	Language and communication deficiency as a 2-way issue: due to colloquialism and accents	Not used to providing basic care to patients; feeling devalued and deskilled: skills not being recognized or utilized	Feeling not being trusted for performing some clinical procedures	Cultural differences between UK and home country; induction not specific to foreign nurses' needs
McGonagle et al. (2004)[b]	Difficulties with language, documentation & terminology (ie, abbreviation and jargon)	Irish nurses less autonomous; less focused on patients' physical needs; confusion regarding intellectual disability and mental illness		Little family involvement in care of sick family members; perception of institutionalization of elderly as uncaring and unjust
Miraflor (1976)	Language and communication ranked as top issue: taking phone orders, intonation, accent, and physician's handwriting	Learning to use modern equipment, machines, and supplies	Being taken advantage of by nursing aides; not respected as team leaders by nursing aides	Buying on credit, fast pace of life; "Dutch treat"; concept of "first come, first served"; American concept of time; open expression of affection; pervasive exposure of sex in media; disrespect for the elderly; direct communication style

(continues)

Table 3. Individual study metaphors as related to 4 overarching themes[a] (*Continued*)

Study	Communication challenges	Differences in nursing practice	Marginalization, discrimination, and exploitation	Cultural differences
Spangler (1991)	Language difficulties: slang, accent; had to talk in native language	Heavy workload; inability to provide adequate care; reducing care to technical tasks and its contribution to noncaring behaviors; impact of bureaucracy, standards and policies of regulatory agencies.	Mistrust by US nurses; had to prove self; had to "put up with a lot"; had to settle for less desirable shifts; prohibited from speaking Tagalog in work area; abuse; manipulated by patients; made to float to other clinical areas more frequently; frustration with heavier work load	Conflicts resulting from cultural differences; differences in interaction and relational style; differences in lifestyle
Withers & Snowball (2003)	Communication issues: idioms, abbreviations, slang, unfamiliarity with British accent	Differences in nurse's role; not allowed to perform certain procedures	Unfair treatment from colleagues and patients; cultural imposition: not allowed to speak own language; exploitation and bullying; fear to report abuse	Unassertiveness
Yi (1993) and Yi & Jezewski (2000)	Language deficiency as most challenging for successful adaptation	Different role of nurse and family; focus of care: needs of patients (Korea) vs diseases (United States)	Difficult relations with patients, peers, nurse aides, and supervisors; not being respected and accepted as leader by nursing aides; nonassertiveness and kind nature being taken advantage of; emotions over unfair treatment affecting health; being reported to supervisor behind back	Difficulty dealing with interpersonal conflicts; different communication styles

[a] ADLs indicates activities of daily living; Tagalog, most frequently spoken native language of the Philippines.
[b] Study took place in a learning disability service clinical setting.

Study Guide for Essentials of Nursing Research: Appraising Evidence for Nursing Practice, 7e

refusals were interpreted by the involved nurses as incompetence to fulfill the basic duties for which they were hired. Moreover, Asian nurses tended to take such events personally because of their cultural upbringing and socialization. What made this feeling of inadequacy even worse was the cognitive dissonance with their self-perceived image as caring, compassionate, and competent professionals.[7,9,24]

Telecommunication as most challenging

Verbal communication over the telephone was reported as the most nerve-racking experiences for Asian nurses. Fear of making medical errors from communication mistakes and from other situational factors such as a medical emergency or talking to an awakening on-call physician at an early morning hour could magnify the experienced stress due to absence of nonverbal cues for validation as evidenced by the following reflexive reaction: "During the first few days on the job, I ran to the bathroom when the phone rang."[9(p93)]

Domino effects of communication deficiency

Language barrier virtually affected every other aspect of Asian nurses' experiences. First, it affected their confidence in themselves and stripped them of their dignity in extreme cases when they felt embarrassed because they could not express themselves adequately.[8-10,24] To save "face," Yi[9] documented that a Korean nurse was too frightened to ask questions, which could potentially cause harm to her patients. Second, it further reinforced the stereotype of Asian nurses that they were shy, unassertive, and not tough enough to be leaders. However, when a Filipino nurse did not fit into the stereotype, she was labeled as un-Filipino because she was "not quiet."[6(p31)] Third, language deficiency had a vicious cycle: the less Asian nurses spoke because of fear of making mistakes, the longer it took for them to develop a command of the language. Further-

more, language improvement was inherently associated with improvement in professional knowledge and interpersonal skills.[9] Unfortunately, some Asian nurses never overcame the language barrier and had to take a lower level position, quit nursing, or even return to their home countries.[7] These outcomes were regarded not only as catastrophic failures to the involved nurses but also as bringing shame to the nurses' families and even home countries.

Accent and communication deficiency as grounds for discrimination

Language was a key factor for distress to Asian nurses because accent was unjustly used as a "social marker" for stigmatization.[12] The intense emotions were palpable in the following comment by a Filipino nurse working in a New Jersey hospital: "They [American nursing staff] hate our accent. That's why they don't want to work with us. Although they don't say that, you just sense it."[7(p84)] Although some Filipino nurses lived and worked in the host country for more than 10 years, they still encountered "accent discrimination."[6(p30)] Being labeled "different" or "difficult" because of an unfamiliar accent or language deficiency was frequently used as a vehicle for discrimination. In some cases, this also gave their Western peers a "legitimate" excuse for not trying to understand.

Clashes between Asian nurses and their Western peers regarding language were constant. In an extreme case, a Filipino nurse had to resort to litigation to regain her civil rights to speak her indigenous language in the staff lounge during breaks.[6] On the surface, communication medium appeared to be the concern; in fact, these conflicts revealed deeper issues—intolerance, imposition, and the seemingly paradoxical coexistence of superiority and insecurity on the part of American nurses.

Lack of communication proficiency also negatively affected Asian nurses' ability to fight for their own rights: "Some people tell us, 'Why don't you speak up?' Maybe because we have a hard time in speaking in

English, that's why."[24(p185)] On the other hand, learning to "speak the same language" facilitated the acceptance of Asian nurses by their Western peers, and hence, their socialization and integration. It also served as an indicator of their acculturation level. For example, when a Filipino nurse expressed frustration with "Oh my god," her American peer was very excited to tell her that she "had become Americanized."[7(p90)]

Theme 2: Differences in nursing practice

Role of the nurse

One of the first differences Asian nurses discovered was the autonomy granted by laws and regulations as well as the accountability in Western nursing.[15] Initially, it was surprising for them to learn that nurses in Western countries functioned much more independently. However, they were also appalled that family members did not provide or assist with activities of daily living (ADLs) at all and depended completely on the nursing staff for meeting such needs.[9–12,15,19,20] Both professionally and culturally, they were not used to providing ADLs because those basic needs were taken care of by families in Asian countries. Asian family members regard providing such basic and intimate care for their loved one as their privilege. Consequently, many Asian nurses perceived providing ADLs as being deskilled, humiliating, demoralizing, and a waste of their education as evidenced by the following statements: "I feel degraded and frustrated having to wash patients"[10(p15)]; "I did not expect that life as a nurse would go around words like pee, loo, and poo."[19(p285)]

In addition, many Asian nurses were not prepared for the physical and psychological demand in taking care of heavy and dependent Western patients, referring to their weight and high acuity.[15] Furthermore, they were highly critical of the approach to nursing where the focus was perceived to be on the disease process rather than on the needs of patients and holistic care. They were frustrated to see nursing being reduced to technical tasks that contributed little to bedside care. To them, the most important role of the nurse was to provide bedside care that incorporated the hands, mind, heart, and soul.[9,24] Nursing was to give hands-on care with compassion, relieve suffering, and help with the healing process. It should never be merely a series of mechanical tasks. For instance, the sampled Filipino nurses in Spangler's study[24] felt an "obligation to care" and emphasized patients' physical comfort as their central concern. To them, caring was expressed by "doing," especially spending time with patients.

Meanwhile, Asian nurses were shocked by the amount of paperwork required institutionally and legally. Not surprisingly, such emphasis on documentation was perceived as "putting the cart before the horse" as criticized by a Filipino nurse: "Nursing is bedside care, not paper work. Here in the U.S. the prestige is when you are away from the bedside. Actual patient care is relegated to the nurses' aide."[24(p206)] Because of fast work pace, heavy paper work, and understaffing, many Asian nurses felt torn between providing quality patient care and getting everything done on time, which often lead to stress, job dissatisfaction, changing job, or even leaving the profession once for all.

Scope of practice

Quickly, Asian nurses learned that some routinely performed procedures in their home countries such as cannulation, venipuncture, and collecting arterial blood might not fall within the legal practice in some Western countries such as the United Kingdom.[15] Consequently, they felt that patients under their care suffered needlessly because of procedure delays. Such restriction also affected their job satisfaction because of the perception of being treated less like professionals.

Technological and legal environment

Asian nurses had to get to know quickly the 3 Ps: protocols, procedures, and policies, as well as new healthcare technologies to adapt to a more automated healthcare environment.[8] While the use of advanced technology was largely true in America, it was disappointing to find that healthcare technologies in some Western countries such as the United Kingdom were not as advanced as expected.[12] On the other hand, the legal framework within which Western healthcare operated was dramatically different.[7,15] For example, the emphasis on documentation took on added legal importance because "If it is not charted, it didn't happen." Given the prevalence of litigation, many Asian nurses quickly learned to practice what this researcher called "defensive nursing" to minimize the margin of error and thus liability for both themselves and their employers. However, during the process, fear, stress, and distress could take their toll: "You have more at stake here. If you administer a medication a doctor ordered and it's wrong, you are liable since you are the one that gave it."[6(p33)] The Western notions of legality and accountability were unfamiliar and even foreign to them at the beginning of their first job.

Theme 3: Marginalization, discrimination, and exploitation
Nursing as a gendered profession

The vast majority of Asian nurses were females (Table 1). Because of the social perception of women as the weaker and less powerful gender, stereotypes of Asian women, and the simple fact of being in a foreign country, Asian nurses were exposed to a host of vulnerabilities and frequently became targets of marginalization, discrimination, and exploitation.[6-7,10-12,16-17,19] On a cultural level, Asian nurses collectively felt "otherness" or a lack of sense of belonging because of cultural differences or lack of sufficient cultural knowledge to fit in; hence, they felt disfranchised from their coworkers.[6,10,11,16] For instance, one Indian nurse related a disheartening experience: "Nobody learned my name for 4 months when I first came, and when they did it. . . they shortened it and pro-

nounced it wrong. I finally stopped correcting them."[16(p26)]

To some degree, the unassertiveness of Asian nurses contributed to what this researcher termed "professional silence and invisibility"—the lack of professional representation and leadership positions in the healthcare hierarchy, and hence the lack of perceived political clout in the collective consciousness of the host country. Asian nurses (and Asians in general) as a group were taught in their home cultures not to challenge authorities or "rock the boat."[7,9,24] They also had high expectations of others and of themselves and expected that their preceptors and supervisors would take on a maternal role, treating them like a *parang kapatid* (like a sister) or an "adopted mother." These "messages" internalized through primary socialization were incongruent with dominant Western values and norms. The following excerpt from a Filipino nurse demonstrated how long she had to suffer needlessly before feeling accepted enough to request what she needed to do her job adequately:

I am only 4'11" and the operating tables were almost at the level of my neck. Even with the use of a stool I could hardly see what was going on with the surgery. I could not anticipate very well the instruments that the surgeons needed. They were frustrated and so was I. After the surgery I would go to the bathroom and cry. It was after 3 years that I felt I really belonged to the OR and therefore I had the right to ask for a higher stool.[7(pp87-88)]

Unfair treatment and lack of equal opportunity

Asian nurses were frequently passed over for career opportunities and believed that race determines promotion.[6,16] In addition, in some situations Asian nurses were paid substandard wages,[6] or unfairly compensated for a lower position while being asked to take on responsibilities of a higher one.[12] Moreover, they felt that they were discriminated against because of their skin color and "foreignness": "We can change some of our outlook, our values, but we cannot change our looks, our accents. No matter how egalitarian

Americans claim to be, we know that they are not color blind. . ."[24(p208)] Although many Asian nurses wanted to fight against injustice, they felt powerless and uncertain about the outcome. Some did fight, but at the expense of personal health.[9]

Bullying and sexual harassment

At times, Asian nurses were taken advantage of by their Western employers, coworkers, and even subordinates.[6-7,9-12,19] Receiving the "worst" patient assignment, being given the most undesirable work shift, and being assigned to work during holidays were not uncommon. In extreme cases, Asian nurses were targets of bullying by prejudicial patients, physicians, peers, supervisors, and even their subordinates. Furthermore, there was outright harassment as Asian nurses were perceived as exotic and sexual objects. One Filipino nurse encountered a white patient who asked whether he could bring her home as a maid with a sexual overtone and profound ignorance that the Philippines was so backward that the entire country was connected by dirt roads. This Filipino nurse fought back courageously by replying with a laugh: "You cannot afford to hire me."[6(p22)] At other times, Asian nurses told stories of being backstabbed such as being reported to management without their knowledge, being policed by their white peers, intentional withholding critical information by white peers, and a lack of appreciation and recognition for what they could contribute.[12] *We Need Respect,* the title of a recent report on the experiences of IRNs in the United Kingdom commissioned by the Royal College of Nursing, projected the voices of these nurses, including those from Asia— loud and clear.[12]

Having to prove self

Asian nurses believed they had to prove themselves to their patients, peers, and supervisors in order to win their trust and support.[10-12,17] Until then, there was frequent doubt about their worth and competence.

Such apprehension and suspicion were particularly hurtful when patients under their care were dubious about the medications given to them and checked with their white peers behind their back.[12]

Theme 4: Cultural differences
Cultural displacement

Asian nurses felt "uprooted" culturally and "being thrown into a different world," especially during their initial transition after arrival.[10-11,16] Meanwhile, they experienced mounting pressure to "re-root"in the new culture. The feeling of being torn between 2 cultures was best captured by the metaphor from an Indian nurse as "a foot here, a foot there, a foot nowhere"[16(p28)] and as a "rupture"[16(p29)] with her homeland. The sense of cultural displacement was frequently made worse by the fact that a majority of Asian nurses left their close-knit families behind. Lopez reported that one Filipino nurse spent an average of $500 monthly on telephone fees to relieve her nostalgia.[7]

Asian nurses were challenged to understand the host culture and adjust to new ways of life.[6-9,24] During this adaptation process, their own values, beliefs, and cultural norms unavoidably clashed with those of Western societies as the 2 systems of thinking were likened to "oil and water."[14(p57)] These cultural differences ranged from different concepts of time (ie, "American time" equaling to "punctuality") to different communication styles, foods, and ways of life and customs such as "Dutch treat" and buying things on credit. In addition, they were not used to the "loose morality"(eg, being naked in the street, permeation of sex in the media), lack of discipline, and the "crumbling" of the family in Western societies.[8]

Negativity toward the elderly

Asian nurses were not prepared culturally for the perceived lack of respect for the elderly such as "Calling elders by their first name"[8(p75)] and for the perceived maltreatment of the elderly.[15] Moreover, they resented what they perceived as the "elder abandonment" when frail parents were institutionalized in nursing homes with few visitations from their families or without family members being at the bedside when they were hospitalized. This perceived lack of family obligation and compassion was regarded as the ultimate shame and social evil of Western societies.

Interpersonal challenge

To a large extent, interpersonal challenge had its "roots" in the cultural upbringing of Asian nurses, who were taught to avoid conflicts at all cost in order to maintain harmony.[7] Culturally, Asian nurses came from collectivistic cultures where "we" and "us" came before "I" and "me." Therefore, to say "No" was socially unacceptable, especially to people with seniority and authority. To challenge physicians when necessary was expected in the Western nursing culture, but very hard to learn for Asian nurses, even though they realized that it was a legal and professional requirement.

In addition, Asian nurses quickly found out that their "all-yes" habitual mentality frequently brought them unnecessary work and even trouble in the real world because their kindness and tendency to accommodate were taken advantage of and even abused. Interestingly, the most intense conflicts were with nursing aides, especially those of African American background, rather than with their peers, supervisors, or physicians.[7,9] Asian nurses were particularly resentful if their subordinates refused to follow their directions because obedience to authority was expected according to the ways they were brought up.[6-9,24]

Inadequate training on leadership and management skills such as delegation and conflict resolution[8] was another barrier to building productive working relationships. In addition, many Asian nurses operated under their culture-based assumption that every employee was motivated, who was willing and ready to carry out duties as specified in one's own job description. Moreover, the cultural

belief that it was an insult to someone if he or she had to be told to perform his or her regular duties also affected Asian nurses' management behaviors. However, frequently this culture-based expectation proved to be a un-starter at Western workplaces, particularly with many less motivated or unmotivated nursing aides.

DISCUSSION

Gender, race, culture, and interpersonal dynamics

Gender, race, and culture are at the crux of one's identity and impact interpersonal interactions profoundly; therefore, they are salient categories of analysis. The lived experiences of Asian nurses working in Western countries cannot be fully understood without looking through these 3 different lenses simultaneously. Essentially, their experiences were framed by these 3 dimensions of one's identity and humanity as well as their intricate interactions in the ever-changing physical, technological, legal, and interpersonal contexts in Western countries. It is from this framing that meanings of their experiences are defined and dynamics of relationships understood.

What Asian nurses went through was a *gendered* experience. Such experiences are crystallized in the metaphoric advertisement: "Your cap is your passport."[14(p61)] The socially constructed image of women in general and Asian women in particular affected not only the perceived status of Asian nurses but also treatment by their Western employers and the people they interacted with. This metasynthesis suggested that as women, Asian nurses were more vulnerable to social injustice and sexual harassment. Moreover, Asian nurses perceived that they had little power to change the status quo, particularly given the foreign contexts. The gendered experiences of Asian nurses in this metasynthesis validated similar experiences by minority foreign nurses documented in numerous Western countries.[11,14,25] Moreover, their gendered experiences were furthermore compounded by race and culture. As Thurston and

Vissandjee pointed out: "...gender interacts with other Symbolic Institutions—in particular race, class, and sexuality—to form hierarchies of inclusion and exclusion, is never seen alone, and is essential to understanding the organization of society."[26(p232)]

What Asian nurses went through was also a *racial* experience. They reported sabotaging attempts aiming to set them up for failure; documented double standards, exploitation, and abuse; witnessed intolerance and unrelenting discrimination; and encountered the "glass ceiling," all because of their skin color. Perhaps, the worst example racial discrimination was against 2 Filipino nurses who were convicted of poisoning, murder, and conspiracy at the Veteran Affairs Hospital in Ann Arbor, Mich, in 1976 and later were acquitted in a sensational national trial. Consequently as a group, Filipino nurses suffered from public suspicion about their professional intentions and even death threat.[14]

Furthermore, the glass ceiling effect was validated by longitudinal data in a study indicating that the vast majority of internationally educated nurses in the United States held staff nurse positions, which increased from 71.2% to 76.7% during 1977–2000, while their proportions in management positions declined from 6.2% to 2.7% during 1984–2000.[27] Hawthorn also found that immigrant nurses from non–English-speaking countries were not only much less likely to advance beyond the entry-level registered nurse position but also disproportionately concentrated in stigmatized geriatric units.[28] The documented experiences of Asian nurses in this metasynthesis revealed that racial equality in Western countries remain merely a myth. In light of the increasing reports of discrimination against nonwhite foreign nurses in Australia, Canada, the United Kingdom, and the United States,[3,12,14,16,25,29,30] one has to conclude that institutional racism still exists.

Lastly, what Asian nurses went through was also a *cultural* experience. The cultural heritage of Asian nurses was a mixed blessing, serving as both a barrier and a resource to their transition. Frequently, Asian nurses were puzzled and frustrated as to what part of "themselves" to give up and what part to retain during the adaptation process. This was an intense, and frequently agonizing, intrapersonal process involving soul searching, resolution of values conflicts, and even self-negation to seek and establish a new personal, professional, and cultural identity. Data indicated that Asian nurses had to change *who they were* in varying degrees in order to adapt successfully to the new culture and work environment. However, changing oneself was a challenge that was at least formidable to some but monumental to others.

Language is one of the most important carriers and exemplars of culture. Essentially, language functioned as both a symbol and a tool for Asian nurses. As a symbol, language and its associated properties such as accent gave away their "foreignness" and frequently served as a social marker, thus offering a handy vehicle for prejudice and discrimination.[28] As a tool, language served as a fundamental instrument for survival and adaptation both at work and in daily life in a new culture.

The meanings and dynamics of the precarious relationships between Asian nurses and African American nurse aides in the US healthcare environment cannot be fully understood unless the frequently cited conflicts are put into the sociopolitical, economic, and cultural contexts.[31] Control of the work environment is at the core of these conflicts. The underlying factors go far beyond the simple explanations of different accents, language use such as "Black English," and ways of relating to one another,[8] as well as cultural differences such as work ethics.[24] On the one hand, African Americans find themselves at the bottom of the American society. The position of African Americans nurse aides in the US healthcare system reflects their socioeconomic status in the American society at large. They often have the most physically challenging jobs but the lowest pay. Many of these African American nurse aides are single parents with limited education and work at multiple jobs to make ends meet. Their work and daily struggles are vividly portrayed in Diamond's classic ethnography of American nursing home care—*Making Gray Gold*.[32] Compounding the situation is the ingrained memory of slavery and the painful fight for civil rights in US history. The feeling that the system has failed them can be overwhelming, often accompanied with a sense of powerlessness and hopelessness. Frequently, a spark is all that is needed to trigger an explosion of their frustration and anger. A simple, delegated task from a newly arrived Asian nurse, who is a "foreigner" with less-than-fluent English and a hard-to-understand accent but a higher position and salary, could well be "the last straw on the camel's back."

On the other hand, several factors on the part of Asian nurses also contribute to the surfacing and development of these conflicts. First, brought up in hierarchical cultures, Asian nurses expect obedience from subordinates. Furthermore, culturally Asian nurses avoid interpersonal conflicts if at all possible. However, oftentimes such avoidance behaviors enable African American nurse aids to become more testy and demanding. Second, they are thrown into the preexisting, predominant black-white racial politics that play out in the workplace daily. However, unaware of the interpersonal dynamics that are affected by the racial politics beyond hospital walls and situational factors, Asian nurses are caught completely unprepared and clueless as to how to effectively handle disobedience and subsequent conflicts. Third, Asian nurses are perceived as having multiple vulnerabilities and weaknesses that have further contributed to their ineffectiveness as team leaders: language deficiency, status as "aliens," job insecurity as contracted foreign nurses, less seniority as new comers, soft voice, and the small physical stature.

Implications for knowledge development, clinical practice, and policy making
Implications for nursing knowledge development

Asian nurses working in Western countries encounter a host of unique challenges that ultimately affect their adaptation as re-ported above. Consequently, the experiences and adaptation of Asian nurses in Western countries are likely to be different from those of non-Asian nurses, at least in some aspects. Consequently, this metasynthesis provides a starting point for the development of a midrange theory regarding Asian nurses' adaptation to the Western healthcare environment. This theory is expected to provide the foundation for theory-based interventions to improve the integration of Asian nurses into the Western healthcare environment. In addition, such theoretical advancement will contribute substantively to the knowledge base related to "transition" as one major area of inquiry in nursing research.[33] Finally, the research on the lived experiences of immigrant Asian nurses has opened new areas of inquiry into the dynamics of interpersonal relationships: How does the "failure" of some Asian nurses affect other immigrant nurses? What are the relationships between native-born Asian nurses and immigrant Asian nurses? How do immigrant nurses from different countries interface with each other? Is there any "reverse discrimination" against white nurses, especially in healthcare settings where immigrant nurses concentrate?

Implications for practice

In light of this metasynthesis, several issues need to be addressed regarding the current orientation and transitional programs for IRNs. First, apart from the general facility orientation, there should be a tailored transitional program for IRNs that specifically addresses their needs such as the differences in nursing practice, with detailed elaborations on legality, policies, and procedures and their implications. The importance of explaining these differences cannot be overestimated because they directly affect patient safety and quality of care. Second, Western healthcare employers need to develop and implement support mechanisms to facilitate the adaptation and integration of IRNs. Such measures should include mentoring programs such as the "buddy system," which proved effective in enhancing the adaptation of Asian nurses, and hence, their retention and success. Third, cultural competence training that facilitates mutual understanding of culture-based values, beliefs, expectations, and behavioral and communication patterns is also needed. For Asian nurses, such training needs to be included in their prearrival recruitment programs.

However, how to prepare Asian nurses to handle inevitable interpersonal conflicts remains a serious challenge, especially when such conflicts are rooted in history and framed by socioeconomic forces that are beyond institutional control. At the minimum, Asian nurses should be made aware of the potential conflicts arising from racial tension in the new country prior to their arrival. In addition, exercises such as role-play to practice how to handle these emotionally charged situations in a high-stress environment will be helpful. A working knowledge of the history, people, and sociopolitical system of the host country and building a repertoire of interpersonal skills will certainly help in dealing with the unavoidable conflicts.

Meanwhile, Western employers need to understand that language acquisition is a lengthy process that takes years of learning and practice. Asian nurses have varying levels of language skills that differ from individual to individual and from one source country to another. For nurses from the Philippines and India, the language issues might be less profound since English is one of the official languages and most nurses from these 2 countries were trained in English nursing programs. However, for nurses from non–English-speaking Asian countries such as Korea, language barriers could be more challenging. Similarly, acquisition of a working knowledge about a new culture also requires years of immersion and accumulation through persistent efforts.

Implications for policy making

The documented experiences of Asian nurses in this metasynthesis underscore the central issue of social injustice and the imperative to address it head-on. The included stud-

ies reported widespread discriminatory practices and behaviors in one form or another. Oftentimes, discrimination was covert and subtle; other times, it was explicit and outright. To a large extent, the prejudice and discrimination against Asian nurses reflect the deeply rooted intolerance for, and injustice against, racial and ethnic minorities in Western societies and nurses from these groups. Although the eradication of racism is a long-term goal in nursing, both Western governments and employers need to determine what more can be done at the societal and institutional levels. Could Western governments make and implement policies on recruitment, credentialing, employment nondiscriminatory to immigrant nurses, including those from Asia? Although many of these policies are already in place, they exist merely on paper in many cases, with wide variations in their interpretation and execution. At the institutional level, can Western employers implement programs on cultural diversity and competence to cultivate a more tolerable, welcoming workplace environment and to facilitate the communication between Asian nurses and those they work with? More importantly, could specific measures be institutionalized to prevent or minimize discrimination in hiring, performance evaluation, compensation, and so forth so that antidiscrimination is not merely empty lip service or calculated political tactic?

CONCLUSIONS

Asian nurses constitute the largest group of immigrant nurses working in Western countries. For the foreseeable future, the number and share of Asian nurses in the global migration of nurses are likely to continue to increase. This metasynthesis of the lived experiences of Asian nurses working in Western countries encapsulates their challenges, agonies, and struggles for personal and professional identity and social justice. To a large extent, the story of Asian nurses is an integral part of the collective experiences of international nurses from other parts of the world and parallels those of immigrant women. The lived experiences of Asian nurses must be first documented and examined before any effective interventions can be designed and implemented to facilitate their adaptation and integration. However, when gender, race, and culture intersect, the dynamics of relationships of the involved groups will inevitably be complex, and defies simple, linear explanations and easy solutions.

REFERENCES

1. Aiken LH, Buchan J, Sochalski J, Nichols B, Powell M. Trends in international nurse migration. *Health Aff.* 2004;23(3):69-77.
2. Buchan J, Calman L. *The Global Shortage of Registered Nurses: An Overview of Issues and Actions.* Geneva: International Council of Nurses; 2004.
3. Kingma M. *Nurses on the Move: Migration and the Global Health Care Economy.* Ithaca, NY: Cornell University Press; 2006.
4. Health Resources and Services Administration. Preliminary findings: 2004 national sample survey of registered nurses. http://bhpr. hrsa.gov/healthworkforce/reports/rnpopulation/preliminaryfindings.htm. Accessed July 6, 2006.
5. Buchan J. Filipino nurses in the UK: A case study in active international recruitment. *Harv Health Policy Rev.* 2006;7(1):113-120.
6. Davison MA. *Filipina Nurses: Voices of Struggle and Determination* [master's thesis]. Los Angeles, CA: University of California; 1993.
7. Lopez N. *The Acculturation of Selected Filipino Nurses to Nursing Practice in the United States* [dissertation]. Philadelphia, PA: University of Pennsylvania; 1990.
8. Miraflor CG. *The Philippine Nurses: Implications for Orientation and In-Service Education for Foreign Nurses in the United States* [dissertation]. Chicago, IL: Loyola University of Chicago; 1976.
9. Yi M. *Adjustment of Korean Nurses to United States Hospital Settings* [dissertation]. Buffalo, NY: State University of New York; 1993.
10. Alexis O, Vydelingum V. The lived experiences of overseas black and minority ethnic nurses in the NHS in the south of England. *Divers Health Soc Care.* 2004;1(1):13-20.
11. Alexis O, Vydelingum V. The experiences of overseas black and minority ethnic nurses in the NHS in an English hospital: a phenomenological study. *J Res Nurs.* 2005a;10(4):459-472.
12. Allan H, Larsen JA. *"We Need Respect": Experiences of Internationally Recruited Nurses in the UK.* London: Royal College of Nursing; 2003.
13. Allan H, Larsen JA, Bryan K, Smith PA. The social reproduction of institutional racism: internationally recruited nurses' experiences of the British health services. *Divers Health Soc Care.* 2003;1:117-125.
14. Choy CC. *Empire of Care: Nursing and Migration in Filipino American History.* Durham, NC: Duke University Press; 2003.
15. Daniel P, Chamberlain A, Gordon F. Expectations and experiences of newly recruited Filipino nurses. *Br J Nurs.* 2001;10(4):254, 256, 258-265.
16. DiCicco-Bloom B. The racial and gendered experiences of immigrant nurses from Kerala, India. *J Transcult Nurs.* 2004;15(1):26-33.
17. Matiti MR, Taylor D. The cultural lived experience of internationally recruited nurses: a phenomenological study. *Divers Health Soc Care.* 2005;2(1):7-15.
18. Mc Gonagle C, Halloran SO, O'Reilly O. The expectations and experiences of Filipino nurses working in an intellectual disability service in the Republic of Ireland. *J Learn Disabil.* 2004;8(4):371-381.
19. Withers J, Snowball J. Adapting to a new culture: a study of the expectations and experiences of Filipino nurses in the Oxford Radcliffe Hospitals NHS Trust. *NT Res.* 2003;8(4):278-290.
20. Yi M, Jezewski MA. Korean nurses' adjustment to hospitals in the United States of America. *J Adv Nurs.* 2000;32(3):721-729.
21. Alexis O, Vydelingum V. Overseas black and minority ethnic nurses: a systematic review. *Nurse Res.* 2005b;12(4):42-56.
22. Sandelowski M, Docherty S, Emden C. Qualitative meta-synthesis: issues and techniques. *Res Nurs Health.* 1997;20:365-371.
23. Noblit GW, Hare RD. *Meta-ethnography: Synthesizing Qualitative Studies.* Newbury Park, CA: Sage; 1988.
24. Spangler Z. *Nursing Care Values and Caregiving Practices of Anglo-American and Philippine-American Nurse Conceptualize within Leininger's Theory* [dissertation]. Detroit, Mich: Wayne State University; 1991.
25. Omeri A, Atkins K. Lived experiences of immigrant nurses in New South Wales, Australia: searching for meaning. *Int J Nur Stud.* 2002;39:495-505.
26. Thurston WE, Vissandjee B. An ecological model for understanding culture as a determinant of women's health. *Crit Public Health.* 2005;15(3):229-242.
27. Xu Y, Kwak C. Comparative trend analysis of characteristics of internationally educated nurses and U.S. educated nurses (1977-2000). *Int Nurs Rev.* 2007;54:78-84.

28. Hawthorn L. The globalization of the nursing workforce: barriers confronting overseas qualified nurses in Australia. *Nurs Inq.* 2001;8(4):213–229.

29. Hagey R, Choudhry U, Guruge S, Turrittin J, Collins E, Lee R. Immigrant nurses' experience of racism. *J Nurs Sch.* 2001;33(4):389–394.

30. Turrittin J, Hagey R, Guruge S, Collins E, Mitchell M. The experiences of professional nurses who have migrated to Canada: cosmopolitan citizenship or democratic racism? *Int J Nur Stud.* 2005;39(6):655–667.

31. McFerson HM. *Blacks and Asians: Crossings, Conflict and Commonality.* Durham, NC: Carolina Academic Press; 2006.

32. Diamond T. *Making Gray Gold.* Chicago, Ill: University of Chicago Press; 1992.

33. Schumacher K, Meleis A. Transitions: a central concept in nursing. *Image J Nurs Sch.* 1994;26(2):119–127.

APPENDIX H

ANSWER KEY

■ Chapter 1

A. CROSSWORD PUZZLE ANSWERS

¹E	V	I	D	E	N	C	E	--	B	A	S	E	²D	
M													³E	B	M
⁴P	A	⁵R	A	⁶D	I	G	M			⁷N	A	T	
I		E		E			⁸H			E		⁹E
R	¹⁰P	O	S	I	T	I	V	I	S	¹¹M		R		X
I	L		C			E		E		M		P
C	I		R	¹²N	C	N	R		¹³T	R	I	A	L
A	C		I			A		H		N		A
L	¹⁴A	P	P	L		¹⁵Q		R		I		N
	T		T		U		¹⁶C	L	U	B	S		A
¹⁷C	L	I	N	I	C		A		H	Y		M		T
O	O		O		L		Y			I
N	¹⁸N	¹⁹I	N	R		I			²⁰B		²¹D		O
T		N			²²T	R	A	D	I	T	I	O	N
R		T			A		A
O	²³D	E	D	U	C		²⁴H		S		²⁵G	E	²⁶N
L		R			²⁷C	A	U	S	E		N		I
		V			R		S		O		H
		²⁸A	S	S	U	M	P	T		S

B. MATCHING EXERCISES

1. a   2. b   3. d   4. b   5. a
6. b   7. d   8. b   9. c   10. a

D. APPLICATION EXERCISES

Exercise 1: Questions of Fact (Appendix A)

a. Yes, this was a systematic study that tested the efficacy of an intervention designed to improve the psychosocial health of chronically ill rural women.

b. It was a quantitative study. The researchers systematically measured several psychosocial outcomes (e.g., self-esteem, empowerment) using scales that yielded quantitative information.

c. The underlying paradigm was positivism/ postpositivism.

d. Yes, the study involved the collection of information through the senses (i.e., through scrutiny of study participants' written responses to series of questions).

e. This study was applied research—there was a practical problem that the researchers wanted to solve (i.e., a problem relating to the psychosocial health of chronically ill rural women).

f. Yes, this study was concerned with evaluating whether the intervention *caused* improvements to the psychosocial health of the women in the study. In this and most studies, the underlying assumption is that phenomena are multiply determined. Thus, women's scores on the various psychosocial scales are *caused* by a number of factors, and the one being tested in this study is whether one of the causes is participation in the intervention.

g. The purposes of the study could perhaps be described as prediction and control: The investigators examined possible methods of controlling (improving) psychosocial outcomes.

Study Guide for Essentials of Nursing Research: Appraising Evidence for Nursing Practice, 7e

h. Yes, this study directly addressed a question relevant to the *treatment* of patients. The results of this study, together with those from other similar studies, could provide guidance about evidence-based treatment decisions.

Exercise 2: Questions of Fact (Appendix B)

a. Yes, this was a systematic study of how young women with diabetes managed turning points and transitions in their lives.

b. This was a qualitative study. The researchers used loosely structured methods to capture—in an in-depth fashion—the experiences of young women with type 1 diabetes.

c. The underlying paradigm is naturalism.

d. Yes, the study involved the collection of information through the senses (e.g., through conversations with young women).

e. This study is best described as basic—to gain a better understanding of the experiences of young women with a chronic health condition. Strategies could, however, be developed to serve better the needs of young women with type 1 diabetes by taking the study findings into account.

f. This study would not be described as cause probing. Its intent is not to explain the determinants of any phenomena, but rather to understand a process.

g. The stated aim of the study was to develop a theory "to *explain* how young women with type 1 diabetes managed their lives when facing turning points and undergoing transitions."

h. This study addresses the EBP question described in the textbook as "Meaning and Processes" (i.e., developing an in-depth understanding of the young women's perspectives, needs, and circumstances).

▪ Chapter 2

A. CROSSWORD PUZZLE ANSWERS

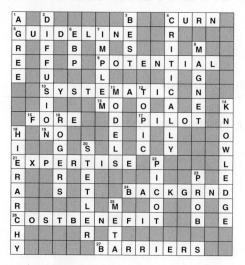

B. MATCHING EXERCISES

1. c	2. d	3. a	4. b	5. d
6. a	7. a	8. b		

D. APPLICATION EXERCISES

Exercise 1: Questions of Fact (Appendix E)

a. There were six authors of this report and, presumably, they were the major team members on this project. Three of the authors (Tracy, Dufault, and Rossi) were faculty in schools of nursing, two (Kogut and Willey-Temkin) were non-nursing faculty, and one (Martin) was a nursing administrator (director of surgical nursing) in a hospital—presumably in the hospital where the project was implemented. It is not unusual for EBP project teams to be composed of researchers and clinical staff, and to be multidisciplinary.

b. The authors described research evidence indicating that "the use of complementary, nondrug strategies is not integrated fully into standard postoperative pain management practices in most hospitals"; that "nondrug methods are underused in the postoperative older adult"; and that "nursing knowledge about pain and pain relief has not improved over time." This evidence supported the need for the EBP project that they undertook.

c. The article indicated that The American Geriatric Society "and other organizations. . . have published pain management guidelines," but the guidelines were not described in the paper. The extent to which these guidelines were used in developing the project protocols was not indicated.

d. The article mentioned some of the same barriers to using evidence in practice that were cited in the textbook, such as organizational climate, clinician attitudes, and nurses' lack of knowledge.

e. The authors indicated that one unique aspect of the CRU model was "the use of nursing students to evaluate the strength of the empirical evidence in the context of their coursework and assist clinicians and scientists in generating best-practice protocols."

f. The team identified five hospitals throughout the state of Rhode Island that were "interested in participating in a *translating best practice in pain management* study." The article did not describe what methods were used to ascertain hospitals' interest. Of the five that were interested, the one selected had "a strong commitment to improving pain management, a well-integrated information system, and established documentation forms for cueing clinicians' pain management practices." The report cited another paper by one of the research team (Dufault) that described these criteria as important to the success of EBP projects.

g. Yes, this project did involve the collection of empirical evidence. The EBP project included a pilot test of the newly developed protocols, which involved collecting information from patients who were exposed to the intervention.

Exercise 2: Questions of Fact (Appendix F)

a. Yes, the article by Lee and colleagues described a systematic review undertaken to summarize evidence on interventions for caregivers of stroke patients. Systematic reviews are a particularly important type of preappraised evidence. The type of systematic review in this example was a meta-analysis.

b. The meta-analysis in this study integrated information from several RCTs, and so evidence from this study would be at the top rung of the evidence hierarchy portrayed in Figure 2.1.

c. The researchers stated the following purpose: "The purpose of this meta-analysis was to examine the effectiveness of interventions for improving the mental health of caregivers of stroke patients by synthesizing across studies."

d. The authors said that their research question was: "What are the effects of interventions on the mental health of informal stroke caregivers?" In terms of the formula for well-worded clinical questions, the *population* was informal caregivers of stroke patients; the *intervention* was not defined, but presumably referred to any systematic protocol or program to assist informal caregivers; and the *outcomes* were mental health outcomes, not elaborated on in the articulation of the question (although well-described later in the paper). The implied *comparison* was no intervention. The time factor was not expressed.

■ Chapter 3

A. CROSSWORD PUZZLE ANSWERS

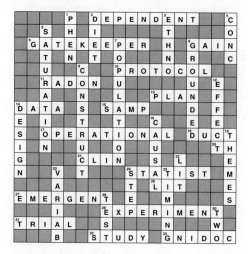

B. MATCHING EXERCISES

B.1.

1. a	2. c	3. b	4. a	5. b
6. c	7. c	8. c	9. b	10. c

B.2.

1. b	2. c	3. a	4. c	5. c
6. b	7. d	8. d		

B.3.

1. a	2. b	3. a	4. c	5. c
6. c	7. d	8. c	9. b	10. a

B.4.

1. c	2. b	3. a	4. a	5. b
6. d	7. e	8. b	9. c	10. d

C. STUDY QUESTIONS

C.2.

a. Independent variable (IV) = participation versus nonparticipation in assertiveness training; dependent variable (DV) = psychiatric nurses' effectiveness

b. IV = patients' postural positioning; DV = respiratory function

c. IV = amount of touch by nursing staff; DV = patients' psychological well-being

d. IV = frequency of turning patients; DV = incidence of decubitus

e. IV = history of parents' abuse during their childhood; DV = parental abuse of their own children

f. IVs = patients' age and gender; DV = tolerance for pain

g. IV = pregnant women's number of prenatal visits; DV = labor and delivery outcomes

h. IV = children's experience (versus nonexperience) of a sibling death; DV = levels of depression

i. IV = gender; DV = compliance with a medical regimen

j. IV = participation versus nonparticipation in a support group among family caregivers of patients with AIDS; DV = coping

k. IV = time of day; DV = hearing acuity among the elderly

l. IV = location of giving birth—home versus hospital; DV = parents' satisfaction with the childbirth experience

m. IV = type of diet in the outpatient setting among patients undergoing chemotherapy; DV = incidence of positive blood cultures

C.5.

a. An ethnographic study would not be experimental—no intervention would be introduced.

b. The independent variable is relaxation therapy (the intervention), and the dependent variable is pain.

c. Grounded theory studies are not clinical trials, which involve an intervention.

d. Study participants would not be exposed to an intervention in phenomenologic studies.

e. In experimental studies, decisions about data collection would be made well before going into the field to implement the intervention.

C.6.

a. Ethnographic   b. Phenomenologic
c. Grounded theory

D. APPLICATION EXERCISES

Exercise 1: Questions of Fact (Appendix C)

a. The researchers were all doctorally prepared professionals affiliated with schools of nursing. At the time of publication, Vollman and LaMontagne were faculty at the Vanderbilt University School of Nursing and Hepworth was affiliated with the University of Arizona.
b. The study participants were adults diagnosed with heart failure.
c. The site for this study was not described in the paper, although it seems likely that it was in Nashville, TN, where two of the researchers were located. The setting for data collection was a heart clinic.
d. The primary independent variable in this study was coping strategies, but the researchers also considered various demographic characteristics, such as marital status and functional impairment. Coping strategies could readily be a dependent variable in a study (e.g., to explore what factors lead to different coping styles).
e. The dependent variable in this study was depression level. This variable is not inherently a dependent variable—one could readily imagine studies that seek to ascertain what effect depression has on other variables (e.g., physical illness, functional ability).
f. No, the report did not actually use the terms "independent variable" or "dependent variable."
g. Depression was operationally defined as scores on a self-report measure, the Beck Depression Inventory. Depression was not conceptually defined; the authors devoted more space to explicating the primary independent variable, coping, and linking it to a theoretic framework.

h. The data in this study were all quantitative.
i. Yes, the researchers investigated the relationship between coping strategies and depression. The report suggests that the researchers were thinking about the relationship in causal terms (i.e., that different coping strategies caused different levels of depression), but—as will subsequently be discussed in Chapter 9—establishing causality with the study design used in this study is tricky.
j. This was a nonexperimental (observational) study.
k. There was no intervention in this study. The researchers captured characteristics of the study participants at one point in time without intervening in any way.
l. The study involved the statistical analysis of data; there were no qualitative analyses.

Exercise 2: Questions of Fact (Appendix D)

a. Three nurses were the researchers for this study. At the time this paper was published, the lead author, Ward-Griffin, was a professor at a Canadian university, the second author (Bol) was a clinical nurse specialist at a health care center, and the third (Oudshoorn) was a doctoral student.
b. The study participants were ten community-dwelling older women with mild to moderate dementia, and their daughters.
c. The setting for this study was in the residences of the older women (i.e., in private homes for some and in retirement homes for others).
d. The key concept was the relationship between the mothers and their adult daughters within the context of the care needed as a result of the mothers' cognitive impairments.
e. No, there were no independent variables or dependent variables in this qualitative study.
f. The data for this study were primarily qualitative, although the researchers also obtained some quantitative demographic information that allowed them to describe the sample (e.g., the average age of the mothers was 88).

g. No, this study did not explicitly study relationships among concepts.

h. This study was not conducted within one of the three main qualitative traditions. It was a qualitative inquiry, but it was neither an ethnography, a phenomenologic study, nor a grounded theory study.

i. This study was nonexperimental.

j. There was no intervention in this study, as is usually the case in stand-alone qualitative inquiries.

k. The study did report a few pieces of statistical information, such as the average age of the mothers. The study primarily involved the qualitative analysis of rich, narrative data.

Exercise 3: Questions of Fact (Appendix E)

a. It appears that there was interdisciplinary collaboration in this project. Four of the project team (four authors) were RNs, three of whom were university faculty. The fourth was the Director of Surgical Nursing at a hospital. A fifth team member appears to have a business background (MBA degree) and a sixth taught in a school of pharmacy.

b. For the substudy described in the report, the study participants were older surgical patients undergoing elective joint replacement surgery at a hospital in Rhode Island.

c. The independent variable was exposure (versus nonexposure) to the pain management protocol. The patients were assessed with regard to outcomes before being introduced to the pain protocol, and then again after the protocol was implemented. The dependent variables in this study were patients' knowledge about, attitudes toward, and use of the three nondrug pain management procedures.

d. According to Table 1, 8 to 12 months were required to implement the protocols, collect data from study participants, and analyze how much change had occurred from before to after the protocols were implemented.

■ Chapter 4

A. CROSSWORD PUZZLE ANSWERS

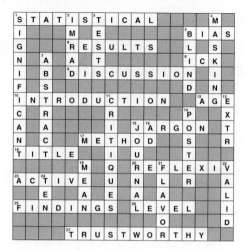

B. MATCHING EXERCISES

1. c	2. d	3. b	4. a	5. c
6. e	7. d	8. b	9. c	10. e
11. b	12. d			

D. APPLICATION EXERCISES

Exercise 1: Questions of Fact (Appendix A)

a. Yes, the structure of the Hill and colleagues' article follows the IMRAD format. The Introduction begins with the first word and includes a subheading called "Background." Then, a Method, Results, and Discussion sections follow.

b. The Abstract is a "new style" abstract with subheadings, as is now required for articles submitted to the journal *Nursing Research,* which published this paper.

c. Yes, the Abstract includes all this information, organized into sections called Background, Objective, Methods, Results, and Discussion.

d. The article is written in the passive voice. For example, the first sentence states that "this research *was approved* and *monitored* through the university's institutional review board." In the active voice, this sentence could be stated as follows: "The university's institutional review board approved and monitored this research."

e. This study is experimental. The researchers intervened by offering a computer intervention to some chronically ill rural women who participated in the study.

f. Yes, although the Abstract does not explicitly mention randomness. In the first paragraph of the Method section, however, the authors stated that "... 120 women were randomized into intervention and control groups. ..."

Exercise 2: Questions of Fact (Appendix B)

a. Yes, the report basically follows the IMRAD format. The first part of the article is the introduction and the next part is called Design and Methods. The "Results" are labeled "Findings" in this paper, and the final section is the Discussion.

b. The Abstract is a traditional narrative style abstract. The journal in which the article was published, *Qualitative Health Research*, requires an abstract of no more than 150 words. This Abstract had 142 words.

c. The Abstract does indicate the study purpose in the first sentence ("to develop a substantive theory to explain. ..". There is little information about the researchers' methods, except to say that they used a grounded theory approach. For example, the Abstract does not indicate how many women were in the sample, how many times they were interviewed, and so on. Most of the Abstract is devoted to a summary of the findings, and the last sentence

noted that the findings have important implications for delivery of health care.

d. The presentation is in the passive voice. For example, the first sentence of the Design and Methods section states that "Grounded theory was used to address the study objectives." In the active voice, this might be stated as follows: "We used grounded theory to address the study objectives."

e. Yes, this study was a grounded theory study, which is appropriate for understanding social processes relating to a phenomenon. Here, the researchers were interested in understanding how young women with type 1 diabetes managed their lives.

■ Chapter 5

A. CROSSWORD PUZZLE ANSWERS

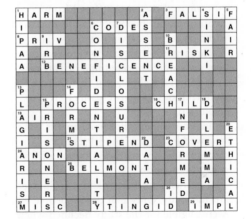

B. MATCHING EXERCISES

1. d	2. b	3. c	4. b	5. a
6. d	7. b	8. a	9. c	10. a
11. b	12. d			

D. APPLICATION EXERCISES

Exercise 1: Questions of Fact (Appendix C)

a. Yes, the report indicated, in a subsection labeled "Procedure," that approval for the study was obtained from an Institutional Review Board, although it did not state *which* IRB was used. The researchers are associated with Vanderbilt University (Vollman and LaMontagne) and the University of Arizona (Hepworth). The site for this study was not stated in the article.

b. No, the subjects in this study would not be considered *vulnerable* in the standard sense. A diagnosis of heart failure is not a criterion for needing special human rights protections.

c. It does not appear that study participants were subjected to any harm or discomfort. It is possible that some of the questions on the psychosocial scales were mildly distressing to those who suffered from depression, but probably no more so than ordinary day-to-day interactions. The researchers took precautions to ensure that data were collected in a private setting within the clinic, and that there were opportunities for participants to rest to avoid fatigue.

d. It does not appear that participants were deceived in any way, nor does there appear to be any methodological advantage of deception.

e. No, participants were asked to volunteer for the study. Only 2 of the 77 people who were eligible for the study declined when invited to participate, and they had other illness that made participation difficult.

f. The article stated that informed consent was obtained. No further details about the informed consent process was provided (e.g., ensuring that all participants could read and properly understand the consent form), but this is typical.

g. The article indicated that data were collected in a private setting. The researchers also took steps to ensure confidentiality.

The article indicated that they used an "anonymous descriptor" to attach to the data and kept the data in a locked file in the principal investigator's office. This does not mean that data were collected anonymously—the researcher personally collected the questionnaires and forms from each participant and, in such situations, anonymity is not possible. Anonymity occurs only when no one can tell who provided information. Nevertheless, the researchers took steps to ensure that the names and identifying information of participants were not attached to the data. The article also indicated that the actual questionnaires were destroyed at the end of the study.

Exercise 2: Questions of Fact (Appendix D)

a. Yes, the authors stated, in a subsection labeled "Recruiting and Sampling Methods," that approval for the study was obtained from "the Ethics Review Board of the affiliated university." Presumably, that meant the University of Western Ontario, the university with which Ward-Griffin is associated.

b. The mothers in the study might be considered vulnerable because of their cognitive impairment, but their scores on a test of cognitive function suggested that their dementia was fairly mild. A cutoff score on the SMMSE—a widely used scale for measuring cognitive function in the elderly—was established, and one criterion for participating in the interview was the women had to demonstrate good verbal and comprehension skills (e.g., state their date of birth). Women with more serious cognitive impairment were not interviewed. The researchers took special steps to "provide support and information during the interview" and to use special strategies, such as visual aids, which have been found useful in interviewing people with cognitive impairments.

c. It appears that the researchers were respectful of the study participants and did not subject them to harm or discomfort. The interviews did arouse the expression of some psychologically difficult emotions (e.g., guilt), but the conversations had the potential to be cathartic and therapeutic as well. The researchers took steps to ensure that the interviews were at a convenient time and place, and also allowed the mothers to decide whether they wanted to be interviewed in private (which was the intent) or in the presence of a relative, usually the daughter. The daughters were interviewed separately. The researchers appear to have taken steps to ensure that the experience for the mothers was a positive one—and one that would give voice to *their* experiences, from their perspective (unlike most research on dementia, which typically gathers information from caregivers). The report specifically noted that a goal was to create "the potential for personal empowerment consistent with feminist goals" and, therefore, it is likely that study participants themselves benefited from participating in this study.

d. Nothing in the report suggests that study participants were deceived in any way.

e. Given the feminist perspective of this research—a perspective that is purposefully respectful of women's autonomy—it is highly unlikely that any of the mothers or daughters were coerced to participate in this study. Indeed, in some families more than one daughter wanted to be included in the study.

f. It appears that both mothers and daughters signed their own informed consent forms. If the daughters had not themselves been participants in this study, it probably would have been advisable to get their consent (or the consent of another relative) on behalf of their mothers. Some might argue that a third party (i.e., not the daughters) should have been asked to give consent for the older women, but that would be an extremely conservative position—a position that the ethical review board apparently did not hold. In most cases, there were two sets of interviews,

and at the second, the assent of each participant was reaffirmed.

g. All participants were assured of confidentiality and, in the report itself, the names of the study participants were not disclosed; pseudonyms were used. Most interviews were conducted in private, except when the mothers expressly requested that a relative be present. Although nonprivate interviews were not specifically sought by the researchers, these joint sessions did allow them to make interesting observations of mother–daughter interactions.

■ **Chapter 6**

A. CROSSWORD PUZZLE ANSWERS

```
          S   R   S   C           M
N O N D I R E C T I O N A L       U
U   A   M   S   A       S   I     L
L   P O P   S   T A T E M E N T
L       L   I           I         I V
  M O R E       S O C I A L       P
    B           T                 L
    J       H   I           B   E R
T H E O R Y     C O M P L E X     E
E   C       P   A   U   F         L
S   T       L   P R O O F         A
T   I       P       P   R         T
  V E R B S       T W O   E       I
    E   O           S             O
D V S   B I A S   Q U E S T I O N
```

B. MATCHING EXERCISES

B.1.

1. b	2. c	3. a	4. b	5. a
6. c	7. b	8. a		

B.2.

1. a	2. c	3. d	4. a	5. b
6. d	7. a	8. c	9. b	10. d
11. b	12. c	13. b	14. a	15. c

C. STUDY QUESTIONS

C.4. Independent variable = IV, dependent variable = DV

2a. IV = type of stimulation (tactile versus verbal); DV = physiologic arousal
2b. IV = infants' birth weight; DV = incidence of hypoglycemia
2c. IV = use versus nonuse of isotonic sodium chloride solution; DV = oxygen saturation
2d. IV = patients' fluid balance; DV = success in weaning patients from mechanical ventilation
2e. IV = patients' gender; DV = amount of narcotic analgesics administered by nurses
3a. IV = prior blood donation versus no prior donation; DV = amount of anxiety during donation
3b. IV = amount of conversation initiated by nurses; DV = patients' ratings of nursing effectiveness
3c. IV = ratings of nurses' informativeness; DV = amount of preoperative stress
3d. IV = pregnancy status of female appendectomy patients; DV = incidence of peritoneal infection
3e. IV = type of delivery (vaginal versus cesarean); DV = incidence of postpartum depression

D. APPLICATION EXERCISES

Exercise 1: Questions of Fact (Appendix A)

a. The first paragraph of this report stated the crux of the problem. Here is one way in which the problem might be summarized:

  Adaptation to chronic disease is a lifelong process that is emotionally challenging. Rural women who are chronically ill have limited access to resources to address their adaptation difficulties; they are typically forced to struggle with the challenges of their chronic illness in isolation. Computer-based support systems are one potential solution to the problem of adaptation to chronic disease within the context of an isolated residence.

b. A purpose statement was presented in the last sentence before the "Method" section. Two purposes are stated, the first of which implies a descriptive intent: to *examine* relationships among various psychosocial indicators. The second purpose is consistent with a study using an experimental design, as this study did: to *determine* the effect of the intervention on various outcomes.
c. The report did not explicitly state research questions, although they were implied by the purpose statement. They might be stated as follows: "To what extent are psychosocial indicators, such as social support, self-esteem, empowerment, self-efficacy, stress, depression, and loneliness, interrelated among rural women who are chronically ill?" and "What is the effect of a computer intervention for chronically ill rural women on these psychosocial indicators?"
d. No hypotheses were formally stated.
e. One hypothesis would be "chronically ill rural women exposed to the computer intervention will have greater improvements to their self-esteem than similar women not exposed to the intervention."
f. Yes, the researchers used hypothesis-testing statistical tests. In fact, they tested the hypotheses we proposed in (e.), along with others.

Exercise 2: Questions of Fact (Appendix D)

a. The research problem is a bit difficult to ferret out in this report; it is not stated in a single paragraph. Rather, it is woven throughout the first four paragraphs. Here is one way in which the basic problem could be stated:

  Diabetes is a significant chronic illness affecting many people. Individuals living with diabetes face many challenges, and some of those challenges are particularly acute during times of life transition. Limited information exists linking people's experience of chronic illness to their life trajectories. Of particular concern, a paucity of evidence describes strategies that young women with type 1 diabetes use to address issues related to the transition to motherhood.

b. Rasmussen and her colleagues summarized the purpose of the study in the last sentence of the Introduction: The aim of the study was to develop a substantive theory of how women with type 1 diabetes managed turning points and transitions in their lives. The phrase used (*to develop a theory*) implies a grounded theory study, which, in fact, this study was.

c. The report did not state specific research questions. Here is a possible research question, which is basically the statement of purposes worded in the interrogatory form: "How do young women with type 1 diabetes manage turning points and transitions in their lives?" Given the redundancy of this question with the statement of purpose, it was not necessary to state both in the report.

d. No hypotheses were stated, nor would one have been appropriate in this qualitative study.

e. No, no hypotheses were tested. Qualitative studies do not use statistical methods to test hypotheses.

■ Chapter 7

A. CROSSWORD PUZZLE ANSWERS

B. MATCHING EXERCISES

B.1.

1. d   2. a   3. b   4. a   5. c
6. b   7. d   8. c   9. b   10. d

D. APPLICATION EXERCISES

Exercise 1: Questions of Fact (Appendix F)

a. This was a systematic literature review—a meta-analysis.

b. Yes, the Introduction described a research problem that the researchers addressed. The problem might be stated as followed: "Researchers have tested interventions designed to improve the mental health of caregivers of stroke patients. However, this body of research has not been systematically evaluated and integrated."

c. Yes, there was a statement of purpose in the first sentence of a subsection labeled *Purpose, Research Question, and Variable Definitions*: "The purpose of this meta-analysis was to examine the effectiveness of interventions for improving the mental health of caregivers of stroke patients by synthesizing across studies."

d. The researchers used two primary databases in their literature search—CINAHL and MEDLINE. They also noted that they did a citation search in the Social Science Citation Index and the Science Citation Index (these are both part of ISI's Web of Knowledge). This suggests they used a descendancy approach, although the specifics of this strategy were not described in the article. It appears that these electronic database searches were supplemented by a search in the Cochrane library, but again not much detail about this strategy was provided.

e. The keywords were: caregiving, stroke caregiver, stroke caregiving, control group, and intervention.

f. Yes, the reviewers restricted their search to reports written in English.

g. The researchers originally identified 30 citations through CINAHL and MEDLINE, and then obtained one additional citation through the citation search strategy.

h. The report identified five specific criteria for including a study in their review: (a) it had to include informal caregivers of stroke patients; (b) the study had to involve an intervention designed to improve the mental health of the caregivers; (c) the mental health outcome had to be measured by a specific instrument, the SF-36; (d) it had to be a quantitative study; and (e) there had to be an intervention group and a comparison group for whom outcome data were available. Studies not meeting these criteria were excluded.

i. Only 11 of the 31 originally identified studies met all the criteria for inclusion in the review.

j. All studies included in the review were quantitative—which is always the case in a meta-analysis.

Exercise 2: Questions of Fact (Appendix G)

a. Xu undertook a systematic review of studies relating to the experience of being an Asian nurse working in a western country. His review was a metasynthesis.

b. Xu began with a problem statement that noted that the nursing shortage throughout the world has resulted in the international recruitment of Asian nurses, but that little is known about the actual experiences of Asian nurses who work in western countries.

c. According to the report, Xu searched five mainstream electronic databases, including CINAHL, Medline, PsychINFO, Sociological Abstract, and ERIC (a database for education literature). He also searched Proquest Dissertations and Theses for nonpublished work. His efforts were not restricted to electronic database searches. Xu also used traditional "ancestry" type searches (i.e., retrieving studies cited in other relevant studies) and hand-searched journals that had a history of publishing research on the topic of interest. Xu also made efforts to interact with original researchers.

d. The keywords used in the search included *Asian nurses, foreign nurses, foreign-born nurses, internationally educated nurse, internationally recruited nurses, immigrant nurses,* and the names of specific Asian countries, such as Korea and Taiwan.

e. The report indicated that the search was restricted to English-language reports.

f. The report did not indicate how many references were initially retrieved using the stated search strategies, nor how many were discarded because they did not meet inclusion criteria. A total of 14 studies were actually included in the review.

g. The studies included in the review were either purely qualitative or there was a qualitative component within a study that included both qualitative and quantitative data.

h. The 14 studies in the review included a grounded theory study, an ethnography, phenomenological studies, qualitative descriptive studies, and some studies that had both qualitative and quantitative components (mixed methods studies).

■ Chapter 8

A. CROSSWORD PUZZLE ANSWERS

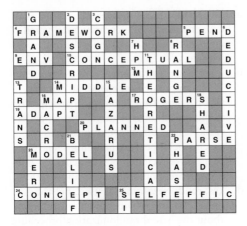

B. MATCHING EXERCISES

B.1.

1. c   2. e   3. d   4. e   5. d
6. a   7. b   8. d

B.2.

1. c   2. d   3. g   4. a   5. f
6. b   7. h   8. e

D. APPLICATION EXERCISES

Exercise 1: Questions of Fact (Appendix C)

a. Yes, the theoretical framework for this study was Lazarus and Folkman's Theory of Stress and Coping.

b. Yes, the authors devoted several paragraphs in the Introduction explaining features of the theory and its relevance to adjustment to heart failure.

c. No, the theory is not a theory of nursing, although the central constructs (stress and coping) are of clear relevance to health care professionals.

d. Yes, the Lazarus and Folkman theory is an example of a theory developed in the con-

text of one discipline (psychology) that has been found to be productive in nursing and other health care disciplines. It is an excellent example of a shared theory.

e. No, the report did not include a schematic model.

f. The report provided conceptual definitions of two important concepts—emotion-focused strategies of coping and problem-focused coping strategies.

g. The authors alluded to, but did not formally state, their hypotheses. They did, however, use statistical tests that are hypothesis-testing analyses.

h. According to the theory, emotion-focused coping would be expected to result in more depressive symptoms than problem-focused strategies.

Exercise 2: Questions of Fact (Appendix D)

a. Ward-Griffin and her colleagues described two theoretical or philosophical perspectives that served organizational and interpretive roles in their study: Feminism and a Life-course Perspective.

b. The perspectives were outlined in a section specifically called "Theoretical Framework." Although the description is relatively brief, it helps to orient readers to the frame of reference for the inquiry.

c. No, the frameworks are not one of the models of nursing cited in the textbook.

d. Both the feminist and life course perspectives have been used in many social science and health care disciplines, and so could be called *shared*. Feminist theory will be briefly discussed in Chapter 10.

e. No, no schematic model was used in this paper.

f. No, the report did not present hypotheses that the researchers wished to test, nor was any hypothesis testing undertaken. Qualitative studies do not test hypotheses; they explore the real-world experiences of people. Qualitative researchers often attempt *not* to have any preconceptions. Their findings sometimes lead to hypotheses, however. For example, based on this study, it might be possible to test whether feelings of "grateful guilt" among mothers with Alzheimer's disease are greater among mothers actually living with their daughters than among those who are not. This would, however, require the development of a formal instrument to measure "grateful guilt."

■ Chapter 9

A. CROSSWORD PUZZLE ANSWERS

```
                              V A L I D I T Y
        C R O S S O V E R     F             S
        A               A T T R       P         P
        S E L E C T I O N     E     F A C T O R
      Q E   O     O       D   R A N     N     N E
        C O N T R O L     O       F     E     L
        O   G   R       M O R T A L I T Y
        N   I   E   M       E
        T   T   L   A   B   P R O S P E C
      G R O U P     T R E N     O       C
        O   D   E   C   T   T       W     O
      T L     X   H A W T H O R N E     O   U
      E       P   I       R               B
      M   I N T E R N A L     E X T E R N A L
      P   F   R   G       A   W             E
      O       I     S E C T I O N A L
      R A N D O M I Z E     O               W
      A       E     L E V E L   R I V A L
      L       N   F   A                 I
        C O U N T E R   T R E A T M E N T
```

B. MATCHING EXERCISES

B.1.

1. b   2. b   3. a   4. d   5. b
6. a   7. d   8. a   9. b   10. d

C. STUDY QUESTIONS

C.2.

2.a. Nonexperimental   3.a. Nonexperimental
2.b. Nonexperimental   3.b. Both
2.c. Nonexperimental   3.c. Nonexperimental
2.d. Both   3.d. Both
2.e. Nonexperimental   3.e. Nonexperimental

D. APPLICATION EXERCISES

Exercise 1: Questions of Fact (Appendix A)

a. Yes, the purpose of the study was to evaluate the effects of a computer-delivered intervention for chronically ill rural women.

b. The design for this study was experimental.

c. The manipulated independent variable was participation versus nonparticipation in the special intervention. The dependent variables included several measures of psychosocial health, including social support, self-esteem, empowerment, self-efficacy, depression, loneliness, and stress.

d. Yes, randomization was used, but the report did not provide much information about the actual randomization procedure.

e. The control group strategy (counterfactual) in this study was the absence of a special intervention.

f. In this study, data were collected from experimental and control group members twice—at baseline and at some point after the intervention. Thus, the specific design was a pretest–posttest (before–after) experimental design.

g. The design is a between–subjects design; the researchers compared outcomes for the experimental and control group members, who were not the same people.

h. It does not appear that any masking or blinding was used in this study.

i. Although data were collected twice (before and after the intervention), the study would not be called longitudinal. If Hill and colleagues had collected another round of follow-up data 3 months later to ascertain long-term effects of the intervention, then the study would be longitudinal.

j. Hill and colleagues used two methods to control confounding variables, the most important of which was randomization to groups. Another method (although this method was undoubtedly not explicitly used as a control method) was homogeneity. All of the study participants were women (not men); they lived in rural areas (not urban or suburban areas) and had a chronic (not acute) illness.

k. Through randomization, virtually all subject characteristics (e.g., age, income, marital status, type of chronic illness) would have been controlled. Through homogeneity, gender, area of residence, and acute versus chronic illness were controlled (i.e., held constant).

l. Yes, there was attrition. As shown in Figure 1, 17 members of the experimental group (28%) did not receive the intervention and 1 additional subject did not complete the follow-up data collection forms. Additionally, 2 control group members (3%) did not provide follow-up data.

m. In this study, it would have been difficult to achieve constancy of conditions. The intervention itself was delivered in a manner that made it possible for women in the treatment group to "participate at any convenient time" (or *not* to participate). Researchers had no control over such factors as privacy, comfort, time of day the intervention was used, and so on. Data were collected via self-administered questionnaire, and again there would have been no opportunity to ensure that conditions were constant or even similar. On the other hand, by having a standardized Internet-based program, the researchers had control over some aspects that would be difficult to achieve if the intervention had been delivered "live" in various community settings.

n. As noted in the previous question, the researchers did not have much control over the intervention, except to offer it to those in the experimental group and withhold it from those in the control group. It would have been possible for those in the treatment group to get virtually no intervention, and it might have been possible for those in the control group to get alternative (and varying) forms of social support and health-related information. Given the decentralized nature of the intervention, this was not an aspect over which researchers had much control.

Exercise 2: Questions of Fact (Appendix C)

a. No, there was no intervention in this study.

b. The study design was nonexperimental.

c. As noted in Chapter 3, the researchers conceptualized coping styles as the key independent variable and depressive symptoms as the dependent variable.

d. No, the researchers could not have experimentally manipulated coping styles. People had previously developed different styles of coping with stress, and "brought" those styles to the study.

e. The researchers did not compare people who could be categorized into distinct groups, as in, for example, a case-control design. Instead, they compared people who had different levels of alternative coping styles. People with higher scores on, for example, the escape-avoidance subscale of the Ways of Coping Questionnaire (WCQ) were compared with those with lower scores on that subscale in terms of their depressive symptoms. The researchers examined whether high scores on all eight subscales of the WCQ correlated with (were associated with) higher scores on the depression scale.

f. The researchers stated that their design was descriptive correlational.

g. No, there was no randomization in this study. Matching was not used either, although technically this would have been possible. That is, people who primarily used problem-focused coping strategies could have been matched to people who primarily used emotion-focused coping strategies in terms of key background characteristics, such as gender, age, marital status, or functional impairment. Homogeneity was used to a certain extent—for example, all study participants were adults who had been diagnosed with heart failure. The analysis section is undoubtedly too complex for most of you at this point, but we can point out that the researchers did use statistical methods to control a few of the participants' background characteristics.

Study Guide for Essentials of Nursing Research: Appraising Evidence for Nursing Practice, 7e

h. No, there was no masking or blinding in this study. Although masking is more common in experimental than in nonexperimental studies, it is possible (and sometimes advisable) to use masking with the people collecting data in a nonexperimental study (i.e., not to tell them the study hypotheses).

i. The study is retrospective. The depressive symptoms had already occurred in the study participants, and the researchers were trying to examine previously established coping styles as potential contributing factors.

j. This study was cross-sectional. All data were collected at a single point in time.

k. The research design was described as *descriptive* correlational, and yet the researchers invoked a theoretical model in which different coping strategies could be viewed as contributing to ("causing") depression. The researchers were aware, however, of the limitations of their design to support causal inferences. The authors themselves noted at the end of their report (under "Limitations") that their research design "restricts the ability to make causal inferences regarding the causal nature of these relationships."

■ Chapter 10

A. CROSSWORD PUZZLE ANSWERS

B. MATCHING EXERCISES

A.1.

1. b	2. a	3. d	4. c	5. b
6. a	7. b	8. c	9. d	10. c
11. a	12. d			

C. STUDY QUESTIONS

C.1.

a. Grounded theory b. Ethnography
c. Discourse analysis d. Phenomenology

D. APPLICATION EXERCISES

Exercise 1: Questions of Fact (Appendix B)

a. The research by Rasmussen and colleagues was a grounded theory study.

b. The researchers used the Glaserian approach to grounded theory. They cited two of Glaser's writings in the section on data analysis.

c. The central phenomenon studied in this project was the self-management of young women with type 1 diabetes during turning points and transitions in their lives.

d. No, the study was not longitudinal. Rasmussen and her colleagues did not follow the young women through periods of transition to observe how these transitions were negotiated and processed. Rather, the young women were asked to give retrospective accounts of their experiences.

e. This study was conducted in Victoria, Australia. Women were recruited through an advertisement in Diabetes Australia newsletters and on a support group Web site. Unfortunately, the report did not actually state where data were collected. It seems likely that the interviews were conducted in the young women's homes, but it is possible that they were conducted elsewhere, such as at a health care facility or at the researchers' university offices.

f. Yes, in the data analysis subsection the researchers stated that "Constant comparative analysis was used throughout the study." No further elaboration was provided.

g. Yes, Rasmussen and colleagues identified the basic social problem as *being in the grip of blood glucose levels*. The basic social process was called "creating stability."

h. Rasmussen and colleagues used a well-suited methodological approach, grounded theory, to get a rich, holistic understanding of the problems that young women with type 1 diabetes faced during life transitions, and the processes used to manage those transitions successfully. Given the researchers' aims, no other qualitative approach would have been as suitable. Other qualitative traditions would not have discovered the major concern of "being in the grip" of blood glucose levels, nor the basic social process (creating stability) that described the young women's manner of addressing it.

i. The methods used in this study were congruent with a grounded theory approach. The researchers conducted lengthy conversational interviews with 20 young women, supplemented by conversations with relatives and health professionals. During the interviews, the researchers made observations of the women and recorded "nonverbal communication." They also analyzed relevant documents and newspapers, although details about these data sources were not provided.

j. No, this study did not have an ideological perspective. Although all of the study participants were female, gender was not a key construct in helping the researchers interpret the data.

Exercise 2: Questions of Fact (Appendix D)

a. The study by Ward-Griffin and colleagues was a feminist study. The report explicitly noted that the researchers were "guided by feminist and life-course perspectives."

An entire section of the report was devoted to explicating these perspectives ("Theoretical Framework."). We did not explain the "life course perspective" in the textbook; it is a method of capturing the ongoing and evolving nature of a phenomenon by eliciting rich retrospective narratives. In this case, the approach was used to focus the conversations on the care relationships between two generations of women as they developed over time and as they shaped the women's sense of well-being.

b. The central phenomenon of this study was the care that women with dementia received from their adult daughters, with emphasis on the women's own perspectives on that care.

c. This study was longitudinal. Mothers and their daughters (sometimes multiple daughters) were interviewed twice, 6 to 9 months apart. The researchers explicitly wanted to capture how the care relationship evolved over time: ". . . We were interested in understanding how the progress of dementia may shape the mother–daughter relationship." They also offered a rationale for the amount of time elapsed between interviews: ". . . We selected an intermediate time frame, one that would potentially capture this aspect of the relationship without risking participant attrition."

d. The research was conducted in an unidentified Canadian community. (It is not uncommon for qualitative reports to avoid mentioning the community name, as a measure to protect privacy and confidentiality.) The researchers offered to conduct interviews in locations that were "mutually convenient," but it appears that all interviews were "held at the mother's residence." The mothers all lived in the community, some in their own homes, some in the daughters' homes, and two in retirement homes.

e. The researchers articulated three research questions. The first, "How do women with AD (Alzheimer's disease) and their adult daughters describe their experiences of receiving/providing care?" is one that could perhaps have been addressed in a phenomenological study. The second question was, "How do women with AD and their adult daughters describe their relationship?" This is a question that appears especially well-suited to a life course perspective, inasmuch as the relationships were continually evolving and ever-changing within the context of shifting life experiences, needs, health, demands, and capabilities. The third question was, "What contextual factors influence the care provided/received?" It is this third question that is especially congruent with a feminist perspective. As the researchers noted, a feminist perspective "views women's everyday caring experiences as inextricably connected to the larger political, social, and economic environment."

f. The in-depth and longitudinal methods used in this study were well-suited to answering the research questions and were congruent with the framework within which the study was conducted. The researchers selected a relatively small sample of families, but these families varied in important ways, such as living arrangements. Both daughters and mothers were interviewed—typically separately, but sometimes the daughters were present for the mothers' interview, which gave the researchers an opportunity to observe interactions between them. Two interviews were conducted with all but two families, which allowed the researchers to capture the evolution of the caring relationship.

▪ Chapter 11

A. CROSSWORD PUZZLE ANSWERS

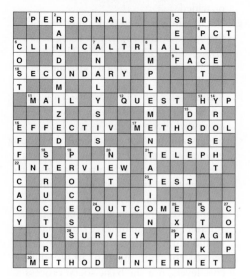

B. MATCHING EXERCISES

1. a, b, c	2. b	3. e	4. d	5. c
6. a	7. b	8. e	9. a	10. f

D. APPLICATION EXERCISES

Exercise 1: All Studies in Appendices

a. Clinical trial
  • The Hill et al. study in Appendix A could be described as a clinical trial: A randomized design was used to test an innovative intervention.

b. Economic analysis
  • None of the studies in the appendices involved an economic analysis (or, if they did, that part of the study was not presented in the reports).

c. Outcomes research
  • None of the studies in the appendices could be described as outcomes research.

d. Survey research
  • The Vollman et al. study (Appendix C) is the closest thing to a survey in the appendices, but it is not really an example of survey research. Surveys typically gather self-report data from a broad population of respondents—as in an opinion poll—rather than from patients with a particular health problem served at a particular institution.
e. Secondary analysis
  • None of the reports in the appendices is secondary analysis.
f. Methodological research
  • None of the studies in the appendices could be described as methodological research.

Exercise 3: Questions of Fact (Appendix E)

a. The overall project involved the collection of both qualitative and quantitative data, but (as described in this paper) the study was primarily quantitative. Narrative information appears to have been used primarily in the development of the project. For example, the report indicated that the principal investigators "conducted interviews at hospitals throughout the state" as part of the site selection process. These interviews were undoubtedly loosely structured and yielded narrative data, although a formal analysis was undoubtedly not undertaken. Then, the researcher conducted group interviews at the study site to identify problematic areas of pain management. Again, these were almost surely conversational discussions that helped to narrow the focus of this EBP project. Although the report did not provide elaborate detail about these aspects of the project, it did illustrate the value of qualitative information in the development of a large-scale study.
b. Yes, this study involved the testing of an evidence-based intervention in a real-world setting. The intervention was the best-practice pain management protocols.

c. Yes, the report mentions that an Audit Instrument was used "to assure that each patient's complementary pain service nurse followed the best-practice protocols." The article later described efforts of the site coordinator to monitor all patients and to measure nurses' compliance with study protocols.
d. Some methodological research was undertaken in developing and refining the instrument that was used to collect pain outcome data—the Non-Drug Complementary Pain Interventions Survey. The original instrument was tested with a small group of adults to ascertain its "readability, user-friendliness, and length." Also, a panel of nursing experts assessed the degree of consistency between the conceptual definitions and the operational definitions of the concepts.
e. The researchers noted that a "primary efficacy study" was underway when this paper was submitted for publication. Although the full research design for the efficacy study was not described in detail, the paper indicated that a "two-group, quasi-experimental design" was being used "to determine the impact of nondrug interventions on pain intensity, functional ability, and patient satisfaction."
f. It is fair to say that the researchers were *evaluating* the effectiveness of their best-practices protocols. The part of the study that received the most attention in this report was the pilot substudy, which is a good example of an outcome analysis. The primary purposes of the substudy were to ascertain feasibility for the primary study and to get preliminary evidence about the effectiveness of the protocols. A simple one-group, pretest–posttest design was used to evaluate changes in patient knowledge and attitudes. The main study (the results of which were not yet available) could be described as an impact analysis; in fact, the researchers themselves used the word "impact" in describing this component. The efforts to monitor intervention fidelity

could be considered part of a process analysis—and, undoubtedly, other steps were taken to document how the intervention actually worked in practice. Cost analysis was not mentioned in this project.

▪ Chapter 12

A. CROSSWORD PUZZLE ANSWERS

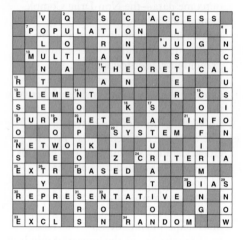

B. MATCHING EXERCISES

B.1.

| 1. c | 2. a | 3. d | 4. b | 5. d |
| 6. b | 7. c | 8. d | 9. a | 10. d |

B.2.

| 1. b | 2. c | 3. a | 4. d | 5. a |
| 6. c | 7. a | 8. a | 9. d | 10. b |

C. STUDY QUESTIONS

C.3.

a. Cluster (multistage)   b. Convenience
c. Systematic   d. Quota
e. Simple random   f. Purposive
g. Consecutive

D. APPLICATION EXERCISES

Exercise 1: All Appendix Studies

a. None of the studies in the appendices used probability samples.
b. It appears that all of the quantitative studies in the appendices (A, C, and E) used convenience sampling, although there is a possibility that a consecutive sample was recruited by Tracy and colleagues (Appendix E). Convenience sampling was also used initially by Ward-Griffin and colleagues to recruit community-dwelling women with cognitive impairment (Appendix D). (Sampling in the study by Rasmussen and colleagues, Appendix B, is discussed below.)
c. Snowball sampling was used in the study by Ward-Griffin and colleagues in Appendix D. Some study participants were referred to the researchers by participants already in the study (their sisters).

Exercise 2: Questions of Fact (Appendix C)

a. The target population for this study is presumably adults diagnosed with heart failure (HF) in the United States. The accessible population was adults with HF in one particular locale. The locale was not identified in the article. (Probably it was Nashville, Tennessee, where two of the three authors teach at a university.)
b. To be eligible for the study, prospective participants had to (a) be able to speak and understand English; (b) be 21 years or older; (c) have an HF diagnosis; (d) not have acute cardiac decompensation; (e) not have any clinically significant psychopathology, other than depression; (f) be able to complete the study questionnaires; and (g) have access to a telephone.
c. According to the paper itself, the sampling method was convenience sampling, a nonprobability method. It seems possible that a consecutive sample *might* have been recruited, but there is insufficient information to make this determination.

d. Participants were patients at a heart institute. Patients who met the eligibility criteria were invited to take part in the study by a physician or nurse practitioner during a routine clinic visit.

e. The article stated that the researchers approached 77 people who met the eligibility criteria for the study, and that 75 of them actually participated. This suggests a very high response rate of 97%. It is not clear, however, whether there were only 77 patients who met the eligibility criteria in the heart institute. It seems more likely that when the physician or nurse practitioner approached potential participants, some of them immediately expressed a lack of interest in participating. In other words, it is probably not possible to calculate a true response rate in this study.

f. The final sample consisted of 75 adults with HF.

g. In the subsection called "Research Design," the researchers indicated that they had done a power analysis for their planned analyses and concluded that a sample of 75 subjects would be adequate for testing the relationships among study variables.

h. The first subsection of the Results section is labeled "Sample Characteristics." The sample was described in considerable detail in terms of age, gender, marital status, ethnicity, socioeconomic status, functional impairment, length of time since diagnosis of HF, and use of antidepressants. Although there was diversity, the "typical" study participant was a white middle-aged, middle-class married man who had been diagnosed with HF about 4 years previously.

Exercise 3: Questions of Fact (Appendix B)

a. Specific eligibility criteria were not stated in this report. We can infer, however, that to be eligible, prospective participants had to (a) be female; (b) have a diagnosis of type 1 diabetes; (c) be an adult (e.g., >18

years of age); and (d) be able to speak and understand English. The title of the article indicates that the focus was on "young women," but the article did not stipulate an upper age limit for eligibility—only that the oldest person was 36 years old.

b. Participants were recruited through advertisements in a diabetes-focused newsletter (Diabetes Australia) and through announcements on the web sites of local diabetes support groups.

c. The article stated that "both purposeful and theoretical sampling procedures were used." As described, however, the primary sampling approach appears to be sampling by convenience. Participants were women who volunteered in response to the recruitment advertisements. It does not appear that the researchers purposively selected particular types of young women, nor sought to maximize variation, select typical cases, and so on. In other words, the only "purposive" aspect of the sampling plan, it appears, is that the researchers deliberately selected young women with diabetes, but their participants were a convenience sample of those who met these criteria. Later in the study, however, the researchers expanded their sample to address theoretical concerns. For example, their theoretical needs led them to interview young women who had given birth, and they also interviewed family members of young women with diabetes and health professionals who worked with diabetes patients.

d. The main sample consisted of 20 women with type 1 diabetes.

e. The report did not mention saturation. (This does not mean that it did not occur.)

f. Sampling confirming or disconfirming cases was not mentioned.

g. Characteristics of the 20 women were briefly described. The young women were, on average, 28 years of age and had lived with diabetes for an average of 17 years. More than half the women had no family history of type 1 diabetes, but one-fourth had immediate family members with diabetes. It appears that all participants were white women of European descent. The marital status, educational background, and employment status of the women were not described. Although the researchers stated that they had theoretically sampled women who had given birth, no information about childbearing histories of the 20 women was provided.

■ Chapter 13

A. CROSSWORD PUZZLE ANSWERS

B. MATCHING EXERCISES

B.1.

1. a, c 2. a, b   3. b, c 4. c   5. b
6. b   7. a, b, c 8. a, b 9. a, b, c 10. a, b

B.2.

1. b   2. a   3. c   4. a   5. d
6. a   7. a   8. b   9. d   10. c
11. c   12. b

D. APPLICATION EXERCISES

Exercise 1: Various Appendix Studies

The studies that used the three major data collection methods (by Appendix and author) are as follows:

- **Self Reports:** Appendix A (Hill and colleagues), Appendix B (Rasmussen and colleagues); and Appendix C (Vollman and colleagues) all used self-reports. Rasmussen et al. collected unstructured self-report data. The studies by Hill et al. and Vollman et al. used structured self-reports, including formal composite scales.
- **Observation:** In the study in Appendix B (Rasmussen et al.), the researchers indicated that they observed nonverbal communication.
- **Biophysiologic Measures:** None of the studies used biophysiologic measures.
- **Records:** Rasmussen and colleagues (Appendix B) indicated that their data included "relevant documents." There was no further mention of these documents, but they might have been existing records relating to the participants' health.

Exercise 2: Questions of Fact (Appendix E)

a. In their substudy, which served as a pilot for a larger, more rigorously designed study, Tracy and colleagues used data collection methods that were high on structure, quantifiability, obtrusiveness, and objectivity. All of the data were collected in a systematic, structured fashion, and in a manner that permitted statistical analysis. The numerical values were derived in an objective fashion. Researchers were "obtrusive"—participants were aware of their "subject" status.

b. Many of the variables in this study were operationally defined using instruments that the researchers developed themselves. The Non-Drug Complementary Pain Interventions Survey (NDCPI) appears to have been previously developed by Tracy, but was pretested and modified for the current study. After the pretest, the NDCPI was shortened and modifications were made to make the survey more "readable." This means that the researchers made efforts to ensure that the wording and sentence structure were easier to read by people with limited reading skills. Study participants also completed another form developed for this study, the Use of Non-Drug Complementary Interventions (UNDCPI) to document their use of the comfort enhancements described as part of the intervention. The researchers did use one existing instrument, the Miller Behavioral Style Scale (MBSS), to assess patients' information-coping style. The scale had been developed in 1987 for another purpose. Researchers almost always borrow or adapt existing instruments, rather than starting from scratch.

c. The primary method of collecting data in this study was via patient self-reports. All three of the instruments mentioned in the previous question—the NDCPI, the UNDCPI, and the MBSS—were structured self-report instruments. Patients recorded their own answers to questions in a paper-and-pencil format. These instruments measured patients' knowledge, attitudes, and prior behaviors regarding the best-practice protocols (NDCPI), as well as their actual use following the intervention (UNDCPI). The MBSS, as noted, was used to assess patients' preferred method for receiving information. This scale incorporated two "hypothetically stressful" vignettes designed to elicit information about patients' mode of dealing with stressful situations.

d. Data were apparently not collected by observation, although observation *was* an option in this study. Observers could have gathered information about the nurses' behavior in delivering the pain treatment plans and protocols, and also about the patients' use of music, imagery, and massage in the period after intervention.

e. No biophysiologic measurements were used in this study. None of the variables of interest were biophysiologic in nature.

f. It does appear that records were used to monitor nurses' adherence to the individualized pain treatment plans and protocols. The report indicates that they developed an audit instrument (an adaptation of a previously used instrument) to extract data about nursing actions from patients' charts.

g. A research assistant explained the project to study participants and gathered baseline data. The report does not specify who gathered the daily UNDCPI data or the NDCPI data on postoperative day 3, but in all likelihood, it was the same research assistant. No information is in the report about how the research assistant was trained, but this is not unusual. Also, no information is provided about whether the research assistant was blinded, but presumably, he or she was not.

h. The report does give some indications that steps were taken to enhance data quality. Commendably, for example, the newly developed instrument (NDCPI) was pretested and modified to accommodate patients with modest reading skills and to make it shorter. Moreover, the instrument was reviewed by a "panel of four nursing experts in complementary methods. . . ." (The concept of content validity is explained in Chapter 14 of the textbook.) Also, in choosing the MBSS, the researchers selected an instrument that had previously been found to be of good quality "in naturalistic, laboratory, and hypothetical settings."

Exercise 3: Questions of Fact (Appendix D)

a. In this study, data collection methods were *mostly* low on structure, quantifiability, and objectivity. The participants were, of course, aware of the researchers' presence and of their own role as study participants. Some data, such as demographic data and the formal instrument to measure level of dementia (the Standardized Mini-Mental Status Examination or SMMSE), were gathered in a formal, structured manner. Responses to the SMMSE questions were scored, and the scores were used in determining eligibility for the study. These structured data were not, however, used in any substantive manner in the study.

b. Most of the data in this study were collected via unstructured self-reports, through personal, face-to-face interviews with mothers and their daughters. Most interviews were individual interviews, between the interviewer and the study participant, but in three cases, the mother required or requested the presence of a third person, usually her daughter. The interviews were described as "focused," or semistructured. According to the article, "the interviewer asked the participant nondirective questions designed to trigger dialogue about her experiences in providing or receiving care, the mother–daughter relationship, and the factors influencing the process of care." The interviews, which lasted about 45 minutes each, were tape-recorded and then later transcribed for analysis. Many participants were interviewed on two occasions, 6 to 9 months apart, to capture the evolution of the mother–daughter caring relationship.

c. The study did not formally gather data via observation (i.e., it was not specifically part of the original plan), but some observations were made and recorded in field notes. For the three mothers who requested or needed conjoint interviews, the researcher was able to observe interactions between mothers and daughters. Even with individual interviewers, the researchers recorded full field notes "to record perceptions, insights, and observations."

d. No, this study did not collect any biophysiologic measures. None of the concepts of interest were biophysiologic in nature.

e. It does not appear that records, documents, or artifacts were used in this study. It is possible that some existing documents could have enriched the study (e.g., diaries of the daughters), but they were not essential to the study aims.

f. The three researchers on this project (Ward-Griffin, Bol, and Oudshoorn) appear to have been the interviewers on this study. No information is provided about their training for the study.

g. The report did mention some steps were taken to enhance data quality. In the paragraph before the subsection labeled "Data Analysis," the paper indicated that "all three investigators strove to build rapport with the participant," a crucial effort in in-depth studies. Without rapport between the interviewers and participants, the data tend to be thin, incomplete, and sometimes inaccurate. The researchers also noted the care they took to use interview strategies known to be successful with people who have Alzheimer's disease.

■ Chapter 14

A. CROSSWORD PUZZLE ANSWERS

¹F	A	²C	E			³C		⁴C	O	N	T	⁵E	N	⁶T	
		V				R						R		R	
⁷C	R	I	⁸T	E	R	I	O	N			¹⁰N		R	U	
¹¹G		E	E			N		¹²M		E		¹³O	N	E	
¹⁴R	U	L	E	S			¹⁵O	B	S	E	R	V	E	R	
O		I	T				A		A		E				¹⁶C
U		A					C		S		R				O
P		B					H		¹⁷P	¹⁸S		¹⁹V			N
S		I	²⁰O	²¹R	D			²²I		R	E	A			C
	²³L		R	A			²⁴I	N	T	E	R	N	A	L	U
	I			T				T		D	S		I		R
	T			I		²⁵L	E		I		I		D		R
²⁶P	S	Y	²⁷C	H	O	M	E	T	R	I	C		²⁸T	W	I	C	E
			U			V		V		T			I		T		N
²⁹F	A	C	T	O	R		E	A					V	Y		T
						L		L					I			

B. MATCHING EXERCISES

B.1.

1. d	2. a	3. d	4. b	5. c
6. a	7. b	8. d	9. c	10. b
11. b	12. a			

B.2.

1. a	2. c	3. d	4. c	5. b
6. d	7. b	8. a	9. c	10. d

C. STUDY QUESTIONS

C.1.

Two of these attributes—attitudes toward abortion and achievement motivation—are sufficiently enduring that they are unlikely to change markedly from one month to the next, unless an intervention was specifically designed to modify them. Thus, the test–retest approach would be an appropriate method of assessing reliability for these two traits. Nursing effectiveness is likely to be fairly stable, but *might* be modified over a 1-month period, depending on the extent of the nurses' experience and any intervening instruction or activities. The reliability of measures of stress and depression should not be assessed with a test–retest method (unless the time frames are quite short) because both these traits can fluctuate and be modified over time.

C.3.

a. High reliability of an instrument is necessary for strong validity, but it does not guarantee it.
b. The internal consistency of an instrument does not address whether it yields stable measurements over time.
c. The low validity coefficient could reflect a problem with the criterion measure rather than with the scale. For example, if the criterion had low reliability, this would depress the validity coefficient.
d. A true score can never be known. A reliability coefficient provides information about how good an approximation a *set* of obtained scores will be, on average, in representing true scores, but an individual true score cannot be inferred.
e. Validation efforts lend evidence in support of an inference of construct validity, but no amount of evidence *proves* construct validity.
f. Expert opinions yield one type of evidence about the validity of a measure, but one person's opinion would never yield sufficient *assurance*.

C.4.

a. The 15-item scale would likely be more reliable; longer scales are usually more reliable than shorter ones.
b. Stress would likely be more uniformly high among patients just diagnosed with cancer; the higher similarity of these scores would tend to depress reliability because it would be harder reliably to discriminate among people with high levels of stress.
c. Nursing knowledge would probably be more varied among seniors (some of whom have mastered nursing content and others of whom have not) than among freshmen. Therefore, reliability would be expected to be higher among senior students.

D. APPLICATION EXERCISES

Exercise 1: Studies in Appendices C and E

The levels of measurement of variables in these two studies are shown in the following table:

Level of Measurement	Appendix C, Vollman et al.	Appendix E, Tracy et al.
Nominal	Gender, marital status, race or ethnicity, diagnosis of depression, antidepressant medication use	Gender, race, marital status
Ordinal	Level of functional impairment (NYHA classification); socioeconomic status (Hollingshead Four-Factor Index)	Education
Interval	Depression (scores on the Beck Depression Inventory); coping (scores on the Ways of Coping Questionnaire)	Knowledge, attitudes, ability (Non-Drug Complementary Pain Interventions Survey); information coping style (Miller Behavioral Style Scale); Audit Instrument; Use of Non-drug-Complementary Interventions Form
Ratio	Age, illness duration	Age

Exercise 2: Questions of Fact (Appendix A)

a. All of the scales used in the Hill et al. study were assessed for internal consistency reliability using Cronbach's alpha, both by previous researchers and by the study team itself. The reliability coefficients were all presented in Table 2, in column 4 as published in other reports ("Reported α") and then in column 5 for this study ("Study α"). As computed using study data, the values of alpha were as follows: The Personal Resource Questionnaire (PRQ2000): .90; Self-Efficacy Scale: .88; Self-Esteem Scale: .87; Perceived Stress Scale: .90; CES-D Depression Scale: .90; and UCLA Loneliness Scale: .94. Several of these measures likely had also been assessed for test–retest reliability, but this information was not presented in the report.

b. The researchers selected instruments that have a strong reputation, but no specific information about validity was provided in the report. The report did indicate that the researchers selected their instruments based "on the strength of their psychometric properties," which suggests that they took validity assessments into consideration.

c. Hill and colleagues reported reliability assessments from other researchers, but they also computed Cronbach's alpha using data in their own study. There was no documentation of validity, either in this study or in earlier research.

d. No, no information was provided about the specificity or sensitivity of any of the instruments used in this study.

e. Levels of measurement for the variables in this study are shown in the following table:

Level of Measurement	Appendix A, Hill et al.
Nominal	Group status (experimental vs. control), time of measurement (baseline vs. 3 months later), ethnicity, marital status, employment status, dropout status, reasons for dropping out of the study
Ordinal	Household income, education, age (if asked in categories, as suggested, rather than as actual age)
Interval	Scores on the psychosocial scales (social support, self-esteem, empowerment, self-efficacy, stress, depression, loneliness)
Ratio	Length of chronic illness, travel distance for routine health care

■ Chapter 15

A. CROSSWORD PUZZLE ANSWERS

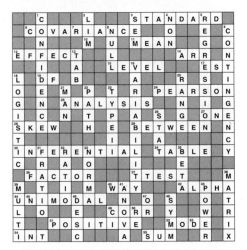

B. MATCHING EXERCISES

1. b   2. a   3. c   4. d   5. b
6. b   7. a   8. a   9. c   10. a

C. STUDY QUESTIONS

C.1. Unimodal, fairly symmetric
C.2. Mean: 81.8; Median: 83; Mode: 84

C.4. Absolute Risk, exposed group (AR$_E$) = .60; Absolute Risk, nonexposed group (AR$_{NE}$) = .90; Absolute Risk Reduction (ARR) = .30; Odds Ratio (OR) = .167
C.7. a. Chi-squared   b. *t*-test
        c. Pearson's *r*   d. ANOVA
C.8. a. Logistic regression   b. ANCOVA
        c. MANOVA   d. Multiple regression

D. APPLICATION EXERCISES

Exercise 1: Questions of Fact (Appendix A)

a. Both in the table and in the accompanying text, Hill and colleagues described their sample primarily using percentages (e.g., percentage older than age 40, percentage married). The only exceptions were that they reported the sample's mean length of time having a chronic illness, and the mean distance they traveled for routine health care. In both instances, the standard deviations were reported, and the range was also mentioned for length of time with a chronic illness. The researchers presumably *could have* reported the participants' mean age—unless they gathered their data as an ordinal variable. That is, if they asked participants how old they were, the responses would yield ratio-to-level data, for which a mean value could be computed. If, however, they asked participants to indicate whether they were 30 to 39, 40 to 49, and so on, this would yield ordinal data, for which percentages in each category would be appropriate. The same is true for the variable *Income*.

b. If a formal statistical analysis of group differences in preintervention characteristics was undertaken, it was not reported. Table 1 could have shown sample characteristics separately for the two groups, so that readers could assess the plausibility that the groups were demographically equivalent. Table 4 *did* present baseline (preintervention) means for experimentals (Es) and controls (Cs) on all the key outcomes, but it did not report whether E and C differences were statistically significant. For example, Table 4 indicates that Es scored higher than Cs at baseline on the Loneliness and Self-Esteem scales, but were these differences significant? In other words, to what extent should readers be concerned that the groups were really not equivalent before the Es received the intervention? Fortunately, the direction of the possible bias (favoring Cs) is opposite to the direction of the research hypothesis (psychosocial outcomes favoring Es). Ideally, however, the researchers would have noted in the report the results of analyses comparing the two groups on demographic characteristics (using χ^2 tests for differences in proportions) and baseline outcomes (using *t*-tests for independent groups).

c. Yes, there was some attrition—only 43 of 61 subjects randomly assigned to the E group provided data for the statistical analyses (29.5% attrition), and 57 of 59 subjects in the C group completed the study (3.3% attrition). Differences between those who completed and dropped out of the study—in terms of baseline and demographic characteristics—were not discussed, and so readers cannot be sure if there were any attrition biases.

d. The researchers used Pearson's *r* and RM-ANOVA.

e. Information relating to hypothesis tests was included, but confidence interval and effect size information was not presented (except that the Pearson *r*s are also effect size estimates). We can, however, compute *d*s (effect size estimates) using data provided in Table 4. For example, the effect of the intervention on empowerment was fairly substantial (estimated *d* = .75), whereas its effect on social support scores was modest (estimated *d* = .31).

f. Referring to Table 3:
- Correlation between depression and self-efficacy scores = −.586.
- All variables *except* depression were negatively correlated with loneliness.
- Stress scores were significantly correlated with all other variables.
- The correlation between stress and loneliness was the strongest (.716).
- The correlation between self-esteem and empowerment was the weakest (.354).
- *All* of the correlations were statistically significant at or beyond the .05 level.
- Pearson's *r*

g. Referring to Table 5:
- The independent variable is treatment group status.
- A significant main effect was seen for time (i.e., overall, empowerment levels improved over time for the sample as a whole), and a significant interaction effect (i.e., the improvement was significantly greater for the intervention group).
- Neither the main effect nor the interaction effect for self-efficacy was significant; neither the Es nor the Cs had a significant change in self-efficacy.
- Changes over time differed significantly for the two groups with regard to self-esteem, social support, and empowerment.
- Significant changes over time were observed for empowerment, depression, loneliness, and stress for the sample overall.
- RM-ANOVA was used and yielded *F*-ratio statistics.

h. No, the report did not indicate that a power analysis was done to estimate sample size needs.

Exercise 2: Questions of Fact (Appendix C)

a. Vollman and colleagues described their sample with various descriptive indexes, including percentages (e.g., percentage married = 44%); means and SDs (e.g., mean length of time since diagnosis = 49.2 months, SD = 14.4), and ranges (range for time since diagnosis = <1 month to 292 months). It might be noted that this information makes it clear that time since diagnosis was positively skewed, with at least one person with a very lengthy time period in the upper right tail of the distribution. The researchers presented all descriptive information in the text. A summary table would have been helpful.

b. The researchers used Pearson's correlation coefficients in their analysis of bivariate relationships. There was no correlation matrix—some *rs* (and associated *p* values) were reported in the text, and several others were mentioned as nonsignificant without specifying the actual values of the coefficients.

c. Information was provided relating to hypothesis tests, but confidence interval and effect size information was not presented (except that the Pearson *rs* are also effect size estimates).

d. Yes, the researchers did multiple regression analyses.

e. Referring to Table 2:
    * The dependent variable was scores on the depression scale (ideally, this information should have been noted in the title of the table). Depression was measured with a 21-item scale that yielded interval-level data.
    * The article was not specific about the number of predictor variables in the initial regression analysis. The text indicated that coping strategies and demographic variables were included in the regression. With regard to coping, as measured by the Ways of Coping Questionnaire, there are seven subscales and so there were presumably seven coping variables used as predictors. With regard to demographic or background factors, the ones mentioned in the text included age, gender, marital status, ethnicity, socioeconomic status, functional impairment status, ejection fractions from echocardiographic or ventriculographic studies, length of time with a diagnosis of heart failure, and use of antidepressant medications—in other words, possibly up to nine additional predictors. We doubt, however, that all were used in the initial regression analysis. In particular, it seems unlikely that prior use of antidepressants was used as a predictor, because if it had been used, it likely would have been found to be a significant predictor of depression scores, and this variable is *not* included in Table 2. Nevertheless, it seems safe to assume that the original regression used about 15 predictors.
    * Only the significant predictors of depression scores were retained in the final analysis. Thus, the four variables shown in Table 2 were significantly related to depression.
    * Neither the text nor Table 2 did a thorough job in indicating how all of the predictor variables were operationalized for the regression analysis. The two coping subscales (Escape-avoidance coping and Planful problem-solving coping) are straightforward—these were presumably the actual interval-level scores on these scales. The problem is with the last two variables in the table, the NYHA functional impairment class, and marital status. In multiple regression, the predictor variables must either be interval- or ratio-level variables (e.g., coping scale scores) *or* dichotomous nominal-level variables. Indeed, the text acknowledges that the researchers dichotomized categorical variables "where necessary in order to meet the critical assumptions of regression

analysis." The researchers did not directly tell us, however, what they did. The variable *marital status*, for example could be dichotomized as (a) currently married and living with a spouse versus (b) not currently married. Alternatively, it could be dichotomized as (a) single, *never* married versus (b) married or previously married. We learn in the Discussion section that the researchers contrasted single and not single people, but it is still not clear whether "single" corresponds to never married, or whether it corresponds to not currently married (i.e., single, widowed, divorced). Similarly, Table 2 provided no information about how the four-category ordinal variable *functional impairment* was dichotomized for the regression analysis. Were classes I and II combined and contrasted with class II and IV? We cannot tell.

- The beta coefficients for Escape-avoidance coping and functional impairment had a positive sign (implied by absence of a minus sign). This means that higher scores on the depression scale were associated with greater functional impairment and with a tendency to use Escape-avoidance as an approach to coping. The two other betas had negative signs: Depression scores tended to be lower for nonsingle people (whatever way that was defined) and for those with a tendency to Planful problem-solving coping.
- With other predictors controlled, the most powerful predictor of depression in this sample of patients with heart failure was scores on the Escape-avoidance coping subscale. This means that regardless of functional impairment, regardless of marital status, and regardless of other characteristics that

were excluded because they were nonsignificant (e.g., age, gender, ethnicity), people who tended to use escape-avoidance as a coping mechanism tended to be more depressed than those who did not.

- The statistic in this table is R^2, which summarizes the aggregate relationship between the four predictors on the one hand and depression scores on the other. The value of R^2 was .40, which means that the four predictors accounted for 40% of the variability in patients' depression scale scores.

f. Yes, the researchers did a power analysis to estimate the number of subjects that they would need to avoid a Type II error. In fact, this study provides a good and fairly simple illustration of how a power analysis works. The researchers estimated, presumably based on their knowledge of the literature, that their variables might be moderately intercorrelated. The effect size indicator for correlation analysis is r itself, and an r of .30 is considered a moderate effect. By estimating the effect that they would achieve, they were able to learn (through power analysis tables or relevant software) that they could achieve a power of .75 with a sample size of 75. This is a somewhat lower power criterion than is considered conventional (.80). To achieve a power of .80, they would have needed a sample of 88 subjects. Put another way, a sample of 75 would have adequate power (.80) for an r of .30, but not for an r of .28. This means that, in their regression analyses, some of the predictor variables might not have had sufficient power to be statistically significant, although in reality they were reliable predictors of depression. Of course, this is always a risk, but researchers try to limit there risk to 20% rather than 25%.

Chapter 16

A. CROSSWORD PUZZLE ANSWERS

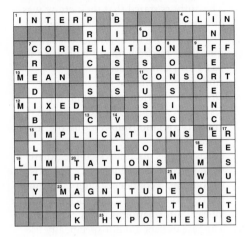

B. MATCHING EXERCISES

1. b   2. a   3. e   4. d   5. c
6. a, d   7. a   8. e

D. APPLICATION EXERCISES

Exercise 1: Questions of Fact (Appendix A)

a. Baseline values on the dependent variables were presented in Table 4 for both experimental and control group members, but nothing was indicated about whether group differences were statistically significant. For some outcomes (e.g., loneliness), the mean differences are not trivial, and so it seems possible that the groups may have differed significantly at the outset.

b. More than one-fourth of those in the intervention group dropped out of the study, compared with fewer than 4% of those in the control group. Hill and colleagues appeared not to have tested for attrition biases.

c. Hypotheses relating to Aim 1 were not formally stated in the introduction, although the authors implied that inter-correlations among psychosocial variables were expected. A statement that the correlations were "in the anticipated direction" (first paragraph of the Results section) confirms this inference. All of the correlations were statistically significant.

d. Hypotheses with regard to the effects of the intervention were not formally stated, although they were clearly implied. Results were mixed; there were intervention effects for some outcomes (self-esteem, social support, and empowerment), but not for others.

e. No, there was no information about the precision of estimates of group differences; confidence intervals were not presented.

f. Effect size estimates summarizing the magnitude of the intervention effects were not presented in the report. Despite this, the authors used language relating to effect magnitude (e.g., toward the end of the Results section, the authors said, "These results suggest that the intervention had an appreciable effect on self-esteem, social support, and empowerment. . ."). As noted in our comments in the previous chapter, it is possible to calculate effect size estimates using information in the article, and when we did this, we found that some of the effects *were* of fairly sizable magnitude (e.g., the intervention's effect on the women's sense of empowerment, with $d = .75$). It is unfortunate that these effect size estimates were not included in the article itself.

g. There was no explicit discussion about internal validity in the Discussion section.

h. In the subsection labeled "Strengths," the researchers noted that the external validity of the study was strengthened by the fact that the intervention was tested among women with a variety of chronic illnesses. The issue of whether the results might be unique to women, or to residents of rural areas, was not raised.

i. Yes, in the subsection labeled "Limitations," the authors noted a potential problem with regard to statistical power as a result of attrition. Other factors that might have reduced statistical conclusion validity, (e.g., a treatment that was insufficiently powerful, problems with intervention fidelity) were not mentioned, however.

j. Yes, considerable space in the Discussion section was devoted to discussing the findings within the context of earlier research.

k. Yes, there was a section on study limitations, although it did not mention several important ones, such as the possible risk of attrition or selection bias, possible problems with intervention fidelity, and so on.

Exercise 2: Questions of Fact (Appendix C)

a. Attrition is not an issue in studies that collect data only at one point in time—except when there is a time lag between when people agree to participate and when they actually provide the study data. In this case, it appears that recruitment, informed consent, and actual completion of the questionnaires occurred virtually simultaneously.

b. If any biases were analyzed in this study, they were not reported. The authors noted that only 2 of 77 eligible potential participants declined to take part in the study. If the number had been greater (e.g., 20 refusers), it would have been possible and desirable to analyze nonresponse bias by comparing characteristics of those who participated and those who did not, but with only 2 refusers, such an analysis does not make sense. The only bias specifically mentioned in the article, which did not involve a formal analysis, was the possibility of sampling bias.

c. Hypotheses were not formally stated in the Introduction of this article, and yet hypotheses were implied and tested. The general (nondirectional) hypothesis is that a relationship exists between a person's coping strategies and level of depression. The authors stated that their study was grounded in Lazarus and Folkman's Process Theory of Coping. That theory, plus prior research, might have been the basis for stating directional hypotheses. And, indeed, the first sentence of the Discussion section implies that the researchers had specific expectations about the relationships among the study variables.

d. Precision was not addressed (i.e., there were no confidence intervals). It is possible to compute a confidence interval around the Pearson r statistic, but such confidence interval information is rarely reported.

e. The researchers did not specifically use effect-size language in discussing their results. But, as noted in the previous chapter, Pearson r values are directly interpretable as effect size estimates. The article, however, did not include a correlation matrix to show how all variables were intercorrelated. Only a few correlation coefficients were directly reported. Only one (the r of .45 between emotion-focused coping and depressive symptoms) was of a magnitude that could be described as fairly large. The correlation between depression and functional impairment was not reported.

f. The article did not discuss internal validity per se, but it did note, commendably, that causal inferences in a study such as this are problematic.

g. The authors addressed at some length the issues of external validity in the Discussion section. They noted that study participants were volunteers recruited from a single comprehensive heart institute within an academic health science center. Such convenience samples, as noted in Chapter 12, could harbor extensive biases. The researchers *could* have explored the nature, direction, and magnitude of such biases by comparing characteristics of participants in this sample with those of other patients with heart failure from more diverse or representative settings—but researchers rarely go to such lengths to understand sampling bias better.

h. The researchers did not discuss potential problems with statistical conclusion validity. Yet they did face a higher-than-desirable risk of a Type II error. The researchers did do a power analysis to estimate the number of subjects that they would need to avoid a Type II error, but they used a criterion of .75 for power, rather than the standard criterion of .80. This means that any correlation of .22 (which is a correlation that is considered in the small-to-moderate range) would not be statistically significant although the correlation might be real and replicable—and possibly of clinical interest.

i. Yes, the researchers did a good job of tying the findings of their study to findings from earlier research.

j. Yes, some important limitations of the study were explicitly noted in the Discussion section. It is noteworthy that the researchers mentioned a key internal validity issue—temporal ambiguity. In a cross-sectional study such as this one, there is no way to know if coping strategies *caused* or influenced depression, or whether long-term depression contributed to the development of different coping strategies—or whether some other factor *caused* or influenced both. As noted, the Discussion also noted potential problems with sampling bias, and made some recommendations for future research.

■ Chapter 17

A. CROSSWORD PUZZLE ANSWERS

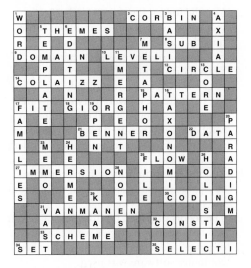

B. MATCHING EXERCISES

1. a, b, c   2. a   3. b   4. a, b, c   5. a
6. c   7. b   8. d

C. STUDY QUESTIONS

C.1.

a. A grounded theory analysis would not yield themes—a phenomenological study involves a thematic analysis.

b. Texts from poetry are used by interpretive phenomenologists, not by ethnographers (unless the poetry is a product of the culture under study, which it is not in this case).

c. Phenomenological studies do not focus on domains, ethnographies do.

d. Grounded theory studies do not yield taxonomies, ethnographies do.

e. A paradigm case is a strategy in a hermeneutic analysis, not in an ethnographic one.

D. APPLICATION EXERCISES

Exercise 1: Questions of Fact (Appendix B)

a. Yes, the formal interviews with 20 young women were audiotaped and then subsequently transcribed for analysis by the first author of the report (Rasmussen). The report did not indicate how many pages of transcription resulted, but it did say that interviews were between 30 and 140 minutes long. This likely resulted in a total of several hundred pages in the data set that had to be read and re-read, coded, and analyzed.

b. Yes, the report indicated that "constant comparative analysis was used throughout the study."

c. The report provided no information about whether manual methods were used to organize and index the data, or whether computer software was used.

d. Rasmussen and colleagues did not use quasi-statistics, but it is important to note that they did engage in (as do most qualitative researchers) a kind of qualitative "accounting." Here are two examples: "*All of the women* described personal interactions and social support as important factors that influenced how they stabilized their lives with diabetes" and "*Some of the women* explained how, when they were young, they met other children at diabetes camps, which they felt contributed to their having a sense of belonging."

e. The report did not explicitly state which grounded theory analytic method was adopted, but it did cite two of Glaser's writings (and none of Strauss and Corbin's writings) and so we assume a Glaserian approach was used.

f. Yes, the report indicated that Rasmussen (the first author) wrote memos throughout the study "to guide her in identifying links between categories, compare and identify differences in the data, develop new questions, and test assumptions."

g. The authors did not say very much about the coding process—but this is not unusual. They indicated that they began with open coding as they read the data line by line.

h. They noted that "Theoretical coding was applied simultaneously and involved connecting the developing categories through open coding with emerging relationships between categories and their properties." The authors did not, however, provide any specific examples of their theoretical codes.

i. The report indicated that the analysis revealed a core category that encompassed three subcategories: (a) the impact of being susceptible to fluctuating blood glucose levels (BGLs), (b) the responses of other people to the women's diabetes, and (c) the impact of the woman's diabetes on other people's lives. Each of these subcategories had further subcategories. For example, *Impact of being susceptible to fluctuating BGLs* itself had three subcategories: Fearing complications, Fluctuating BGLs and entering the workforce, and Fluctuating BGLs during pregnancy and in transition to motherhood.

j. In this study, the core category was the basic social problem, being in the grip of blood glucose levels. The core category was the basic social process (BSP) "because it accounted for the greatest variation in the data, was related to all of the other categories in the data, and accurately described the problem the women experienced during transitional periods."

k. This report did not include a figure depicting the grounded theory and relationships among the categories.

Exercise 2: Questions of Fact (Appendix D)

a. The report indicated that the interviews were audiotaped and transcribed. There was no information about who did the transcriptions. The report also did not indicate how extensive the data set was, but it appears there were nearly 40 interviews (about 10 in each wave with both mother and daughters) that lasted an average of 45 minutes. Our rough estimate is that this would have yielded more than 200 pages of transcriptions. The report also suggested that field notes were fairly detailed, thus adding to the extensiveness of the data set in this study.

b. The report did not indicate the researchers' strategy for data management. It did not specifically mention computer software being used in managing or analyzing the data, and we suspect (although we cannot be sure) that a computer was *not* used.

c. No, the report did not describe the process of developing a category system or coding the data.

d. Nothing in this report suggests explicit quantification, but (as is typical), the researchers did do some loose tabulations, as suggested by the following quotes: "*Most of the mothers* asserted that they continued to live independently" and "*All mothers* spoke of feeling grateful for the care received." It might be noted that the researchers hinted at a more explicit quantification that they would report in a separate paper: "A full account of the different types of mother–daughter relationship, using the dyad as the unit of analysis, will be published elsewhere."

e. Yes, the report indicated that the researchers wrote full field notes after each interview "to record perceptions, insights, and observations." Then, "As data analysis proceeded, memos or notes were used to keep track of the researchers' insights and included justification for making analytic decisions."

f. The researchers did not use one of the approaches described in the textbook. They used a team approach that sounds similar to Diekelmann's team strategy. Each of the three interviewers independently read transcribed interviews and "made a preliminary data analysis" that was then reviewed by the team. Ward-Griffin, the lead researcher, then "explored the connections among the themes and prepared an overarching conceptual interpretation" that was subjected to team review. (The researchers used an analytic approach suggested by Loftland and Loftland, who offer a fairly generic approach to analyzing qualitative data.)

g. The two thematic levels in this study are as follows: The first level captured aspects of the mothers' receipt of care from their daughters, and involved four themes: Doing care, Accepting care, Undemanding care, and Determining care. The second level is more conceptual and concerns "two major underlying ideologies" that appeared to be at the root of the mother's experience of *Grateful guilt* in the care they received. Those ideologies were individualism and familism.

h. Yes, the report is full of rich quotes that supported the thematic analysis.

i. The researchers developed a figure that both describes the mother's experience of being cared for by their daughters, and serves as a metaphor. They embedded their findings into the Alzheimer disease logo, the forget-me-not, which "was purposely selected to depict how mothers managed their contradictory experience of needing care."

▪ Chapter 18

A. CROSSWORD PUZZLE ANSWERS

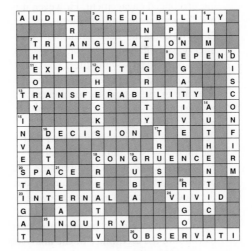

B. MATCHING EXERCISES

1. a   2. c   3. b   4. d   5. a
6. b

D. APPLICATION EXERCISES

Exercise 1: Questions of Fact (Appendix B)

a. Yes, a specific section of the report was labeled "Rigor and Credibility." It was a subsection of the "Design and Methods" section of the report.

b. The researchers used method triangulation: Their main data source, formal interviews with 20 young women, was supplemented with "informal interviews, relevant documents, newspapers," and observations of behaviors during the interviews, as recorded in field notes. The report did not mention that investigator triangulation was used, but—given that there were multiple authors—some level of investigator triangulation likely occurred.

c. Strategies used that were mentioned in the report:
- Prolonged engagement: The report specifically indicated that there was "lengthy contact with the women," and noted that this was designed as a method of achieving prolonged engagement. However, it is not clear what the authors meant by "lengthy contact." Each participant was interviewed only once and the interviews lasted only 30 to 140 minutes. That data were collected over a period of 1½ years does not in itself speak to "prolonged engagement"—it may reflect only the pace of recruitment into the sample.
- Peer review: The report indicated that the theory was "validated by peer review throughout the research process." They cite, as an example, that the study Abstract was peer reviewed for conference presentations. This does not strike us as a good manner for peers to validate the credibility of the analysis and interpretation, because the reviewers would have no access to the actual data or categorization process. Perhaps other forms of peer review were undertaken, but not described, that offered further opportunities for validation.
- Member checks: Member checking was not mentioned.
- Search for disconfirming evidence: If this strategy was used, it was not explicitly mentioned.
- Researcher credibility: The credentials of the researchers were not fully spelled out—we know only that they are doctorally prepared faculty at Deakin University in Australia. In fact, they are on the nursing faculty, although this was not mentioned. There is also no mention of the personal relevance of diabetes to any of them—that is, whether they or any family member has type 1 diabetes. The report did indicate, however, that the lead author had previously undertaken research on the topic of diabetes.

d. Criteria addressed:
- Dependability: Method triangulation enhances the reliability of the data and interpretation, but it does not appear that Rasmussen and colleagues used formal approaches to enhancing dependability, such as would be achieved with an inquiry audit.
- Confirmability: An inquiry audit is a key approach to enhancing confirmability, but this does not appear to have been used. Investigator triangulation may have been used, but was not discussed. Peer review and debriefing, if done more formally than what was described in the report, would also have contributed to confirmability.
- Transferability: The report provided a good description of the young women who participated in the study, and offered many good verbatim quotes, but perhaps a bit more about the context of their lives would have been helpful—especially, about the specific kinds of transitions with which they were faced and how many of the participants faced them.

- Authenticity: The report used rich verbatim quotes (made possible because the researchers had audiotaped and transcribed the interviews), and these strategies contribute to authenticity. As noted earlier, it is difficult to assess the extent to which prolonged engagement (another strategy for enhancing authenticity) was actually achieved.
- Explicitness: This criterion is primarily about auditability, and it is difficult to assess whether the researchers took steps to document decisions carefully. The report did indicate, however, that the researchers produced memos throughout the study and these would have had information about key decisions. The researchers are to be commended for having a section of their report devoted to quality-enhancement issues, although a bit more information would have been helpful.

Exercise 2: Questions of Fact (Appendix D)

a. This report did not have a separate section devoted to strategies used to enhance integrity and trustworthiness. Various pieces of information about their efforts were scattered throughout the Method section.

b. A fair amount of triangulation was used in this study. In terms of data triangulation, the researchers gathered information from both mothers and daughters (and in some cases from multiple daughters in a single family). They also interviewed family members on multiple occasions. Method triangulation was also used; the data for the study came from interviews and the researchers' observations. Investigator triangulation was also used. In the subsection labeled *Data Analysis*, the authors noted that "individual researchers read the transcription and independently made a preliminary data analysis." Then the team finalized the analysis together.

c. Strategies used that were mentioned in the report:

- Prolonged engagement: The report explicitly mentioned both prolonged engagement and persistent observation (last paragraph in the *Data Analysis* subsection). It is apparent that the investigators spent a lot of time in the field with these families. Both the mothers and their daughters were interviewed twice in the mothers' homes, which would have yielded ample opportunity to "get close" and better understand family dynamics.
- Peer review: The report did not state that external peer reviewers were used to "validate" the analysis and interpretation.
- Member checks: Member checking was not mentioned.
- Search for disconfirming evidence: As in the previous study, this strategy was not explicitly mentioned.
- Researcher credibility: Information about the researchers' backgrounds is limited to a brief note at the end indicating their professional affiliations as faculty and students at a school of nursing. There was no mention of the personal relevance of dementia, although it is probably safe to assume that at least some of the researchers were the daughters of aging mothers.

d. Criteria addressed:

- Dependability: Method and investigator triangulation, both of which were used in this study, enhances the reliability of the data and interpretations.
- Confirmability: It does appear that the authors maintained careful documentation about their thoughts and their decisions. The report indicated that they maintained "an extensive audit trail."
- Transferability: The report provided an excellent description of the characteristics of the study participants, and their personal and family contexts. There was considerable "thick description" in the presentation of the findings, and many excellent verbatim quotes from the mothers, whose voices have seldom been heard in reports about women with dementia.

- Authenticity: As in the previous study in Appendix B, this report used rich verbatim quotes (made possible because the researchers had audiotaped and transcribed the interviews), and these strategies contribute to authenticity. Authenticity was enhanced through persistent observation and the researchers' prolonged engagement doing fieldwork with these families.

- Sensitivity: The report did provide evidence that this research was undertaken with considerable sensitivity. For example, the report was explicit about the care taken to build rapport: "All three investigators strove to build rapport with the participant and to provide support and information during the interview. Guided by clinical evidence in dementia care, the research team employed additional interview strategies for use with individuals with AD. . . Thus, the study sought to include people with dementia in research about their experiences, creating the potential for personal empowerment consistent with feminist goals."

■ Chapter 19

A. CROSSWORD PUZZLE ANSWERS

¹F	A	I	L	²F	³R	E	⁴Q	U	E	N	C	Y
O				R	X		F					⁵R
⁶R	A	N	D	O	⁷M		T		F			A
E				O		E		R		⁹M		T
S				B		T	A		¹⁰S	C	A	L	E		I
¹¹T	O	L	E	R	A	N	C	E			¹²T	W	O
	I			S		T		¹³N			H	
¹⁴E				T		U		¹⁵S	U	B	¹⁶G	R	O	U	P
N				M			L		R		D	
¹⁷C	O	R	R		¹⁸M	O	D	¹⁹E	L		E		²⁰C	²¹I
O				A		X		Y			N	T
²²D	I	²³F	F	E	R	E	N	C	E		²⁴Q	U	T	E
E		I		Y			L		²⁵P		U		I
		X				²⁶P	U	B	L	I	C	A	T	N
	²⁷S	E	N	²⁸S	I	T		D		O		L	S
		D		I			E		T		I		I
				Z					T		T
	²⁹H	E	T	E	R	O	G	E	N	E	I	T	Y		Y

B. MATCHING EXERCISES

1. c   2. d   3. b   4. a   5. b
6. a   7. d   8. b

D. APPLICATION EXERCISES

Exercise 1: Questions of Fact (Appendix F)

a. The purpose of this review was "to examine the effectiveness of interventions for improving the mental health of caregivers of stroke patients by synthesizing across studies." The independent variable was receipt versus nonreceipt of a special mental health intervention, and the dependent variable was mental health—specifically, scores on a particular measure of mental health, the Short Form Health Survey (SF-36).

b. The main databases were Medline and CINAHL, and the Social Sciences Citation Index, Science Citation Index, and Cochrane library database were also used. Keywords included caregiving, stroke caregiver, stroke caregiving, control group, and interventions. The authors specifically noted that no effort was made to retrieve unpublished studies (grey literature) because such reports would not have undergone peer review.

c. The paper states that searches were limited to articles published in English.

d. A total of 31 studies were initially retrieved and reviewed against the inclusion criteria: (a) population was caregivers of stroke patients; (b) involved an intervention to improve caregivers' mental health; (c) outcomes were measured using the SF-36; (d) the study was quantitative; and (e) the study design included a comparison group. Of the 31 studies retrieved, 11 met these criteria. Of the 11 studies, 7 were eliminated for a variety of reasons, including insufficient information to calculate the necessary effect size statistics. Thus, only 4 studies were in the meta-analysis. (Note that meta-analysts often write to authors requesting more information that would allow the calculation of the effect size indexes. It is not clear whether Lee and colleagues did this.)

e. No, if an intervention study used a different measure of mental health than the SF-36, the study would not have been included. It is not typical that meta-analysts insist on a particular method of measuring outcomes. The calculation of an effect size is specifically intended to eliminate the need for a uniform metric.

f. The article indicated that all four studies used a randomized design (i.e., all were experimental).

g. Yes, each study was subjected to a quality appraisal, using an instrument that rated study aim, randomization, blinding, attrition, statistical testing, and quality of the discussion section. Scores could range from 0 to 16. All studies were independently rated by two researchers, and their initial rate of agreement was 90%. After discussion, total consensus was achieved.

h. A study was considered *low quality* if it had a score lower than 10. Only one of the four studies was considered low in quality, but the researchers did not eliminate the study based on its quality.

i. The standardized mean difference, or *d*, was calculated for each study. The raw effect sizes were weighted for sample size, so that studies with larger samples "counted" more.

j. The article stated that statistical heterogeneity was formally assessed using a Q statistic; heterogeneity was found to be significant. The forest plot (Figure 1) shows that effect size estimates varied from a low of 0.0 to a high of .92.

k. The report did not indicate whether a fixed effects or random effects model was used.

l. In all studies combined, there were a total of 718 study participants (Table 2).

m. The effect size was largest in Grant's tudy, $d = .922$; this was significant at $p = .001$.
   • The effect size was smallest in the van den Heuvel study, $d = 0.0$, which was nonsignificant.

• Aside from the van den Heuvel study, the effect size was also not significant in Rodger's study ($p = .24$).

• For the four studies combined, the mean weighted effect size was .277, which was highly significant. This effect size suggests that, on average, the special interventions helped to improve caregivers' mental health (scores on the SF-36) by about one-quarter of a standard deviation.

n. Yes, subgroup analyses were undertaken to explore the heterogeneity of effects across studies. The dimensions included type of intervention (education versus support), whether the intervention was theory-based or not, and location of the study (Europe versus the United States).

o. Yes, Lee and colleagues did a sensitivity analysis to test whether study quality affected the results. The three high-quality studies had an average effect size of .34, whereas the low-quality study had an effect size of 0.0. The authors concluded that "Results indicate that interventions in high quality studies that used blinding were significant in improving mental health of stroke caregivers whereas the low quality study did not."

p. Yes, the authors addressed the issue of publication bias. The fail-safe number was calculated to be 13—that is, the number of studies with an effect size of zero that would reduce the value of *d* to a level of nonsignificance. The tolerance level in this meta-analysis was 30 (i.e., $(5 \times 4) + 10$), which the fail-safe number did *not* exceed. Thus, the authors concluded that publication bias might well be possible. And, in fact, the authors did not search for unpublished studies.

Exercise 2: Questions of Fact (Appendix G)

a. Xu stated that the purpose of his meta-synthesis was to provide insight into the experiences of Asian nurses who practice nursing in Western countries. The central phenomenon was the "collectively lived experiences" of these Asian nurses, who were defined as nurses whose home countries are in Asia.

b. Xu used a wide variety of approaches in searching for and identifying relevant studies. In consultation with a health sciences librarian (an excellent strategy), he searched CINAHL, Medline, PsychINFO, Sociological Abstract, and ERIC (a database for education literature). He also explicitly searched for nonpublished literature through Proquest Dissertations and Theses. Search terms included *Asian nurses, foreign nurses, foreign-born nurses, internationally educated nurse, internationally recruited nurses, immigrant nurses,* and the names of specific Asian countries, such as Korea and Taiwan. In addition to electronic searchers, Xu used traditional "ancestry" type searches (i.e., retrieving studies cited in other relevant studies) and hard-searched journals that had a history of publishing research on the topic of interest. Moreover, commendably, Xu made efforts to interact with the original researchers when, in several instances, he had questions about whether the primary study findings were applicable equally to Asian nurses as to other foreign-born nurses. One study had to be omitted because he did not get a response.

c. Xu explicitly stated that type of qualitative study had no bearing on his decision to use the study in the metasynthesis. In fact, he used data from mixed method studies, as well as data from purely qualitative studies—although his metasynthesis ignored any quantitative findings because they were not relevant to his inquiry. His metasynthesis includes grounded theory studies, an ethnography, phenomenologic study, and qualitative descriptive studies.

d. The final sample for the metasynthesis was 14 studies. These studies were nicely summarized (in terms of sample size, sample, characteristics, country, research tradition, and disciplinary orientation) in Tables 1 and 2.

e. The report did not indicate whether studies were appraised for quality. It is unlikely that any studies were excluded because of poor quality. Xu provided excellent information about his sampling decisions, and had there been exclusions, he likely would have mentioned this.

f. The data in the primary studies were obtained through interviews, focus-group interviews, open-ended questions in written questionnaires, and (in the case of one ethnographic study) observation.

g. Xu used Noblit and Hare's approach to doing a meta-synthesis. He provided an excellent description of the seven phases of the approach, Xu stated a "detailed table of metaphors, themes and concepts from the 14 studies was constructed and translated into each other" and he shared this table in the report (Table 3).

h. No, a meta-summary is a strategy developed by Sandelowski and colleagues, and Xu did not follow this approach.

i. In all of the 14 studies combined, a total of 587 Asian nurses served as study participants—a substantial number for a metasynthesis.

j. Xu identified four overarching themes: Communication as a daunting challenge; Differences in nursing practice; Marginalization, discrimination, and exploitation; and Cultural differences.

k. Xu included some powerful quotes from primary studies in support of his thematic integration. Many were small snippets of quotes, but a few were more extensive—for example, the quote from the nurse who had difficulty because of her short stature.

l. Xu's paper concluded with an excellent discussion section that provided a summary and a series of implications for knowledge development and future research, for nursing practice, and for public policy.

RRS1008